D0828611

WASTE OF A NATION

Waste *of a* Nation

GARBAGE AND GROWTH IN INDIA

ASSA DORON · ROBIN JEFFREY

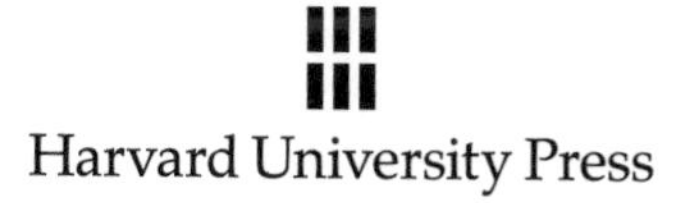

Harvard University Press

Cambridge, Massachusetts, and London, England

2018

Printed in the United States of America

First printing

Library of Congress Cataloging-in-Publication Data

Names: Doron, Assa, author. | Jeffrey, Robin, author.
Title: Waste of a nation : garbage and growth in India / Assa Doron, Robin Jeffrey.
Description: Cambridge, Massachusetts : Harvard University Press, 2018. | Includes bibliographical references and index.
Identifiers: LCCN 2017041557 | ISBN 9780674980600 (cloth : alk. paper)
Subjects: LCSH: Refuse and refuse disposal—India. | Salvage (Waste, etc.)—India. | Sewage disposal—India. | Caste—India. | India—Population.
Classification: LCC HD4485.I4 .D67 2018 | DDC 363.72/88—dc23
LC record available at https://lccn.loc.gov/2017041557

CONTENTS

LIST OF MAPS, ILLUSTRATIONS, AND TABLES

Maps

Illustrations

Tables

PREFACE

This book began one day in 2012 when Doron took a taxi to Seelampur. We were interested in mobile phones and were curious about what happened to them when they died. Seelampur is a neighborhood in the northeast of New Delhi that specializes in electronic waste. Doron's visit made a big impression on him. The immense volume of thrown-away electronic gadgetry and the people—women and children, old and young—engaged in breaking it down and segregating materials provoked nagging questions. Doron returned from his visit declaring, "We've got to do a book about garbage."

To our eyes, what Doron had seen was "garbage." But Seelampur does not deal in garbage; it deals in thrown-away things that can be turned into something else—"recycling." We soon began to realize that "waste" was "a little complicated," a phrase that keeps cropping up in this book. We found ourselves trying to understand the complications and then articulate our understanding to ourselves and others. In the course of the four years that we have grappled with garbage, we have realized how much other people know about the many dimensions of waste and how much has been written about it. We have incurred debts to many people who have shared their experience and detailed knowledge to try to improve ours. The Acknowledgments at the end of the book recognize some of those debts. In the book, we occasionally use pseudonyms when there is a possibility that an informant might be embarrassed to be identified.

If there are, as the Paul Simon song says, fifty ways to leave your lover, there are almost as many ways to study waste in India. You could focus on a particular commodity, as Kaveri Gill focuses on plastic. You could study a single city, as Urvashi Dhamija studies New Delhi. You could take your cue from the powerful work of Bhasha Singh and write about the occupation of a single group—the lowest-status Dalits, locked into collecting human excrement. As a passionate activist, you could produce an evocative photo study of a single landfill and its residents, as Dhrubajyoti Ghosh did by photographing the Dhapa site in Kolkata, or as Sudharak Olwe and Atul Deulgaonkar did when they recorded the activities of sewer workers of Mumbai. You could, like Diane Coffey and Dean Spear, focus on toilets and defecation and the effects on public health, or trace the development of national policy about waste and sanitation, as Susan Chaplin has done. You could follow the lives of a few families who draw livelihoods from waste in a single locality, as Katherine Boo did. Or like the scholars, journalists, and activists of the Centre for Science and Environment, you could prepare a report that takes a snapshot of waste in India at a particular moment.[1]

Among scholars, problems of waste have attracted geographers particularly, such as Vinay Gidwani and Colin McFarlane, who have written with energy and insight for many years about the people who make waste, those who recover it, and the social structures that sustain those roles. Historians such as David Arnold, Mark Harrison, Sandhyal Polu, and Mridula Ramana have traced public health and sanitation from British times. Scholars of cities—sociologists and economists, such as Isher Judge Ahluwalia and Asher Ghertner—have viewed waste in the context of urbanization and the contests between middle-class aesthetics and survival strategies of the poor. Less often, policy makers like the late K. C. Sivaramakrishnan have treated public sanitation as a central element in attempts to improve urbanization processes.[2]

The authorship of the book is as "joint" as such a project, we think, can be. One of us starts a chapter, sends it to the other one, who adds, subtracts, multiplies, and divides, and sends it back. In such prose ping-pong, it becomes difficult sometimes to know whose words were originally whose. And of course it doesn't matter, but readers may wish to know that Doron is a card-carrying anthropologist and Jeffrey began working life as a sports writer. We have an implicit intellectual debt to D. A. Low, whom we both knew quite well, and B. S. Cohn, whom neither of us ever met. They both liked the idea of bringing together the techniques of anthropology and history. So do we, although we can't claim to have done so as elegantly and diligently as they.

Minnie, Itai, and Tomer tolerated Doron's infatuation with waste, and his fondness for stories from landfills, open dumps, and recycling sheds. He could not have done it without them. Lesley Jeffrey endured another scholarly folly of the kind she has had to put up with over the past forty years, for which her devoted *folly-ista* thanks her.

Doron is grateful to the Australian Research Council for supporting his Future Fellowship and for the encouragement of colleagues in the College of Asia and the Pacific and elsewhere at the Australian National University. Jeffrey has been fortunate to have had regular periods at the Institute of South Asian Studies at the National University of Singapore, and he greatly benefited from the institute's support and the companionship of its scholars.

NOTE ON TRANSLITERATION

We have not used diacritical marks for Indian words. We show long vowels by repeating the letter (for example, "aa"), except at the end of words, in which case they are simply "a." For widely used words, we follow common spellings. A "wala" (or wallah) remains a "wala," although a more pedantic transliteration would have "vaala." Direct quotations retain original spellings. We do not differentiate between retroflex and dental sounds, although in Hindi, for example, *thela,* a "cart," has a retroflex "th" and *thali,* a "plate," has a dental "th."

WASTE OF A NATION

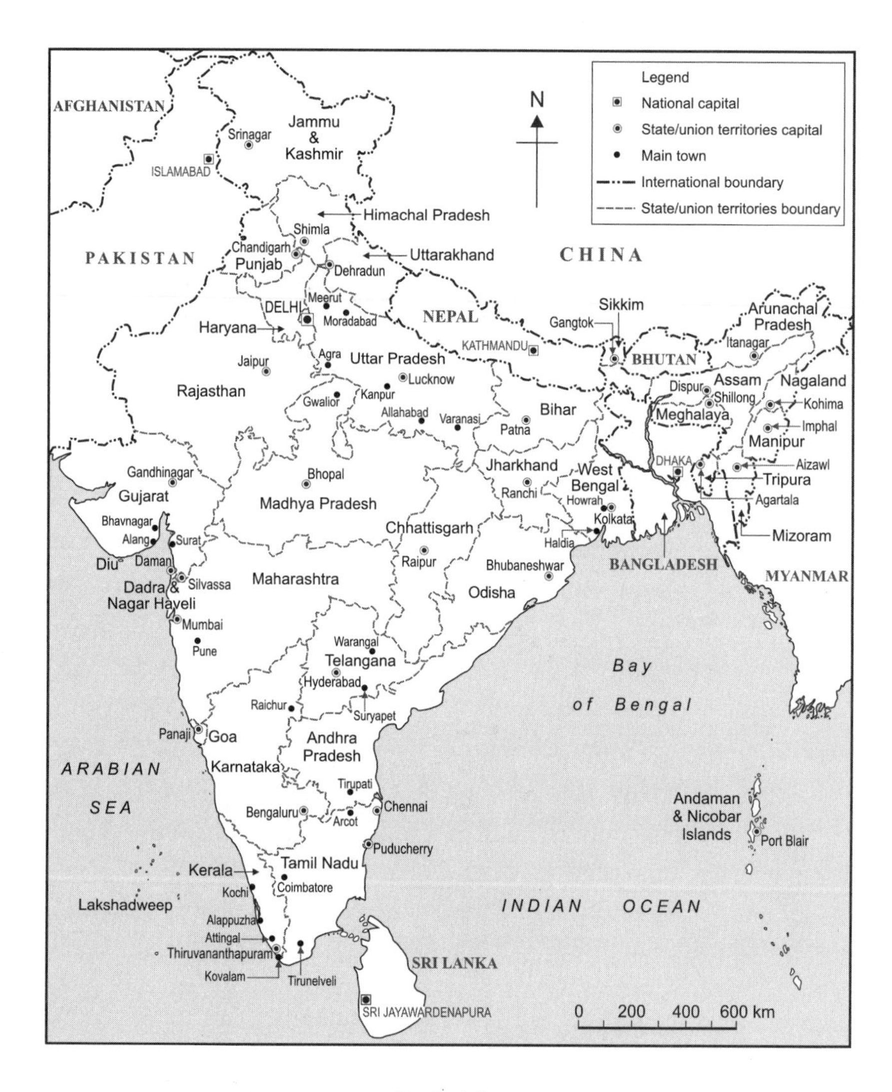
AFGHANISTAN
PAKISTAN
CHINA
NEPAL
BHUTAN
BANGLADESH
MYANMAR
SRI LANKA
ISLAMABAD
KATHMANDU
DHAKA
SRI JAYAWARDENAPURA
Legend
National capital
State/union territories capital
Main town
International boundary
State/union territories boundary
N
Jammu & Kashmir
Srinagar
Himachal Pradesh
Shimla
Chandigarh
Punjab
Uttarakhand
Dehradun
DELHI
Meerut
Moradabad
Haryana
Rajasthan
Jaipur
Agra
Uttar Pradesh
Lucknow
Kanpur
Gwalior
Allahabad
Varanasi
Bihar
Patna
Sikkim
Gangtok
Arunachal Pradesh
Itanagar
Assam
Dispur
Shillong
Meghalaya
Nagaland
Kohima
Imphal
Manipur
Aizawl
Tripura
Agartala
Mizoram
Jharkhand
Ranchi
West Bengal
Howrah
Kolkata
Haldia
Gujarat
Gandhinagar
Bhavnagar
Alang
Surat
Diu
Daman
Dadra & Nagar Haveli
Silvassa
Madhya Pradesh
Bhopal
Chhattisgarh
Raipur
Odisha
Bhubaneshwar
Maharashtra
Mumbai
Pune
Telangana
Warangal
Hyderabad
Suryapet
Raichur
Goa
Panaji
Karnataka
Andhra Pradesh
Tirupati
Chennai
Bengaluru
Arcot
Puducherry
Tamil Nadu
Coimbatore
Kerala
Kochi
Alappuzha
Attingal
Thiruvananthapuram
Kovalam
Tirunelveli
Lakshadweep
ARABIAN SEA
Bay of Bengal
INDIAN OCEAN
Andaman & Nicobar Islands
Port Blair
0 200 400 600 km

Map I.1 India

INTRODUCTION

Assa Doron knows a young man in Varanasi whose name is Mallu. *Mal* in Hindi means "feces" or "excrement." Doron once asked Mallu's mother how he got such a name. She explained that by the time Mallu was born, all three of her older children had died from disease. None had lived past the age of three. When her fourth child was born, elders advised her to place the child briefly in the open drain that ran beside their hamlet. By doing so, she would be acknowledging that this child was no better than excrement and therefore of no interest or value to the gods. Repelled by this repugnant child, the deities would leave him with her. From that day, he was known as Mallu, a name he still carries as an adult with three children of his own.

The story of Mallu's name is not unusual. A practice, sometimes followed by lower castes anxious to prevent the death of a treasured baby boy, is to give the child the name Kachra (rubbish).[1] As an infant, he is removed from the home and placed on a rubbish heap. A Chamarin ("untouchable" woman) picks up the child, because she has the right (*haq*) to take anything left on the rubbish heap. The mother then buys back the child for a symbolic price. The baby has become a worthless object purchased from someone of the lowest caste and unlikely therefore to be desired by malevolent gods. Such practices display an alternative, and perhaps surprising, attitude toward the act of throwing away. Being rubbish brings a kind of power: the power to ward off infant mortality.

How we think about waste is grounded in social relations and everyday fears.[2] In India, attitudes about ritual purity and pollution often collide with scientific understanding of waste and dirt and of sanitation and hygiene. Some local people and many pilgrims in Varanasi bathe in the polluted Ganga and rinse their mouths beside outlets for untreated sewage. Devotees are unperturbed. They may be aware of the physical pollution of the Ganga, but pollution does not compromise for them the river's sacred and purifying properties.[3] Their understanding of waste generally distinguishes between waste as dirt or filth (*gandagi, aswatchhta*) and the pollution associated with religious impurity (*ashuddha, apavitra*). The first pair of words commonly refers to the external forms of waste produced by a society undergoing rapid industrialization and urbanization. The second pair refers to the ritual impurities incurred in the course of daily life, which must be ritually removed to regain purity.[4] Thus, the well-washed hand of a human being may be spurned. Even the cup that such a hand touched may be thrown away as *ashuddha*—something touched and therefore tainted—but brown Ganga water may be used to ritually cleanse the mouth.

Ideas and practices of caste haunt India's efforts to cope effectively with the waste of a vast, urbanizing population. Discrimination based on untouchability was banned in the constitution of 1950. The postindependence governments led by Jawaharlal Nehru developed a system of affirmative action intended to benefit the lowest castes (so-called untouchables, or Dalits) and the tribal people living in remote areas and not part of mainstream Hindu practices. Seats in the national and state legislatures were reserved for them, as well as jobs in government departments. Scholarships and fee waivers were given to students from these groups. The numbers are large—15 percent of the population is officially classified as "Scheduled Castes" and 7 percent as "Scheduled Tribes." In 2018, they total about 280 million people.[5]

Dalits—the preferred term today for Scheduled Castes—form a disproportionate number of India's poorest people and especially of those who perform the most dangerous and unpleasant tasks in dealing with waste. Dalits are not a homogeneous group. Their subcastes (or *jatis*) number hundreds, they speak different languages in different parts of India, and they have among them a tiny middle class and a sprinkling of senior public figures, including India's president in 2017. But the vast majority are poor. In the languages of north India, they are sometimes called the offensive name of *achhuut*—"not to be touched, not touchable." That some human beings are judged to be tainted and believed to transmit pollution merely by touch complicates India's confrontation with growing volumes of thrown-away things. It hinders cooperation and fosters feelings that removing noxious materials is someone else's job—even by virtue of birth.

"Why Is India So Filthy?"

The Ugly Indian, a masked man who presented a TED Talk in Bengaluru, poses a raw, rude question.[6] He tells the audience, "My name is *anamik nagrik* [anonymous citizen]; I am a proud Indian, and I have a problem with my country. And the problem is, Why is India so filthy?"[7] He represents a movement of the same name—The Ugly Indian—that aims to clean up India through the public-spirited actions of individual citizens. It's a theme V. S. Naipaul dwelt on in the 1960s and one that Florence Nightingale, as we shall see, pursued with the British government in the 1860s and after.[8]

The "Clean and Green" India that governments, gated communities, and people who give TED Talks aspire to is distant from the experience of the less well-off and the poor.[9] For them, daily life is a project of survival, punctuated by illness, poor sanitation, and material insecurity.[10] Their existence and experience reflect such uncertainty: disease and deprivation displace ideas of a sanitized modernity. Years ago, when Dipesh Chakrabarty reprimanded a small boy in Kolkata for littering, his target replied defiantly, "You like to think . . . we live in England?"[11]

Nineteenth-century England was no stranger to sanitation issues. Even wealthy families were affected by terrible drains, sewers, and cesspits that dealt with the household's human waste. The Thames River itself was an open sewer. When it flooded, it left raw sewage on the lawns. Queen Victoria herself had typhoid at sixteen, her eldest son almost died of typhoid, and her husband, Prince Albert, may have died of it at age forty-two.[12] One could imagine something similar, yet fundamentally different, in India today. Think of a magnificent mansion in New Delhi built within sight of the Yamuna River, or in Varanasi, within eyeshot of the Ganga. The stench from the river might, on bad days, waft into the house on the breeze, but household sewage would be whisked away by flush toilets, drawing on water from storage tanks to wash excrement off the property. It would then, of course, probably end up in the river to add its mite to the megaliters of effluent that India's rivers receive each day. But the residents of the house would know they were protected from infectious diseases by vaccination and water-purifying systems. Unlike Queen Victoria and her family, who had to share the perils of many diseases with their poor subjects, India's middle classes can protect themselves from most of these afflictions. What they cannot shield themselves from, however, is the visual disorder they see every day. And those who think about health and environment also worry about growing garbage mountains, toxic emissions, and polluted waterways.

The story about Queen Victoria and her family emphasizes one aspect of India's confrontation with the detritus of mass production: India is not alone. Other countries have been there in the past or are in similar circumstances today. And every country, in a world that has quadrupled in population in 110 years (from 1.6 billion in 1901 to 7 billion in 2011), faces immense problems in managing its waste. India can draw on certain assets, such as the scientific advances of the past hundred years and practices of frugality and husbanding that were once, in less prosperous and profligate times, widespread.

In the twenty-first century, however, the problems that accompany consumer capitalism, economic growth, and urbanization confront India inescapably. The economic liberalization that accelerated in 1991 created new volumes of waste from mines, factories, and agricultural industries. This was compounded by an increase in solid waste from homes and businesses and liquid waste, sewage, and industrial effluent dumped into lakes, rivers, and the ocean from expanding towns. The Solid Waste Management Rules, an admirable code for managing waste, were formalized only in 2000, after four years of legal pressure from middle-class activists who were alarmed and offended by uncontrolled dumping and polluted bodies of water. The magnitude of waste in India is complicated by population growth, economic expansion, eager consumerism, and cultural prejudices regarding caste, gender, and class.

What Is Waste?

Discussion of waste and garbage can lead to questions of deep culture or high philosophy. In 1966 the English anthropologist Mary Douglas published *Purity and Danger,* which has become a standard reference for global reflection on the meaning of waste. The book shows, writes Gay Hawkins—herself a scholar of waste and its significance—"how the structuring capacities of culture come to classify things as waste."[13] Ideas about what is pure and impure are often based on custom and belief, rather than on anything intrinsic to the objects involved.

To understand what makes something waste is a trickier exercise than it may first appear. Of course, anything that we don't want anymore, especially if it smells or disintegrates, is waste, junk, or garbage. In English, *waste* can be a noun, an adjective, or a verb. We may see a pile of wastepaper in an office or waste wood on a building site. Children are admonished not to waste food or money. And a person is sometimes said to be wasting away. A Marxist view of waste sees the bodies of laborers "used up or wasted at accelerated rates in order to secure the most profit" and emphasizes an expandable, unorganized labor force whose lives are locked into dealing with waste materials.[14]

What constitutes waste is also in the eye of the beholder. Your waste may contribute to my wealth: long ago in the Netherlands, China, or Japan, enterprising people bid for the right to carry a town's feces to the countryside to sell as fertilizer to eager farmers. Waste is a thing, but the creation of waste is a physical and psychological process. Unless waste is contained in some way, it confuses and contaminates the surroundings of the people who created it. And people who regularly deal with waste, if the work is especially dangerous, loathsome, or stigmatized, may find their lives shortened and made miserable—laid waste, wasted away.

For people who work in public sanitation or administration, waste can be too general a term. In the United States, people who deal with waste professionally use four terms—*trash, garbage, refuse,* and *rubbish.* Trash is dry, garbage is wet, refuse is both, and rubbish is refuse "plus construction and demolition debris."[15] In India, authorities recognize categories requiring special treatment—medical waste, construction and demolition waste, and hazardous waste. And then there is sewage. Sewage is a different category altogether, and some scholars and practitioners would prefer to discuss waste and sewage separately. But sewage in our view is liquid waste, and in India, human waste excites especially charged feelings of revulsion. Creating a clean India requires, among other things, the construction and habitual use of millions of sustainable toilets, but it also requires suppression of prejudices based on caste.

Clean India—*Swachh Bharat*

Cleaning up India became a top priority for officials and elected representatives in 2014 after the election of a national government led by the Bharatiya Janata Party (BJP), with Narendra Modi as prime minister. "Toilets first, temples second" (*pehle shauchaalaya, phir devaalaya*), he declared during the election campaign, and on October 2, 2014, Mahatma Gandhi's birthday, Modi announced the Clean India campaign—*Swachh Bharat* in Hindi.[16] The goal was to make India clean, by providing, for example, toilets convenient for every Indian, by Gandhi's 150th birth anniversary in 2019. There had been programs to encourage public sanitation in the past, but previous prime ministers had not shown Modi's enthusiasm.[17] He lined up celebrities and businesses to support the campaign, and crores of rupees (hundreds of millions of dollars) were committed to fund it. Modi and anyone else who wanted to make friends with the new government were happy to be photographed wielding a broom and doing their symbolic bit to achieve Swachh Bharat.

Why would a new prime minister, elected with a surprising majority, choose to stake so much of his reputation on a program as difficult as cleaning up India? We asked that question of the prime minister in 2017. His reply is reproduced in the Appendix. Two experiences in his native Gujarat, he wrote, influenced his attitude toward social change and san-

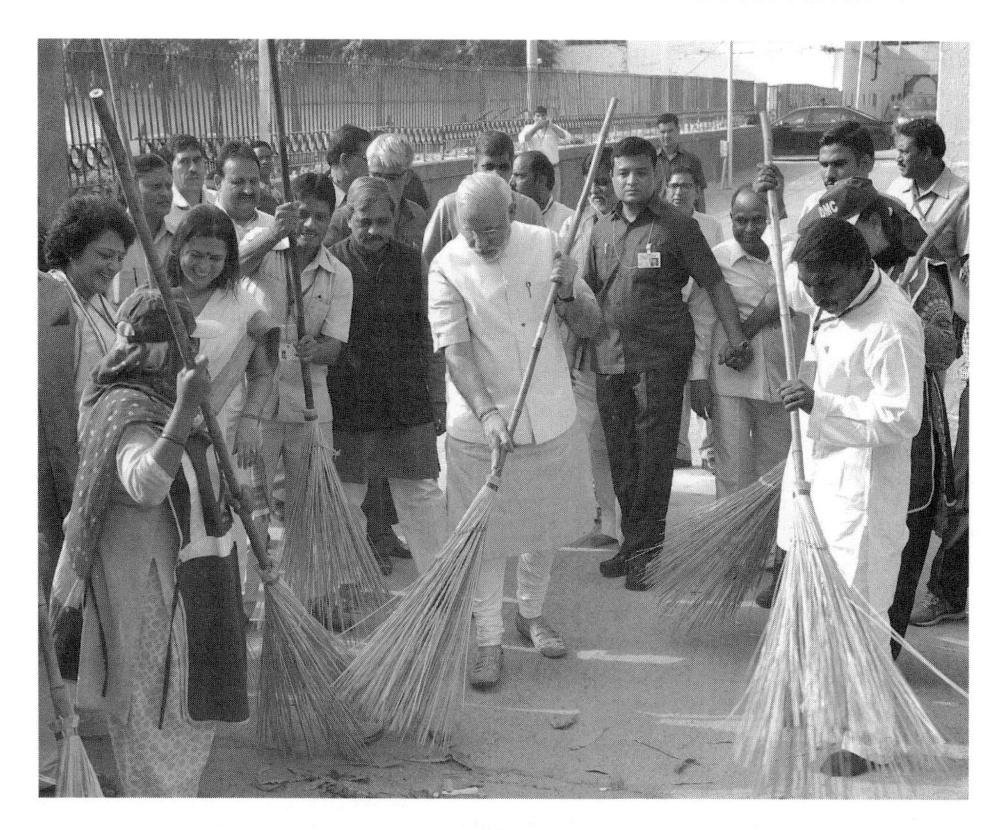

Fig. I.1 **Sweeping all before him. Prime Minister Modi launches the Swachh Bharat campaign in Valmiki Basti, New Delhi, October 2, 2014.** Press Information Bureau, Government of India, Prime Minister's Office. CNR 60274. Photo ID 57537.

itation: the Morbi dam disaster of 1979 and the panic over bubonic plague in the city of Surat in 1994. In the case of Morbi, a badly built dam collapsed during heavy monsoon rains. The town was inundated without warning. Officially, 1,800 people died; researchers later suggested that deaths "may have exceeded five thousand."[18] Modi was at that time a twenty-nine-year-old worker in the Rashtriya Swayamsevak Sangh (RSS), a Hindu-chauvinist organization. "A huge cleaning up operation was undertaken," he wrote, "and I was part of it. We . . . ensured that the town was restored to pre-disaster levels and an epidemic was averted."[19]

By the time the plague panic hit Surat in 1994, Modi was a political organizer, an RSS strongman recently returned from a tour of the United States, and by year's end, state general secretary of the BJP.[20] Armed with his experience of Morbi, Modi said that, on reaching Surat in 1994, "I went around meeting people and encouraging them to stay and not to run away. I told them that there was no need to panic." Modi took the opportunity to educate people "not only about personal hygiene but also about social hygiene. The Plague incident was a game changer as far as Surat is concerned. People's sensitivity towards hygiene increased. The Municipal Corporation's [the local government] decision making capacity improved." If change could happen in Surat, it was possible elsewhere.

The Clean India campaign also had political attractions.[21] It emphasized patriotism, aligned the legacy of Mahatma Gandhi alongside that of a BJP government, and appealed to millions of overseas Indians, many of whom were supporters of Modi and who squirmed at the state of public sanitation when they visited with children, friends, and associates. Clean India would also give daily visibility to the can-do reputation of the prime minister and to promises of *vikas*—development—which had figured prominently in the election campaign. Themes of the campaign suited a BJP agenda. The private sector, through public-private partnerships, was expected to provide many of the solutions to waste management and public sanitation. And the drive to eliminate open defecation, often portrayed as a campaign to protect women—our mothers, sisters, and daughters—suited patriarchal tendencies of the BJP's rhetoric and actions.[22]

A Binding Crisis: Surat, 1994

The horror that the word *plague* evokes put the city of Surat in Gujarat on a global stage in 1994. It provoked stories in media around the world, including *Time* and *Esquire* magazines, and it generated scholarly studies and discussion of plague in Surat in best-selling books about disasters.[23] The author-physician Abraham Varghese wrote in *Esquire*, "When plague broke out in Surat, the shock waves reached as far west

कब तक घर
की ही सोचोगे?
थोड़ी शर्म कर लो,
सोच स्वच्छ कर लो!

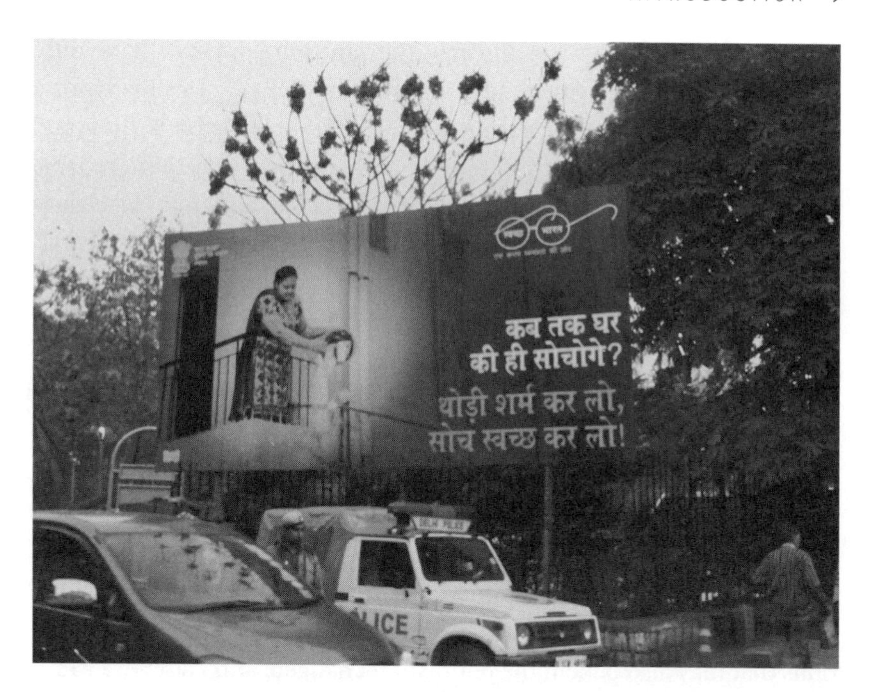

Fig. I.2 The father of the nation is watching. Gandhi's spectacles peer down on a householder dumping kitchen scraps. "How long will you think only of the home? Have some shame. Clean up your thinking!" Photo © Assa Doron, 2015.

as El Paso, Texas."[24] The *Organiser,* the English-language weekly of the RSS, splashed "The Killer Plague" across the front page of its edition of October 9, 1994, and commented at length on "the growing decay of the big cities of India."[25] About a third of Surat's population fled, and there was "panic throughout the nation." Although only eighty deaths were recorded, the event "created worldwide panic."[26]

Later, of course, it appeared not to have been bubonic plague at all. It was a misdiagnosis.[27] What was important, however, was the blind, widespread terror and what came afterward, confirming the politician's maxim "Never let a good crisis go to waste."[28] In 1994, Surat was described as "India's dirtiest city."[29] Within three years, it was described as one of the cleanest, a rank it has largely retained even as it has grown.[30] The shock of "the plague"—whether it was plague or not—galvanized a city's population. "Waste management . . . changed overnight," wrote a woman who was a medical officer at the time. This was partly because "the public who felt helpless [during the outbreak] . . . was ready for a change."[31] A hard-driving municipal commissioner led a willing and wealthy city to institute thorough waste collection and more reliable sewage and drainage. Surat's *binding crisis,* a crisis that unites all classes of citizens in their response to disaster, provoked rigorous and welcomed policy. The city changed its habits and became noticeably cleaner.

Most disasters are nothing more than pure misery. They destroy lives and livings. People die, and the poor come out of them worse off than before. Hurricane Katrina in New Orleans and the Union Carbide disaster in Bhopal further marginalized the poor and dispossessed.[32] Ideally, a binding crisis does minimum harm and generates maximum response. The plague in Surat was democratic: it appeared anyone could catch it. The rich seemed in as much danger as the poor, and only by improving conditions for all could life be made more certain. Such a crisis gives the wealthy immediate, convincing reasons for taking actions that may also benefit the poor. Surat changed, and Narendra Modi had been close at hand to see it. A website sympathetic to the RSS proudly notes that, among its achievements, it had "fought the 1994 outbreak of plague in Surat."[33]

There are celebrated examples from the nineteenth century of binding crises elsewhere. The Great Stink in London in the summer of 1858 was at its worst under the noses of Parliament, and legislation for London's great sewer system quickly followed. Hamburg's reputation for a "progressive stance in sanitary matters" in the mid-nineteenth century was one of the "direct consequences" of the citywide fire of 1842, "and without it they [reforms] would certainly not have occurred so quickly or so comprehensively." Hamburg's notorious cholera epidemic of 1892 enabled Robert Koch to demonstrate conclusively that his theories about the cause of cholera were correct. Governments across Europe and North America could no longer shirk their responsibility to purify water for their citizens. "It needed a terrible catastrophe," a German orator declared, "before the Senate would cast a glance at the poverty in the city."[34] In U.S. cities in the nineteenth century, "the epidemics . . . which originated and garnered momentum in the crowded slums, spread eventually to cleaner and less crowded areas; the problem of the tenements concerned every city dweller."[35] Even Bombay's plague outbreaks of 1896 "forced municipalities . . . to increase their spending on sanitation."[36]

India in the twenty-first century is a far cry from other countries in the nineteenth, however. For a start, the population in India in 2011 (1.2 billion) was not far from the population of the entire world in 1891 (about 1.5 billion). Moreover, disasters that have provoked policy and cultural changes—binding crises—have usually been dramatic, sudden, and narrowly focused. The environmental crises that India faces in the twenty-first century are slower moving and farther reaching. We allude to two possible binding crises in this book. One is air pollution, which even the wealthy and powerful find difficult to escape. Air pollution links inextricably to waste—to the ash produced by coal-fired power plants, the random fires that burn on landfills or are lit by citizens disposing of garbage, and the field stubble burned by farmers because it is cheaper than harvesting it for fodder or compost. As the toxic air that cloaks India's cities worsens, the connections between the coughing rich and the choking poor may grow more obvious. A shared interest in investing money and abandoning old practices may produce a binding crisis that generates profound cultural change. But air pollution is different from a flood, an earthquake, or a disease that kills in hours. It lacks immediacy: responses can be put off; bucks can be passed.

Poor sanitation that impedes children's growth might have been another crisis to bind social classes together in their response, especially in rural north India. The connections between open defecation, intestinal parasites, and childhood mortality, stunting, and ill health are now well established and acknowledged by the very highest levels of government. Prime Minister Modi was quick to announce his flagship campaign to clean India—Swachh Bharat—as he came into office. It was an unprecedented operation. "Various studies," Modi told us, "have shown that open defecation and unsanitary practices are linked to several diseases, especially among children, which lead to high infant mortality and impairs the growth and development of children."[37] If it became common knowledge that open defecation endangered the lives and the well-being of children both rich and poor, the demand for effective toilets, and their use and maintenance, would grow. But this crisis isn't a binding crisis: it lacks the clarity and immediacy of a terrifying threat, such as a wall of water or a neighbor covered in pestilential boils.

The experience of Surat in 1994 suggests that a binding crisis may generate change. And the transmission of ideas in 2018 has never been more possible, pervasive, and democratic (some might say promiscuous). India had 1.15 billion mobile phone subscribers at the end of 2016, a teledensity estimated at 90 percent.[38] This did not mean that almost every citizen owned a mobile phone, but even among poor and marginalized people, phones were within reach and could be borrowed, shared, and wished for. It is possible to transmit messages relentlessly to very large sections of the population, as Modi and his party know well after their remarkable victory in the 2014 elections. The prime minister's bitterest critics would not deny his deftness in the use of media.

Getting to Know Garbage

If India's encounter with the detritus of consumer capitalism is a jigsaw puzzle, the following chapters are pieces of the puzzle, intended to fit together to form an interlocking picture. We aspire to understand and explain cultural beliefs and practices relating to waste, technical and policy nostrums deployed to deal with the perils of pollution, and the political compulsions that drive decisions and programs. Aspiring middle classes seek world-class cities, but proposed solutions often leave the urban poor alienated and dispossessed. India's density of population, intricate cultural practices, and pulsating politics make it essential for successful programs to respond to local needs when (and if) they adopt technical and managerial practices from elsewhere. Simple solutions may appeal to neoliberal ideas and entrepreneurial spirits, but ground-level experience tells a more complicated story of how people think about and experience waste. Existing systems of waste recovery feature an array of actors—scavengers, waste-pickers, garbage buyers, and a host of processors and receivers. They are all linked to each other by an internal logic dictated by economic, social, and cultural relationships.[39]

In the industrialized world, technology mediates and mitigates the relationship between people and waste. Recycling, for example, can be portrayed as a moral act—the redemption of rejected things. In India, however, garbage, refuse, and waste are commonly identified with the *people* who handle them, usually in haphazard, unsystematic ways. To experience waste is ritually polluting, potentially contaminating, and physically risky. Caste prejudice compounds widespread discrimination against a "wasted" underclass of Dalits, landless migrants, and poor Muslims. These heterogeneous groups constitute an almost inexhaustible supply of unskilled laborers who often live in settlements near the piles of rubbish generated by a burgeoning consumer middle class.[40] Waste is therefore not only about economic practices and political compulsions but also central to cultural beliefs, especially the interplay of relations among genders, classes, and castes.

Questions of social class have teased administrators, social scientists, Marxists, and marketers for more than a hundred years. From the 1920s, India's communists struggled to build class-based movements to advance the revolution, adhering to the ideas of Marx and Lenin and following instructions from the Soviet Union. They rarely succeeded. From the 1990s, capitalists and their marketing directors identified "India's growing middle class" as an aspirational group with varied levels of disposable income, defined by their desire for consumer goods and the resulting garbage they produced.[41] But what defines the Indian middle class, and how many people constitute it? Estimates and definitions vary widely.[42]

For purposes of highlighting the magnitude and growth potential of India's waste born of prosperity, a few estimates of consumer goods will serve. In 1996, about 6 percent of Indian households were estimated to have a refrigerator and 23 percent a television set. Estimates in 2015 put TV households at 63 percent and refrigerator households at 29 percent (Table I.1).[43] "There is a huge market being created for the white goods and automobile makers" a scholar at the National Council for Applied Economic Research concluded when one of the council's surveys suggested the middle class amounted to 160 million people, or 13 percent of the population.[44] Such figures represent vast numbers of material goods to be manufactured, supplied with energy, repaired, and ultimately discarded—about 80 million refrigerators for a start. And that 70 percent of households do not have a refrigerator and more than 30 percent lack a television set suggests that many more are waiting. Mass-produced, manufactured things generate waste not merely in themselves but in the

Table I.1 Television and Refrigerator Households, 1996 and 2015

	1996	2015
Number of Households	171 million	277 million
Television households	23 percent	63 percent
Refrigerator households	6 percent	29 percent

Source: Telecom Regulatory Authority of India, *Annual Report, 2014–15* (New Delhi: TRAI, 2015), p. 6, "PRICE, Household Survey on India's Citizen Environmental and Consumer Economy," https://goo.gl/DiR1GH.

processes that make them, the construction of the buildings that produce them, the roads that distribute them, and the energy necessary to dispose of them.

Contemporary India must redefine its relationship with waste. India is not alone in facing expanding towns and cities, mountains of consumer and industrial waste, and rivers of sewage, and India can learn from other countries' experience (Chapters 1 and 2). India's task, however, is uniquely difficult: nowhere, not even in China, have the volumes of waste and the density of human population been so great.

India faces a second extraordinary challenge in addressing the cultural relationship between waste and caste. We touch on aspects of caste throughout the book, but they receive extended treatment in Chapter 3. Ideas of "pure" and "impure," which have little to do with scientific principles of hygiene, continue to inform everyday practice among large sections of Hindu society. Although untouchability has been illegal for more than three generations, 190 million people born into this group are still stigmatized by other people's belief that they are polluting. The most polluting of all are those who deal with human waste and refuse.

Despite these problems, India has a marked advantage in waste management compared with other industrialized countries: its cultural and institutional traditions of reuse and frugality (Chapter 4). The *kabaadiwala*—the rag-and-bone man, the door-to-door purchaser of unwanted items—has been part of India for as long as anyone knows or remembers. The networks of *kabaadiwalas* provide pathways and examples for today's recyclers.

In a number of Indian traditions, austerity and self-denial are valued as examples of virtuous conduct, and Gandhi, the father of the nation, preached simplicity and self-sufficiency as essential elements of a free and fulfilled India. But effective capture, reuse, or disposal of discarded things requires more than reliance on old—and attenuating—ways. It requires systematic thoroughness, technical innovation, realization of an urgent need to change, and respect and fair reward for workers at all links of the waste chain.

Effective recycling of vast quantities of materials, many of them new and volatile, requires both labor, which India has in plenty, and appropriate methods (Chapter 5). Around the country, authorities search for large-scale, technical remedies to solve all their problems. But there are no single-shot solutions—technologies suitable for local conditions are essential.

India's local governments, charged with much of the responsibility for keeping their jurisdictions clean, are underpowered and ill equipped (Chapter 6). Revenue-collecting is underdeveloped, elected councillors are underprepared, and well-trained, committed officials are scarce. Coordination among local governments is difficult, and the temptation to treat local governments as mere tools and instruments of state governments is immense.

Across the country, however, there are remarkable examples of local governments that function well, of competent toilet building, of water management that protects the environment, of effective nongovernmental organizations and community groups, and of projects, large and small, that contribute to a cleaner India (Chapter 7). Successes result from the efforts of skilled individuals who draw their strength from cooperation. Respect, reward, and hope for improved futures are at the heart of successful, sustained programs. Accumulated actions add up to substantial change in behavior and practice. If a Swachh Bharat (Clean India) is to be achieved, it will be a place where the waste of a nation does not include poor and marginalized *people* but is restricted to inanimate *matter*—minimized, collected, neutralized, and reused in ways that provide models for other places in an environmentally fragile world.

1

TIME AND PLACE

FLORENCE NIGHTINGALE (1820–1910) never went to India. When people recall her today, they probably think of the lady with the lamp moving among wounded British soldiers during the Crimean War of 1853–1856. But Nightingale had a special interest in India and in modern notions of public sanitation and control of filth, as she called it. Her advocacy and notoriety focused British officials on a problem they were loath to admit: appalling sanitation practices undermined both the health of British soldiers and any moral case justifying British rule.

Independent India in 1947 inherited attitudes and practices relating to public sanitation developed during British times. The nationalist movement sometimes challenged those attitudes but in ways that celebrated an idealized rural life rather than recognized the needs of a changing urban India. For their part, British governments invested sparingly in public sanitation. They aimed primarily to protect European soldiers and civilians and to prevent international shipping bans based on a reputation that ships from India carried deadly disease. Officials often met even these pressures with the response that widespread public sanitation measures were too expensive and disruptive to undertake. At times of epidemic, panicky and heavy-handed enforcement of quarantine and vaccination further alienated the rulers from the ruled and became a notable element in the nationalist movement.

Analyzing the foundations of public sanitation and comparing it with Indian experience across time and space clarifies India's advantages and handicaps as it confronts unprecedented volumes of waste in the twenty-first century. India has the benefit of drawing on the public-health science of 150 years. But no other country has faced India's density of population, volumes of waste, and the cultural minefield of caste belief and practice.

Sanitation and the State

Florence Nightingale was a product of a modern age of industrial production, urban life, scientific inquiry, fact gathering, and mass media. She earned fame during the Crimean War when the *Illustrated London News* (circulation one hundred thousand) ran an artist's engraving showing her tending the wounded, oil lamp at hand. She returned to Britain in 1856 as a national hero. In the following year the Great Revolt began in India. Two years later, when it was over and authorities counted the casualties, nearly 10,000 soldiers on the British side had died. But fewer than 1,500 Europeans were killed in action; more than 8,500 died of disease. "It was disease, and not the enemy that killed [the British soldier]."[1] This recognition was so startling that a parliamentary commission was set up "to inquire into the Sanitary State of the Army in India."[2] The imposing report of 1863 marked a first attempt in India to deploy modern ideas, based on the science of the time, about waste and sanitation.

The Sanitary Commission went about its work in a manner familiar to employees of any twenty-first-century organization: it conducted a survey. It circulated a questionnaire on sanitation to 175 military centers in India and got a remarkable rate of 117 responses, "more or less fully given." It sent the replies to be analyzed by the most celebrated sanitation personality of the day—Florence Nightingale.[3] Her findings were scathing:

> The description given of the native towns is astonishing. . . . So [far] as one can judge from the evidence, the sanitary state of entire large cities is as bad as, if not worse than, was the state of

> the worst parts of our worst towns before there was any sanitary knowledge in the modern world at all.[4]

The outcome of the commission's report and Nightingale's devastating critique was the realization, as David Arnold writes, "that the health of European soldiers and civilians could not be secured through measures directed at their health alone."[5]

The evidence presented to the commission illustrated the embryonic knowledge of microbiology in the 1850s, particularly among British officials long in India. Commenting on the "endemic" nature of diarrhea, the deputy inspector-general of hospitals conceded that "the quality of the water might have something to answer for, but I am inclined to believe that the well known cause of this complaint everywhere, viz., *suppressed perspiration* [italics in the original], is principally to blame." He advised that the solution—"the grand prophylactic"—was "flannel, and especially the broad flannel abdominal binder worn next the skin."[6] Another medical witness thought that "impure water" seemed to lead to "worms and bowel affections [*sic*]." Others, however, were aware of the discovery made during the cholera epidemic in London in 1854 that dirty water and cholera went together. But precisely why dirty water could lead to cholera was not known, nor was the connection between contaminated water and cholera universally accepted.[7]

On the matter of personal hygiene, witnesses agreed that Indian soldiers were "generally cleanly" and that, for a Hindu solider, "cleanliness is one of the injunctions of his religion."[8] On the other hand, "the natives have no idea," another medical witness submitted, "of taking sanitary precautions. . . . A man will eat and drink and perform his evacuations actually on the very same foot of water, standing in it, or close to it; he has no idea of impurity as long as it happens to be Ganges water." A commissioner asked whether European enlisted men "drink water from these tanks?" The witness replied, "Yes, there is nothing else for them."[9] European enlisted men also "adhered to the good old English custom of washing the face and hands once a day, and the feet as seldom as possible."[10] Global cleanliness campaigns awaited the flowering of nineteenth-century imperialism and the advertising of the great soap industries from the 1880s on.

Florence Nightingale rounded with gusto on the conditions existing in soldiers' barracks and the towns and cities where they were stationed. "If there be an exception," she began one blistering attack,

> *i.e.*, if there be a single station in India with a good system of drainage, water supply and cleansing for itself and its bazaars . . . , these remarks do not apply. But I have not found it. Everywhere there lie grievous sanitary defects, which . . . can lead only to sickness and loss of life. . . . The practical result . . . is that safe water supplies are yet to be found both for Indian cities and British cantonments; and that many sources [of drinking water] . . . would in England be scouted as infallible causes of cholera.[11]

Her critique of the conditions in military towns dripped with irony:

> The system of water supply and drainage in India may be briefly defined as follows: they draw water from a well, not knowing whence it comes, and if there be any means to drain off water it is into a cesspit, or into long, open, pervious drains, not knowing whither it goes. Where this is not done, all the fluid refuse is collected in open cesspits, and carried away by hand labour or carts. Or else it is allowed to dispose of itself in the air or earth as best it can.[12]

India became a focus of Nightingale's work for the next forty years, and her advocacy sometimes attracted attention and led to action. British policy, however, was driven by self-interested economics. Sick soldiers and officials were costly. Only if it preserved the well-being of the rulers and their associates was public sanitation likely to warrant investment.[13]

Nightingale's fame coincided with discoveries related to hygiene and disease. Studying the cholera outbreak in London in 1854, John Snow established the connection between cholera and contaminated water. Nightingale was aware of the connection, but she came to appreciate germ theory only near the end of her life.[14] It was not clear what specific characteristics of bad water caused devastating diseases like cholera.

In 1884 the German microbiologist Robert Koch (1843–1910), using much-improved microscopes and making conclusive discoveries in Calcutta, identified the cholera bacillus, the comma-shaped organism that transmitted the disease, usually through infected water.[15] It took more time to prove that the cholera bacillus *caused* cholera and was not simply *produced* by cholera. However, by the 1880s, Koch and many other scientists were convinced: physical organisms—germs—visible under the microscope caused cholera, not bad air.

Koch's well-publicized work did not translate immediately into policies and public works to protect water supplies of towns and cities. One of the last great cholera epidemics in Europe was in Hamburg in his native Germany in 1892. More than 8,500 people died from sewage being pumped into the River Elbe upstream and becoming part of the water supply of Hamburg downstream.[16] The epidemic, however, produced further evidence, and by 1893, "Koch's theory came to command almost universal assent among medical men in Europe."[17]

If the findings of Koch, a celebrated hero of German science, were slow to provoke government action for public sanitation, it is not surprising that acceptance of germ theory among British officials in India came even more slowly. Official careers had sometimes been founded on arguing for miasma as the cause of deadly diseases: the idea that bad air made people ill. Many British officials and medical people resisted germ theory until the 1890s. The "conservative Indian Medical Service" took until 1908 to accept that fleas were crucial in the transmission of bubonic plague, although authorities elsewhere had recognized the connection nearly a decade earlier.[18]

Florence Nightingale was perceptive. "In India," she wrote, "as at home, no good will be done unless it be made some competent person's express business to look at these things."[19] The fixing of responsibility for making towns and cities clean remains even today at the heart of public sanitation, as we try to show in Chapter 6. Responsibility for waste management is like waste itself: tempting to leave to others. But as Nightingale said, someone must be made responsible and trained to fulfill those responsibilities.

The Sanitary Commission of 1863 led to improved conditions in and around army barracks. Wider understanding of the dangers of tainted water brought modest sewerage improvements and water supply to cities like Calcutta in the 1860s.[20] But only in the 1890s, when self-interest coincided with slow acceptance of medical science, did British government in India begin to "recognize a greater practical responsibility for the health of its subjects."[21]

Other imperialist powers viewed the British as incapable of curbing the threat of infectious disease carried from Indian ports. In a world of steamships, ever-growing international trade, and the Suez Canal (completed 1869), rival powers in Europe, plus the United States, could treat India under British rule as a sink of disease and British ships as potential carriers of cholera, typhoid, and bubonic plague. Cholera in India in 1882 brought quarantines and "the threat of international sanitary sanctions against India."[22] For the rest of the century the British in India were viewed by other imperialist powers as unreliable caretakers of a place from which diseases could spread and whose ships should be strictly monitored. At times of epidemics, British rivals suggested that British ships should be excluded from European ports.

In the 1890s, bubonic plague wove health and sanitation into the fabric of modern Indian nationhood. Once it was widely accepted in Europe that people carried germs and germs carried disease, pressure increased on the British in India to ensure that goods, ships, and people from India did not bring disease to Europe and the United States.[23] Those outside the British Empire had reason for apprehension, because the Government of India had been wedded to the story that India was uniquely mysterious and unhealthy and that it was India's climate and environment, not microbes, that made it so. India's diseases, this fantasy contended, were so exotic that they could survive only in India. After that interpretation was discredited, foreign powers focused on ships originating from India as disease carriers. When the much-feared black death—bubonic plague—circulated widely beginning in 1896, Britain was under intense international pressure to do something. Ian Catanach captured the mood: "The outbreak of plague . . . provided other colonial powers with a pawn in the imperial game."[24]

The Government of India passed legislation that gave officials and the police the right to enforce strict quarantine rules and to enter, and even demolish, houses that might harbor the disease. In doing so, the government put public sanitation and Western medical science near the center of the nationalist movement for the next fifty years. Intrusion into people's homes, including the women's quarters, was passionately resented, especially by higher castes.

Such intrusions led to the murder in Pune in June 1897 of Walter Rand, the European plague commissioner, and a younger officer, by two brothers, Damodar and Balakrishna Chapekar.[25] The British caught the Chapekar brothers, tried them, hanged them, and brought charges of sedition against the editor and social activist Bal Gangadhar Tilak (1856–1920). Tilak's newspapers had supported the agitation against the government's intrusive plague measures. Sentenced to eighteen months for sedition, Tilak became a national hero, dubbed Lokmanya—"honored by the people." Public health and sanitation became an explosive element in the chemistry of nationalism.[26]

Tilak's resistance to government violation of hearths and homes clashed with medical science, but it was anchored in time-honored practices and ideas of ritual purity and pollution. Tilak presented the tension as a conflict between the dignity of India and the blundering ideology of an arrogant West. For Mohandas Karamchand Gandhi, the father of the nation, reconciling Indian custom with medical science became a lifelong concern. Gandhi opposed vaccination on religious grounds and for the harm inflicted on animals in preparing vaccines.[27] By 1930, he grudgingly accepted the theory of germs: "Experts on hygiene have demonstrated through numerous experiments how poisonous germs are born in such water [of an uncontrolled village pond] and diseases like cholera result from drinking it."[28] However, his suspicion of Western medicine and distaste for urban life colored the ideas of the Congress Party during the independence movement and after. Improving India's towns and cities was not a Congress priority; perfecting the village was. British governments welcomed this indifference because it made it easier to shrink budgets and curtail or abandon public sanitation projects.[29] Local governments, even under elected Indian control, had little incentive to think about, or capacity to act on, the needs of their towns or cities. "Very few" local governments during the 1920s and 1930s "were persuaded of the need for sewerage schemes or thorough arrangements for refuse disposal. Conservancy [waste management] methods hardly made any advance."[30] In 1947, India's national and state governments inherited colonial diffidence about urban and rural sanitation. Local governments were weakly supported, and the attitude of the Congress Party toward public health and urbanization was ambivalent.

Sanitation in the World

People in other places and times have confronted the bloating mountains of detritus that consumer capitalism and urbanization produce, and in the nineteenth century India's sanitary practices were not markedly less hygienic than elsewhere in the world. The "sanitary knowledge" that Florence Nightingale referred to in the 1860s was little more than a generation old in Britain and existed more in theory than in practice. "The 1848 Public Health Act," says the website of today's British Parliament, "was the first step on the road to improved public health."[31] The landmark research that documented the foulness of Britain's growing industrial cities was Edwin Chadwick's *Report on the Sanitary Condition of the Labouring Population,* "a masterpiece of protest literature," published in 1842, which led to parliamentary inquiries and legislation.[32] The evidence gathered in Britain described conditions that were similar in India. In Manchester's slums,

> whole streets . . . are unpaved and without drains or main-sewers, . . . and are so covered with refuse and excrementitious matter as to be almost impassable from depth of mud, and intolerable from stench. . . . Privies in the most disgusting state of filth, open cesspools, obstructed drains, ditches full of stagnant water, dunghills, pigsties, &c., from which the most abominable odours are emitted. . . . The doors of these hovels very commonly open upon the uncovered cesspool.[33]

The industrial towns of Continental Europe and North America offered many examples of their own. A celebrated newspaper engraving of 1859 by the American artist Winslow Homer is titled *Scene from the Back Bay Lands* and shows more than a dozen men and women scrabbling for valuable waste on a garbage dump in Boston.[34] The streets of New York in the second half of the nineteenth century steamed with "the pervasive rot and muck that had come to be called 'Corporation Pudding,'"[35] in reference to the local government, which was unable to remove the daily waste. New York City in the 1890s had more than 130,000 horses, each of which produced up to thirty-five pounds of manure and more than one quart of urine on the city's streets each day.[36] In the 1880s, fifteen thousand horses died on the streets of New York every year, along with countless pigs, dogs, cats, and rats.[37] In 2013, the city of Ahmedabad coped each day with ten metric tons of animal carcasses, including cows, buffaloes, donkeys, and occasionally camels.[38] Effective urban sanitation grows out of local needs, changed behavior, and political and administrative persistence. It takes time.

The American historian Martin Melosi has charted the changing methods over the past 150 years that North America and Europe have used to try to tame waste. Large settlements dumped waste into lakes, rivers, or the sea or onto unwanted land on the periphery of a town—the sort of thing Winslow Homer depicted outside Boston. In the 1870s, Britain's growing industrial cities set up giant furnaces to burn waste. "Hailed as a technological panacea," the incineration system spread to Europe and the United States.[39] U.S. cities also experimented with "reduction," by which garbage was compressed to extract "oils and other by-products" that could be sold "as lubricants, perfume bases or fertilizers." But the expense of the process and the resulting "foul odours" and filthy runoff led to it being quickly abandoned.[40] In the twentieth century, local governments began to transform dumps into sanitary landfills (sometimes referred to as "scientific" landfills), places where the daily addition of garbage was covered to control smells and pests, leachate was drained off, and methane gas controlled.[41] A lot went wrong with early sanitary landfills.[42] But since the 1970s public pressure and improved science have reduced defects. When a sanitary landfill is full, it is covered over and turned into land for public purposes, becoming a park or even a housing development. In their idealized form, sanitary landfills become land reclamation projects. That is the cheerful story, and some

Indian cities, such as Ahmedabad, Surat, Delhi, and Hyderabad, have landfills that aspire to sanitary standards, although not necessarily successfully.[43]

Definitions are significant. "Dumpsites," the authors of *Waste Atlas: The World's 50 Biggest Dumpsites—2014 Report* emphasize, "have nothing to do with sanitary landfills."[44] Sanitary landfills, when executed properly, are carefully designed and regulated. Built in suitable geological locations on prepared foundations, they sit on an impermeable plastic blanket to capture and drain off leachate, the liquid that seeps from the festering mass. Sanitary landfills capture the methane gas (CH_4) produced by rotting garbage and either burn it off or use it to make electric power. Released into the atmosphere, methane contributes twenty times more to global warming than an equal amount of carbon dioxide (CO_2).

At their idealized best, sanitary landfills act as recycling centers, control leachate, generate electricity from methane, work closely with neighbors, and have lecture halls for school groups and tour parties. The goal is to minimize what actually gets buried. Canada's favorite retirement city, Victoria, British Columbia, has a sanitary landfill, where views of the snow-capped Olympic Mountains are worthy of a postcard and nearby homes are worth a million dollars.[45] But to make such centers work, appropriate technology, political negotiation, relentless maintenance, and sustained connections with communities are essential, as Chapter 5 investigates.

The largest and best-known of North America's old-style dumps was Freshkills, located on the outskirts of New York City. ("Kill" comes from an old Dutch word, *kille,* meaning "stream.") Started in 1947 and closed in March 2001, Freshkills had to be temporarily reopened to take debris after the destruction of the World Trade Center in September 2001. Freshkills covers nearly 900 hectares (2,200 acres) and rises to 68 meters (225 feet).[46] Robin Nagle, an anthropology professor who took students there when it was a working landfill, describes "bulging hills [that] seemed to go forever . . . a concentrated manifestation of immense material might."[47] In 2008, "the transformation of what was formerly the world's largest landfill into a productive and beautiful cultural destination" began, according to the website of the Freshkills Park Alliance.

The park will eventually become "a symbol of renewal."[48] The website tells a happy story, in which an old dumpsite is made beautiful through planning and investment.

Such portrayals, however, sweep alternative versions of the Freshkills story under its pretty new carpet. Turning dumpsites and landfills into attractive landscapes is never free of politics and powerful interests. For much of its life, Freshkills was a simple dump, an area of wetland far enough away from New York City to offend fewer people than alternative sites would have done. It is not chance that its international twin park partner is the Hiriya landfill, now Ariel Sharon Park, outside Tel Aviv in Israel. The Hiriya landfill was set up in the late 1940s on land Arabs were driven from during the war that created the state of Israel in 1948.[49] The waste that used to go to Hiriya now goes farther south, where Bedouin communities have little scope to object or resist.[50] In the management of waste, human beings themselves are too often transformed into waste, expendable in the cause of some greater aesthetic or hygienic good. India is no different from other places in this respect, but deeply embedded practices related to caste make India's confrontation with consumerist garbage particularly difficult, as we explore in Chapter 3.

India's dumpsites are not the biggest in the world or the worst. To be sure, Mumbai's Deonar site is a small mountain of garbage and ranks as a *Tyrannosaurus rex* among dumps. It captured global attention in February 2016 when parts of its 130 hectares (320 acres) caught fire, and Mumbai coughed and choked more than usual for six weeks.[51] One survey ranks it as the eighth largest, well behind the leader, Apex Regional, which occupies 890 hectares (2,200 acres) on the outskirts of Las Vegas, Nevada.[52] The *Waste Atlas* report identifies "the world's 50 biggest dumpsites," seventeen Asian sites among them. In India, they include only Deonar and the relatively small (30 hectares) Ghazipur site in east Delhi.[53] An attempt by an American ecology writer to pinpoint "15 of the world's largest landfills" lumped various dumps into single sites in both Mumbai and Delhi, and the combined data put the two in the featured fifteen sites. But Apex Regional in Las Vegas again stood out as the largest.[54] Apex Regional, however, is not a dump; it's a "sanitary landfill."

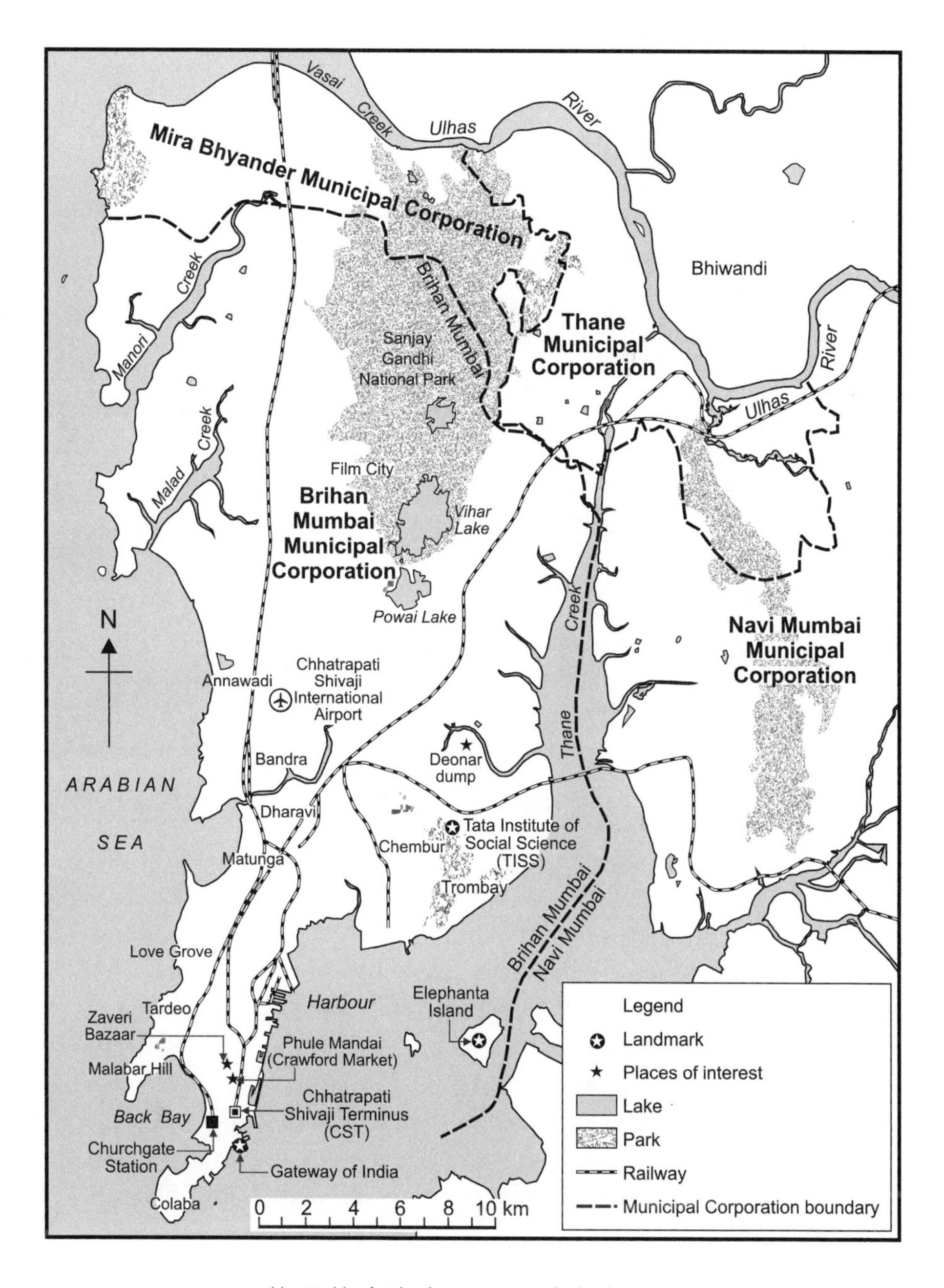

Map 1.1 Mumbai: local governments and select locations

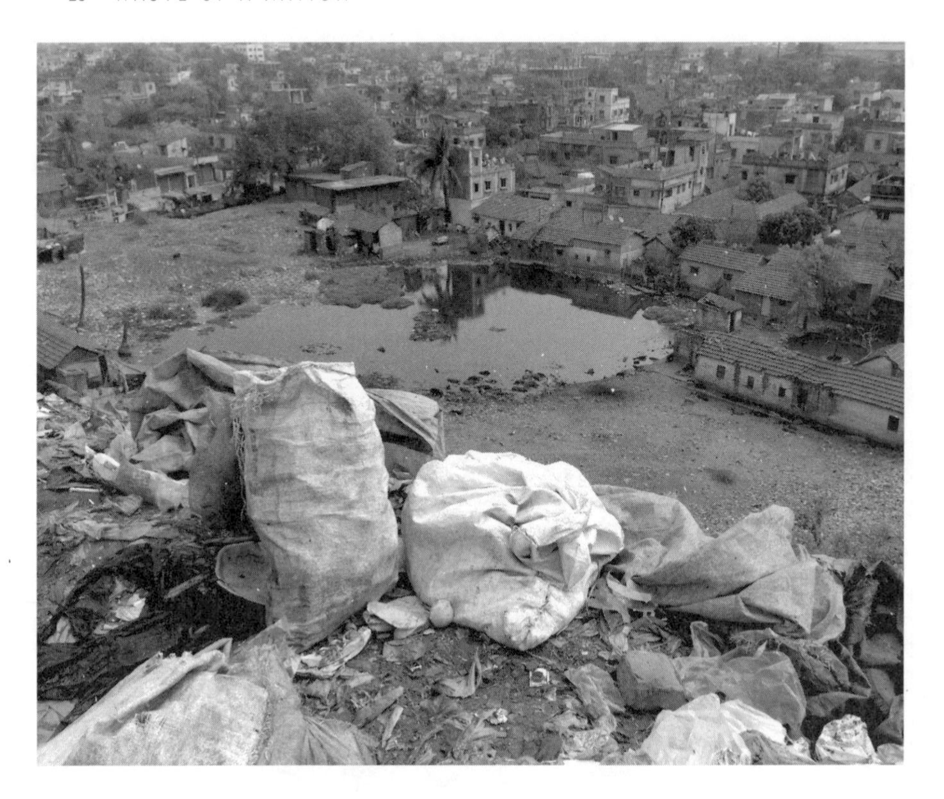

Fig. 1.1 **Landfill at Belgachia, Howrah, West Bengal. A section subsided into villages below in 2009.** Photo © Robin Jeffrey, 2015.

Apex Regional landfill illustrates the complicated relationships between governments and private companies that arise in attempts to manage waste. The Nevada site is owned by Republic Services, a Fortune 500 company with annual revenue of $8.4 billion. It is one of the two largest waste management companies in the United States.[55] The company is licensed to use Apex Regional, which is expected to have an operating life of a hundred years, as a sanitary landfill. Republic Services' major rival, Waste Management, probably the biggest waste company in the world, also owns landfills—including three of the largest in the United States. It operates (but does not own) two other very large landfills on contracts from local governments.[56] Governments decide whether allowing a private company to buy a landfill site or leasing land to a company to operate a site is more beneficial to citizens. In China, the country's largest landfill, Laogang on the southeastern outskirts of Shanghai close to the sea, is owned by the local government but managed by the French waste management company Veolia on a twenty-year agreement. In 2016, Veolia ran twenty waste sites and landfills in China, including some that generated electricity from methane or incineration.[57]

These public-private partnerships (PPP) are a popular management device worldwide. "The Government of India was for a time "actively encouraging PPPs," according to its website.[58] There is caution, however, on both the public and the private sides. Only about forty PPPs for waste management have been notified to the Government of India, and half of these provide little information. The outsourcing of solid waste management to private enterprise, with promises of technical rationality and efficiency, has repeatedly proved a disappointment in India. In Europe and North America, the PPP model appears to have worked much better, because "state services were already a 'going concern,' with near universal coverage. The state had a strong institutional capacity and the private sector was mature and large."[59] Neither condition characterizes India. Local governments are underpowered, and their efforts in waste management and public sanitation have often been half-hearted at best. Private industry has been reluctant to enter the business of waste management. India had no more than half a dozen substantial companies dealing in waste in 2016, and none had managed the high levels of profit achieved by international corporations that work with waste. No major international company had entered India to undertake waste management, although Veolia had PPP agreements for water supply in Maharashtra and Karnataka.[60]

In surveys of notorious dumps of the modern world, a few names regularly appear. The Bordo Poniente dump in Mexico City covered 600 hectares (1,500 acres) and was closed in 2011.[61] Bordo Poniente ranked third in size worldwide, according to Chris Mills's calculations (although a number of the world's legendary dumps missed out on his list).[62] Manila once had the infamous Smokey Mountain, whose successor at Payatas produced a garbage-mountain avalanche that swept three hundred people to their deaths in 2000. By 2014, however,

Manila's dumps had acquired a more benign, although still dubious, reputation.[63] Nairobi's well-known and overflowing Dandora dump covers a mere 13 hectares (about 30 acres), although its public health consequences may be out of proportion to its size.[64] Cairo was said to have been kept tidy by the *zabaleen,* Coptic Christians whose pigs helped contain organic waste. But the authorities hired private companies to collect waste, the pigs were made to disappear, and the city's waste management deteriorated. Egypt has the questionable advantage of vast deserts on the western side of the Nile, where garbage can be dumped in remote corners. But the hard waste of modern life—plastic, glass, paper, medical, electrical—disrupts delicate ecosystems and resists even the hottest sun for a very long time. The most effective mitigation of Cairo's waste was when *zabaleen* were collecting it, sorting it, and selling it for reprocessing.[65]

The countries of the European Union, especially Germany, the Netherlands, and the Nordic countries, have reputations for having the most rigorous and successful waste management programs in the world. On the other hand, the most notorious dump in Europe is on the outskirts of Rome. The Malagrotta landfill covers 240 hectares (600 acres) and was officially closed in 2013. Its owner, Manlio Cerroni (1926–), was dubbed by journalists the King of Landfills. He faced criminal charges in 2014, and the Malagrotta landfill was targeted by the European Commission for flouting EU standards. Italy was estimated to have a thousand illegal dumpsites, sometimes controlled by organized crime.[66]

Crime and garbage often go together, including big-time crime. In Sweden, garbage is imported from other European countries to feed incinerators that generate heat and electricity. When Doron asked a Swedish waste manager why Italian garbage was not part of the Swedish imports, the manager replied, tongue barely in cheek, "I don't want to get killed." In two dense books, Harold Crooks, a Canadian author, describes the competition and crime that have characterized the development of the garbage industry in North America. In San Francisco a hundred years ago, "the typical garbage contractor [went] about his business with a horse, a wagon and gun."[67] A 1986 report to the legislature of New York State began with the statement that "there is overwhelming evidence . . . that organized crime is a dominating presence in the solid waste disposal industry in New York State."[68] Elizabeth Royte traces the contests between organized crime and the city and state of New York. When New York City under Mayor Rudolph Giuliani confronted garbage mafia in the mid-1990s, the result was indictments of more than twenty companies, charges of arson and assault, the enforced closing of about two hundred shady "garbage-hauling companies," and fines totaling $43 million. New York City garbage eventually came to be collected by great corporate entities listed on stock exchanges. One smaller-scale garbage collector tells Royte, "The only difference between the majors [the big corporations] . . . and boys [the crime-based collectors] . . . is that the majors don't actually kill you."[69]

Garbage-related crime in India appears to be common but not at the scale or for the high stakes of North America and Europe. That's not surprising, because Indian capitalists have not yet found ways to turn waste into a large-scale, high-value activity. However, when fires burned out of control on the Deonar dump in Mumbai in 2016, journalists encountered "powerful 'garbage-mafia' gangs" who divided the site to share recyclables said to be worth Rs 6 million ($100,000) a day. The gangs had their own teams of up to a hundred waste-pickers protected and supervised by the gang's own toughs. Gang-employed waste-pickers could earn a reasonable income in return for docility, long hours, and productivity. Turf wars and murders were part of the Deonar scene, as Doron was told when he visited Deonar in 2016.[70] In Bengaluru, people complain of "garbage mafias" who control routes and demand ransom from local governments and community groups.[71] In Kerala, truck drivers are paid to dump waste in a neighboring state.[72] In other cities, waste-related crime may extend to the corrupt award of local contracts, theft of equipment, and struggles to dominate branches of the recycling market.[73]

In its struggle to improve public health and sanitation, India therefore shares characteristics with other places in the world. But cultural practices and demography present it with exceptional challenges.

Sanitation and Society

Manlio Cerroni, the Italian garbage king, found himself stigmatized in his early days in the business: "Those of us who worked in the garbage business had troubles even finding wives, because we were considered trash ourselves."[74] Such feelings are even more deep rooted in India. Caste—ideas, beliefs, and practices associated with one's birth and with ritual purity and pollution—complicates India's confrontation with waste. Some people are thought to be impure merely by virtue of their caste, and groups associated with waste are treated as if they themselves were waste—not to be associated with or touched and in some places, not so long ago, not even to be seen. "The Untouchable is dirt," writes Gopal Guru, "and . . . dirt is the Untouchable, both completely indistinguishable from each other."[75]

More than 180 million people, or 15 percent of the population, are officially designated Scheduled Castes—once referred to as untouchables and today as Dalits. Even among Scheduled Castes there is ranking; some are held to be more impure than others, and at the bottom are those who deal with human waste.[76] In 2013, an estimated 600,000 dry latrines in India were still cleaned each day by human hands. A former minister put the number at 2.6 million.[77] Ancient texts provide justification:

> The dwellings of "Fierce" Untouchables and "Dog-cookers" should be outside the village. . . . Their clothing should be the clothes of the dead, and their food should be in broken dishes. . . . They should not walk about in villages and cities at night. They may move about by day to do their work, recognizable by distinctive marks . . . ; and they should carry out the corpses of people who have no relatives.[78]

To be sure, caste relations have changed across time and place. Yet enduring ideologies of caste still loom large when it comes to occupations associated with handling waste of any kind. In the twentieth century, literature and film captured the inhumanity of many practices. A short story, "Sadgati" (Deliverance), by Premchand, one of the greatest Hindi writers, published in 1931 and made into a film by Satyajit Ray fifty years later, dramatizes the beliefs that enabled some people to treat others as unclean. In the story, the untouchable, forced to work on his Brahmin master's land, dies exhausted on the Brahmin's doorstep. In protest, other untouchables refuse to remove the body. Ultimately, the Brahmin himself is forced to drag the body to the outskirts of the village; he purifies himself and the tainted ground by performing rituals. Mulk Raj Anand's *Untouchable* (1935) is a similar outraged work that captures the degradation of manual scavenging by following a day in the life of an untouchable boy.[79] Although these writings (both by authors from upper castes) were products of the 1930s, when socialist realism was in vogue, the circumstances they describe are still found in twenty-first-century India. In 2016, when Dalits in Gujarat were assaulted by higher-caste Hindus who accused them (wrongly) of killing cows, Dalits replied by refusing to remove dead animals from public places.[80]

J. C. Molony, president of the Madras Municipal Corporation from 1914–1918, gives us an engaging account of the problems of caste, local government, and waste. The sweepers in Molony's time dumped their collection on the fringes of the city. Molony identifies enduring aspects of waste collection. "Sweepers, who handle dust-bins and rubbish-carts," he writes, "are low caste people, and high caste people must keep aloof from that which the sweeper has defiled by his touch. Accordingly, the Madras householder, having collected his rubbish, was wont to sling it broadcast into the street."[81] Sweepers are "at the bottom of the social ladder," he continues,

> and must for ever remain there. They accepted their fate, and made the best of it. They kept very much to themselves (this is understandable), and they resented the interference of outsiders in their arrangements. . . . They swept well enough . . . ; but I do not think that it occurred to them that there was any reason, other than the whim of an insane master, for sweeping at all.[82]

Even today, when politicians, policy makers, nongovernmental organizations, and ordinary citizens look for ways to improve public sanitation, they confront the prejudices of caste and varying beliefs about what makes objects clean or pure.[83]

India's encounters with waste have similarities with earlier agonies experienced in Europe, North America, and Japan. As cities grew, people flowed to ill-equipped slums, poorly prepared settlements, and harsh factory life. The most striking contrast, however, is how human waste—feces and urine—has been dealt with in different places and times. The cultural differences are remarkable. Chadwick in his 1842 British report celebrated the Chinese for the value they placed on feces and urine as fertilizer and asserted that the Dutch, like the Chinese, used human waste systematically in ways the British shunned. In the Netherlands, the containers in which household urine was kept were removed each day "with as much care as our [British] farmers remove their honey from the hives."[84] In French towns, as late as the 1880s, "men . . . crisscrossed the city in wagons with barrels that they filled with [human] waste purchased from housewives and servants and then resold to farmers for fertiliser."[85] Night soil was sometimes used in British farming but in a haphazard and ugly way. Deep inside a slum in Glasgow, Chadwick's informants found that

> there were no privies or drains there, and the dungheaps received all the filth which the swarm of wretched inhabitants could give; . . . a considerable part of the rent of the houses was paid by the produce of the dungheaps. *Thus,* worse off than wild animals, . . . the dwellers in these courts had converted their shame into a kind of money by which their lodging was to be paid.[86]

Rural India did not face such unpalatable choices. Rather, as India's deputy inspector-general of hospitals told the Sanitary Commission in its 1862 inquiry, "to relieve the calls of nature," Indians preferred

> some waste piece of ground. . . . The ordure is thus scantily spread over a large open surface; much is quickly removed by the pigs and kites, and in the hot and dry seasons what remains soon dries up and becomes inodorous. In the rains such "public fields" are necessarily much more offensive, but at all times they

> are less [so] than if the same quantity of ordure were collected together in common moist heaps.[87]

The preferences of much of rural India were similar in the twenty-first century. Open defecation—or random defecation, as it is sometimes called—remained common, as we discuss in Chapter 3.

It is not the openness but the randomness that is interesting for comparative purposes. In India, it was rare for human waste to be systematically collected and used for agriculture.[88] Human waste deposited in this way no doubt enriched the soil, but carelessly. Feces and urine decomposed wherever they were deposited. This was in marked contrast to places like the Netherlands. And investigation of the use of human waste in China and Japan uncovers a literature rich with earthy titles, such as "'Nightsoil Lords,' and Street Corner Urinators in Republican Beijing" or "Treasure Nightsoil as if It Were Gold."[89] Susan Hanley, the distinguished American scholar of Japan, explains practices prevalent in East Asia:

> The most important difference between waste disposal in Japan and in the West was that human excreta were not regarded as something that one paid to have removed, but rather as a product with a positive economic value. The night soil of Japanese cities—and Chinese as well—was long used as fertilizer.[90]

Hanley continues, "As the price of fertilizer rose . . . farmers from neighboring areas were forming associations for the purpose of obtaining monopsony rights to purchase night soil from various areas of Osaka. Eventually fights broke out over collection rights and prices."[91] China was similar, although night soil appears to have been even more valued in southern China, where the climate was "milder and damper" than the north's.[92] One account from Jiangxi Province, which lies between Hong Kong and Shanghai, noted that "the value of night soil can be illustrated by the expression, 'night soil is money.'" A study of hygiene in China found that in some areas "all toilets . . . were built in order to strike deals with local peasants."[93] In towns and cities, "night soil delivery businesses were ubiquitous, operating in the form of cooperative societies."[94]

The actual collectors of night soil might not have been regarded as social leaders, but whatever stigma attached to their occupations was outweighed by the income they derived. As we contrast this with India, it is ironic that, after the Boxer Rebellion of 1900, "the Chinese government . . . hired twenty Indian patrolmen and fifty Indian patrol police to watch over street cleaning tasks and sanitation."[95]

India has not been alone in having specific groups condemned by birth to do repugnant tasks. In Japan, of course, a stigmatized category of people—*burakumin,* numbering perhaps three million people—still experience discrimination stemming from their role in previous times in dealing with dead animals, leather, tanning, death, and excrement. Their place in Japanese society, according to the scholar Timothy Amos, is "undeniably similar in some very important respects" to that of Dalits in India.[96] However, the thrust of Amos's book is to argue that the term *burakumin* is relatively fluid and has come to "categorize a number of diverse *socially* distinct populations (as opposed to *biologically* distinct populations) into one common group."[97]

In parts of coastal West Africa, people from poor regions migrate to wealthier places to scrape a living by doing the dirty work that locals shun. In Dakar, the capital of Senegal, young men were prepared to work in waste collection if the wages were regular and reasonable. But they were "embarrassed at first" and "even covered their faces so as not to be seen by their girlfriends." Garbage workers were "seen as crazy, dirty, or even criminal."[98] In southeastern Ghana, three thousand kilometers (1,900 miles) from Dakar, the Akan people are punctilious about personal cleanliness but careless in their disposal of human waste. An experienced Dutch anthropologist confessed to his own "toilet phobia" because the toilets even of individual households were so noxious. The Akan people with whom he lived occasionally for many years evinced some characteristics seen in India. The left hand was used for all unclean tasks, regular daily bathing was essential, constipation was greatly feared, and low-status people—migrants "from the North"—removed overflowing toilet buckets in the night and carried them to cesspits on the outskirts of the town.[99]

Sewage workers in the industrial West have legal remedies and regulatory protection. A sewage worker drowned in Melbourne, Australia,

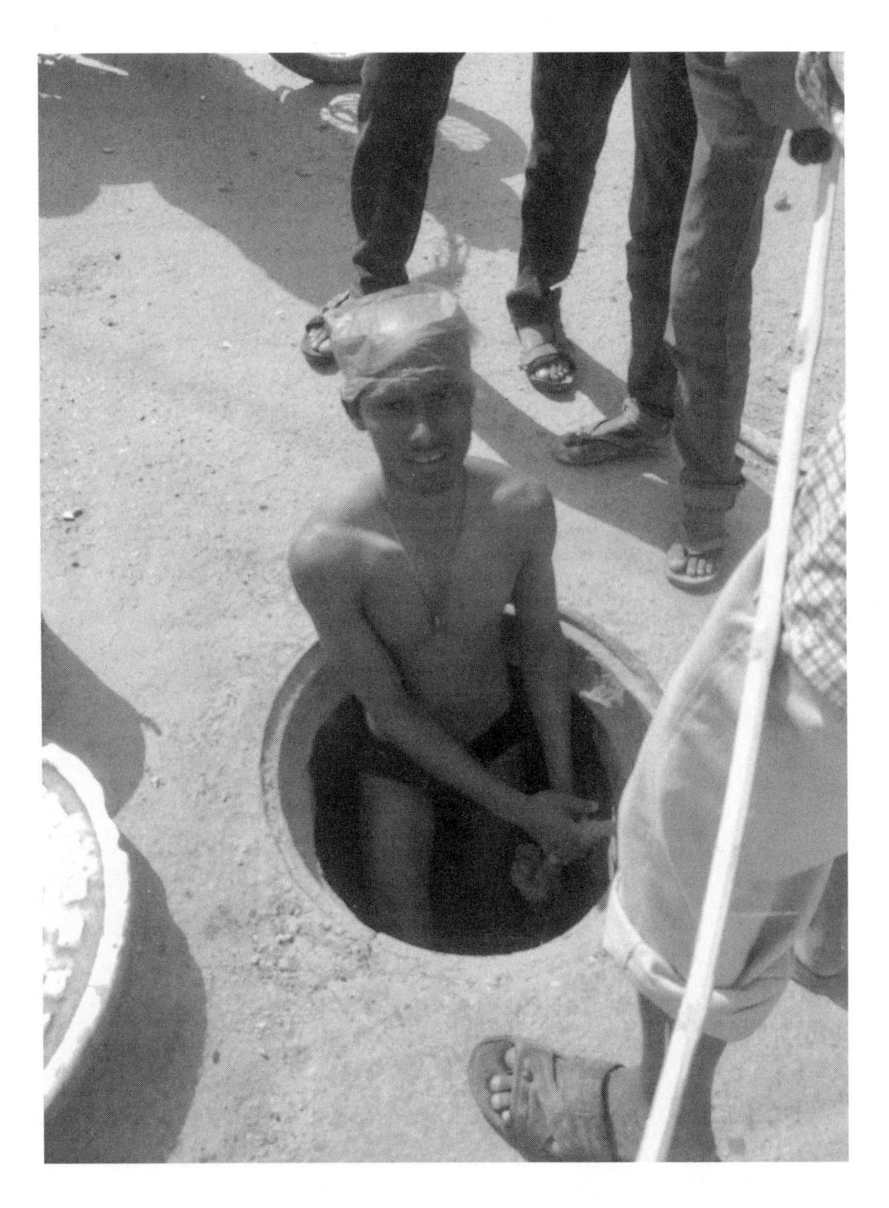

Fig. 1.2 Sewer diving in Varanasi. The plastic bag on the young man's head is pink and protects a good haircut. Photo © Assa Doron, 2014.

in 2011, and his employer was fined A$400,000 for failing to provide a safe workplace.[100] Sewer workers in Europe, North America, and Australia wear the elaborate equipment of a space traveler, which the author Rose George requires a paragraph to describe.[101] But London, New York, and Melbourne sewer workers too must endure the public's distaste for their occupation. George recounts an anecdote about a London sewer man trying to pick up a girl in a pub. He tells her what he does. "Does it involve feces and such?" the girl asks. "I'm glad I didn't get you to buy me a drink, then." George says that the young woman's "disgust [was] genuine."[102] But these sewer workers are moderately well paid and do not go into sewers and cesspits in shorts, a T-shirt, and bare feet. In India, some sewer workers intoxicate themselves before descending into the sewers. "It gives us courage," one man told Doron before he disappeared into a sewer in Varanasi wearing nothing but underwear and a pink plastic bag to protect his hair.

Indian attitudes to feces and urine contrast strikingly with practices and attitudes elsewhere. "The caste system," Bhasha Singh wrote in 2014 in her remarkable book *Unseen,* "aids the belief that all work associated with filth is the lot of the Dalits."[103] Ideas about ritual purity and pollution anchored in the religious practice of large numbers of Hindus pose special problems for an urbanizing, consuming India. Loathsome tasks have been performed by people who are born into subcastes—*jatis*—deemed to be at the bottom of a Hindu hierarchy. Such hierarchies are sometimes replicated among Muslims, Christians, and Sikhs. Manual scavenging is illegal but still done by Dalits in hundreds of localities. "Manual scavenging" means scraping feces from a cement or packed-earth floor (a dry latrine) using a metal or wooden scraper, transferring the excrement to a basket, placing the basket on one's head, and moving along the lane to the next latrine and repeating the process. The contents are eventually dumped into a sewer, drain, or convenient body of water.

The introduction to a book by photojournalist Sudharak Olwe describes conditions of Mumbai conservancy workers, or sweepers, in 2013:

> All 30,000 of them are Dalits, belonging to the lowest rung of the Indian caste system. . . . Without exception, all of them de-

> spise their work. They are either completely ignored or looked down upon with disgust by the rest of society. They . . . work in the midst of filth, with no protective gear, not even access to water to wash off the slime. . . . Alcohol becomes their near and dear friend.[104]

Sudharak Olwe's photographs on his website and in his book *In Search of Dignity and Justice* will make a viewer sitting at a desk in a comfortable room retch.[105] In cities, when drains and cesspits need cleaning, it is overwhelmingly Dalits who do the work and Dalits who die when things go wrong.[106]

More than a hundred years ago, innovations of the modern world, such as railways and growing urbanization, posed challenges to the exclusion and debasement that accompanied caste practices. Within two months of the opening of India's first railway line in 1853 between Bombay and what is now the satellite city of Thane, the objections of higher-caste Hindus led "the Railway Company not to allow persons belonging to the sweeper caste [Dalits] to take a seat in the railway carriages." *Prabhakar,* a Marathi-language newspaper, denounced such "*dhong* or hypocrisy" and pointed out that higher castes now had to reconcile themselves "to travel in the company of Mahars, Chambhars, &c. [Dalits], who, according to the Hindu sacred books, are unclean, and their very presence contaminating." The railway company tried to assuage higher-caste objections by ruling that low-status people would be permitted to travel in the carriages—but not to sit down.[107] Attempts at discrimination on the railways did not last. They were superseded by distinctions of Victorian capitalism—first-, second-, and third-class carriages, according to what a traveler could afford to pay.

A hundred and fifty years later, Chandra Bhan Prasad, a Dalit writer and activist, argues that the spread of capitalism and urbanization undermine much caste-based discrimination. "The sweeper or toilet cleaner in the [modern] mall," he writes,

> becomes a "housekeeper" or "janitor" for a host of reasons. The broom s/he uses is a near-machine, distinct and different from the traditional broom; . . . these workers use gloves, wear a full uniform, complete with trousers, shirt, cap and shoes. Along

> with a new tool which neutralizes caste, the sweeper turns into a housekeeper, looking more like a paramedic than a traditional sweeper. In one stroke, the market has liberated the broom from its caste identity, and the occupation has become caste-neutral.[108]

It would, however, be extremely rare to meet a member of the upper castes engaged in a polluting occupation, such as that of a sweeper or a waste-picker at a dumpsite. Lower castes and poor Muslims, particularly from West Bengal, Bihar, and eastern Uttar Pradesh, are most likely to be found in such roles.[109]

Doron experienced the ambivalence of such change. Early in fieldwork he was doing in Banaras, he engaged a man from a trading caste (*baniya*) to help with research among the boatmen who operate the boats that work on the Ganga. The young man was uncomfortable in the company of low-caste boatmen, some of whom performed polluting jobs, such as carrying dead bodies and carcasses on their vessels for immersion in the river. He said that for this reason he could not continue to assist Doron. Surprisingly, Doron then met a man from a Brahmin *jati* who was willing to assist him. This man had grown up alongside boatmen on the ghats and was undeterred by ritually polluting occupations, even though his parents were unhappy that he fraternized with lower castes. But boatmen too were sensitive about ritual status and pollution. The more powerful boatmen, who could afford to be selective, avoided dealing with corpses, even though they said that it was their *haq* (right or duty) to perform such tasks. They preferred to assert a ritual and social supremacy by not engaging in this stigmatized activity, and they delegated these tasks to poorer boatmen.[110]

At the beginning of the twenty-first century, 150 years after the *Sanitary State of the Army* report, the hands-on work of keeping India clean remained overwhelmingly a task of the lowest castes, the poorest Muslims, and landless people seeking some sort of living in the cities. When Kaveri Gill studied waste-pickers who collected plastic in Delhi, a valuable commodity there, she found that 86 percent were Dalits. "In caste," she writes, "lay the key to the social relations underlying the plastic scrap trade in Delhi."[111]

India enjoys some advantages in its confrontation with consumerism, growth, and the thrown-away things that go with an urbanizing, capitalist-driven world. Its garbage dumps, although large and mostly uncontrolled, are not the world's worst. Indian waste management has not been taken over by a few large corporations that can dictate terms to governments and citizens. Big-time organized crime of the kind seen in parts of Europe and North America has not yet seen profit in Indian waste. India has a tradition of husbanding, repairing, and reusing that goes back to its villages and was a hallmark of M. K. Gandhi and the nationalist movement. Those ideals and practices of frugality were once deeply rooted. And the closed economy that prevailed until the 1990s means that India in 2017 has experienced for only a generation a growing middle class that has wallowed in the dangerous delights of the throw-away life. Acute poverty and long-standing practices of reuse create intricate networks for collection, classification, and recycling of waste. Consumer goods in India embark on complex and unexpected journeys involving street-side repair, disaggregation, and reaggregation (i.e., part swapping and substitution), restoration, recycling, and decomposition. An object's life and journey are rarely as predictable as they are in the developed world.

Writing of nineteenth-century Germany, Richard Evans sums up the processes going on in an urbanizing world: "What was bearable or imperceptible in the small town of the pre-industrial era quickly became obnoxious when multiplied a thousand times in the rapidly expanding urban centres of the industrial age."[112] Unlike rural settings, where there may not be much to throw away, and where there is usually somewhere to throw it and domestic animals to eat it, towns and cities need to dispose of growing quantities of things that their crowded residents discard.

Evans's remark is apposite for India over the past two generations, but three things make India different. On the positive side, India benefits from more than a hundred years of health science and urban experience from around the world, and India has its own traditions of frugality to draw on. But India has also to cope, as other places do not, with the prejudices and preconceptions of caste, most vividly revealed in matters of sewers, toilets, and human waste. Third, the magnitude of India's population—and of its concomitant and growing capacity to make waste—is much greater than anything seen in the industrialized world. This magnitude is the subject of the next chapter.

2

GROWTH AND GARBAGE

NEVER IN HISTORY HAVE so many people had so much to throw away and so little space to throw it as the people of India in the second decade of the twenty-first century. True, China has more people, and Americans make more waste. China had a population of about 1.40 billion to India's 1.27 billion in 2016. But population density was three times greater in India—445 people to the square kilometer (1,157 to the square mile) to China's 147 (382 to the square mile).[1] The United States made more waste—about 250 million metric tons a year, according to Environmental Protection Agency—far surpassing India's high-end estimates of its own waste of 65 million tons.[2] The average American created 150 times more waste each year than the average Indian.[3] But in the United States there were only 35 people to the square kilometer (91 to the square mile): one American could stretch out in an area that accommodated 12 Indians. Wealthy countries like the United States, Canada, and members of the European Union also had the malicious luxury of being able to ship some of their waste to poorer places.[4]

These rough numbers underline the magnitude of India's challenges as it grows, urbanizes, and attempts to satisfy the aspirations of its citizens for the comforts of life elsewhere. By a conservative estimate, India's middle class—people who live in some comfort—amounts to 15 percent of the population, or between 180 and 200 million people, most of whom live in towns and cities. But in 2016, urbanization was modest compared to places elsewhere. Only about one-third of Indians lived in a town. In 1947 when India became independent, its middle class might have reached 30 million, and town and city dwellers were 17 percent of the population. The country then was overwhelmingly rural, agricultural—and frugal. Even for the better-off, there was not a lot to throw away. And cities like Chandigarh, today's capital of the states of Punjab and Haryana, simply did not exist.

Change in Chandigarh

In 1967, the city of Chandigarh was barely ten years old. It grew out of the plains of Punjab, a silhouette seen through a curtain of gray haze as Haryana Roadways buses lumbered their diesel-spewing way from Ambala fifty kilometers (thirty-one miles) to the south. Chandigarh then had a population of about 200,000. The city was a symbol of a new India, designed by the Swiss planner Le Corbusier (1887–1965), and built as a triumphant replacement for Punjab's legendary capital, Lahore, which became part of Pakistan at independence in 1947.[5]

If you had been a foreign teacher or nurse in those days, you might have shared a house with one or two people like yourself, hired as your cook a retired soldier from the Indian Army, and had your first experience of Indian solid waste management. Your cook would not have swept floors, cleaned bathrooms, or carried out kitchen scraps; for that, he would have engaged a sweeper. She would have been a young woman, almost certainly a Scheduled Caste, or *harijan,* formerly an untouchable and a Dalit in the language of the twenty-first century. She would have come on most days to push dust around floors, slosh water in the bathrooms, and carry out waste, mostly food scraps. These would have been wrapped in a single sheet of yesterday's newspaper. Plastic bags did not come to India in a major way for another twenty-five years, and clean newsprint was valuable and could be resold to the *kabaadiwala,* the equivalent of the British rag-and-bone man, who bought household discards to resell.

Chandigarh is a rigidly planned city, laid out in sectors on a rectangular grid. In 1967, houses, shops, and offices were being built in empty fields. Single structures stood here and there with vacant lots between them. The house where you lived might have been like that.

Holidays were common, occasioned by a local religious event or the unexpected death of a politician, and on such a day, you might have found yourself at home in the morning when the sweeper came. You would have watched her perform her work, then pick up the parcel of kitchen waste and leave the house. If you had strolled out after her, you would have seen her go into the vacant lot next door and spill the parcel on the ground, near the remnants of previous days' donations. Dogs, birds, and free-range cows and goats stopped by to nose for edible items, and anything left over would wait for wind, sun, and rain to complete the management process for solid waste in India's newest city.

By 2017, Chandigarh's population had quintupled to more than a million, and it generated 135,000 metric tons of waste a year, collected and measured (most of the time) by the Chandigarh Municipal Corporation.[6] Chandigarh's waste was no longer overwhelmingly edible. Animals still foraged, but they now risked blocking their intestines by eating plastic bags and other indigestible hazards. Only about half of Chandigarh's waste was reckoned to be organic. Most of the rest was made up of plastic (7 percent), paper (6 percent), cloth (4 percent), glass (1 percent), and inert matter (road dust and sweepings; about 20 percent).[7] Waste management was no longer the preserve of crows, cows, and goats. It had become a national campaign, driven by the new prime minister and the pledge to create a Swachh Bharat—a Clean India—by 2019.

The building of Chandigarh embodied independent India's ambivalence about urbanization. When Jawaharlal Nehru inaugurated construction in 1952, he described the plans for the new city as "the first expression of our creative genius, flowering on our newly earned freedom . . . unfettered by traditions of the past." He said, "The site chosen is free from the existing encumbrances of old towns and old traditions, and an expression of the nation's faith in the future."[8] The two dozen villages on the plain where Chandigarh was to be built had a population of less than twenty-five thousand.

Nehru died in 1964, Punjab was divided into two states (Punjab and Haryana) in 1966, and Chandigarh became a centrally administered capital of both states. By 1967 the new city supported a population nearly ten times greater than the villages it had absorbed. But much of the hope of newly independent India had dissolved. Slow economic growth, a disastrous war with China in 1962, and drought and food deficiency in 1965–1966 left a sense of despondency, which even a relatively successful war with Pakistan in 1965 did not dispel. Urban India had received little attention in those first twenty years of independence. National and state governments focused on industrial development and, from the late 1960s, on agriculture and the green revolution to increase production of food grains.

India then was a remarkably frugal place. Most of what households threw away was biodegradable waste of the kind that animals and weather could deal with. In rural India, everyday throwing away commenced with a ritual act, as Sushila Raja who grew up in rural Rajasthan in the early 1960s recalls. "The first roti of the day was given to the cow, and the last one to the dogs. Any extra, uneaten rotis were given to Dalits, the sweepers, or those who worked in cleaning the cowsheds." All rubbish in the village was biodegradable, and leftovers—unused cow dung and food (*juutha*, or touched)—were thrown into a small corner in the village. Sushila recalls her memory as a six-year-old of packaged food: "When my brother-in-law who worked in the city used to bring us packages of Britannia Biscuits, it was so beautiful, wrapped in crisp paper and very tasty."[9]

Takeout food came in packets made of leaves, newspaper, or the pages of an old student exercise book. Bottled drinks were rare and came in glass bottles that got reused relentlessly. If they contained soda, they had a ball forced into the neck to seal in the fizz, and the pressure made them into modest explosives when shattered at the feet of police during demonstrations. Tea and coffee were served in heavy white cups that resisted breakage but cracked and chipped readily. Medical waste was limited. Syringes were always reused and sometimes sterilized. Because towns and cities grew slowly, construction and demolition waste was limited and readily seized for reuse. Writing of the 1960s, an economic historian concludes that "even the production of bicycles, which are of great importance in India, remained rather modest." In 1960–1964, when industrial growth was greatest, bicycle production reached 1.4 million a year in a country then approaching 500 million people.[10] When bicycles broke and tires punctured, they were mended by roadside repairmen or

Table 2.1 Population Growth, 1901–2011

Year	Pop. in millions	Additional pop. millions	Growth (%)
1901	238		
1911	252	14	6
1921	251	–1	0
1931	279	28	11
1941	319	40	14
1951	361	42	12
1961	439	82	23
1971	548	109	25
1981	684	136	25
1991	846	162	24
2001	1,029	183	22
2011	1,210	181	18

Source: 8th Five Year Plan, vol. 2, table 1, accessed 31 March 2016, http://planningcommission.nic.in/plans/planrel/fiveyr/8th/vol2/8v2ch13.htm.

Note: Population figures attempt to exclude districts that became East and West Pakistan in 1947.

a local welding shop. Socks were darned, shirt collars turned, and shoes patched and resoled. No nurse, teacher, or humble middle-class family in Chandigarh in 1967 owned a refrigerator. Television was unknown and reached no more than a few thousand homes in all of India until the late 1970s.

Population

If waste did not grow greatly in these years, population did. The results of the 1961 census sent Indian governments, and aid donors from foreign countries, into a frenzy of family planning campaigns. In the 1950s, the country added what then seemed to be an astonishing 82 million people, and population grew at about 2.3 percent a year. On the basis of previous Indian censuses, this was unprecedented. The annual growth rate in the strongest previous decade (1931–1941) had been only 1.4 percent.[11]

Books like Paul Ehrlich's *The Population Bomb* dwelt sensationally on India's apparently unsustainable population growth—and proved to be

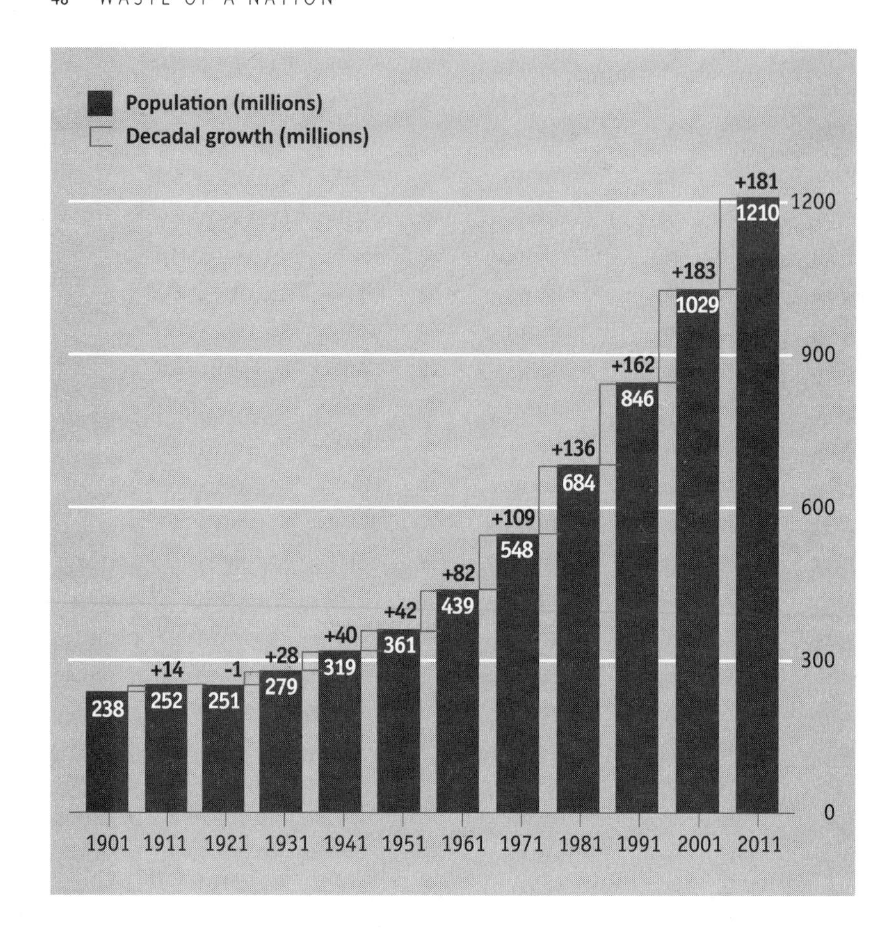

Fig. 2.1 **Population of India, 1901–2011, growth in each decade**

spectacularly wrong. "The battle to feed all of humanity is over," Ehrlich's 1968 book began:

> In the 1970's the world will undergo famines—hundreds of millions of people are going to starve to death in spite of any crash programs embarked upon now. . . . We can no longer afford merely to treat the symptoms of the cancer of population growth; the cancer itself must be cut out. Population control is the only answer.[12]

India took much of the blame. "I came to understand it [the population problem] emotionally one stinking hot night in Delhi. . . . People, people,

people, people. As we moved slowly through the mob, hand horn squawking, the dust, noise, heat, and cooking fires gave the scene a hellish aspect."[13] Not surprisingly, with the 1961 census providing evidence and professors like Stanford University's Ehrlich predicting imminent doom, foreign donors and Indian governments poured money into family planning and efforts to enthuse people about limiting the number of children. *Do ya teen bacche, bas*—"two or three children, enough"—was the modest slogan of those days, giving way later to a more ambitious *hum do, hamare do*—"we are two, we have two." This emphasis on family planning continued until the blundering and callous forced sterilizations and vasectomies driven by Sanjay Gandhi during the state of emergency, the authoritarian rule under his mother, Indira Gandhi, from 1975 to 1977. The resulting mistrust and suspicion left a difficult path for government-sponsored family planning, and India's population grew at more than 2 percent a year until the twenty-first century. It was about 500 million in 1967 when Chandigarh was being built; it exceeded 1.27 billion in 2017.

Towns and Cities

Despite population growth, two characteristics lessened the growth of waste. First, urban growth was relatively slow. Second, most of what people consumed in the market economy—even urban people—were things that land, water, and weather had absorbed for generations. However, as population grew so did the volume of waste. It became more difficult for time-honored natural practices to cope with the new magnitudes, even of biodegradable material and especially of excrement from humans and animals.

Because of their gentle growth, the shocked response to the 1961 census results did not focus on towns and cities. Urban India grew by less than 1 percent a year in 1951–1961, and only 18 out of every 100 Indians were urban in 1961 (Table 2.2). More than 80 percent of the country still lived in its villages, where vaccination campaigns and a DDT-led war on malaria during the 1950s improved life expectancy.

India's governments were in two minds about urbanization. On one hand, the Nehruvian dream was a modern, industrial India, and

Table 2.2 Rural and Urban Population Growth, 1951–2011

Year	Total pop. (millions)	Rural pop. (millions)	Rural pop. growth (millions)	Rural pop. growth (%)	Urban pop. (millions)	Urban pop. growth (millions)	Urban pop. growth (%)	Urban population (% of total)
1951	357	295			62			17.3
1961	439	360	75	22	79	17	27	18.0
1971	548	439	79	22	109	30	38	19.9
1981	684	524	85	19	160	51	47	23.1
1991	844	627	103	20	217	57	36	25.5
2001	1,029	743	116	19	286	69	32	27.8
2011	1,210	833	90	12	377	91	32	31.2

Source: Statistical Outline of India (Mumbai: Tata Services).

such an India had to have substantial cities with great factories. On the other hand, M. K. Gandhi's rejection of urban life was an essential element of his vision. Although Gandhi's philosophy was honored more in word than deed, his ideas about an idealized rural life and the dangers of urbanization affected policy for fifty years after independence.

Gandhi had no doubt about the evils of the city. "I regard the growth of cities," he wrote eighteen months before his death,

> as an evil thing, unfortunate for mankind and the world, unfortunate for England and certainly unfortunate for India. The British have exploited India through its cities. The latter have exploited the villages. The blood of the villages is the cement with which the edifice of the cities is built. I want the blood that is today inflating the arteries of the cities to run once again in the blood vessels of the villagers.[14]

Gandhi's political and philosophical vision was of a free India that aimed for perfection of the village. Life was to be decentralized, based on agriculture and crafts, and hundreds of thousands of villages would achieve meaningful work for all their people through self-sufficiency. Urban India as it had grown under the British was a place of poverty, crime, alienation, and glaring divisions of class. Villages, even as they stood in Gandhi's lifetime, could be portrayed as warmer and more secure—settlements where people knew they had a place. If their residents acquired respect, a tolerable standard of living, and spiritual fulfillment, the Gandhian idea would be realized.

Gandhi's vision of a decentralized polity got scant consideration in the drafting of the constitution of 1950. Some of his ideas about self-sufficiency were packaged to give the appearance that Gandhian ideals supported policies of state ownership of key industries and restrictions on foreign imports to encourage Indian products. And there were sops like the Khadi and Village Industries Commission set up in 1956 to promote rural industry and the manufacture of *khadi* (homespun) cloth.[15] The late K. C. Sivaramakrishnan, a prophet of urban government and planning, writes,

> In the first two decades after Independence, public policy in India favoured containment and restriction of metropolitan growth and specifically discouraged new investments. The aphorism "India lives in its villages," rightly or wrongly attributed to M. K. Gandhi, captured India's negative attitude towards cities.[16]

Gandhian ideals were reflected in a romantic vision of village life and a suspicion of the corrupting effects of the city.

Such attitudes were common among governments and policy makers and appear to have been widely held at all levels of society. One of the best-loved Hindi films of the postindependence era was *Shri 420,* "Mr. 420," so-called for Section 420 of the criminal code relating to shysters and con artists. In the film, the innocent country lad falls prey to the temptations of the city and "the corruption of the urban rich."[17]

At the level of policy, development of towns and cities drew only sporadic attention. "Of the first 10 Five Year Plans between 1951 and 2006," writes Sivaramakrishnan, "the word 'urban development' occurs for the first time as a chapter heading only in . . . 1974."[18] There was a view that urban development would lead to undesirable migrations from country to town. Until the 1970s, the goal of many politicians and planners had been to stem the tide and to keep people in the villages where the

Gandhian idyll might one day be enacted. A document circulated as part of discussions of economic policy in 1977 summed up this attitude: "Development in the telecommunications infrastructure has tended to intensify the migration of population from rural to urban areas. There is need to curb growth of telecommunication infrastructure, particularly in the urban area."[19]

The Ministry of Urban Development was not created until 1985. The Five-Year Plans that embodied government aspirations emphasized "a well considered and articulated urbanisation policy . . . for disease surveillance, epidemic control and urban solid and liquid waste management" only in the Ninth Plan of 1997–2002.[20] By 2001, however, 286 million people lived in towns and cities. (Table 2.2 and Figure 2.2.)

People leave the countryside for a town because they have no option or because they hope for a better life.[21] Some may find it, and when they do, that better life often means the ability to consume more and to have more to throw away. Even poor people in cities contribute substantially to waste, because they must buy what they need, increasingly in packages and invariably in small day-to-day quantities. This was true in the United States in the 1990s when poor people threw away "more packaging per ounce of useful product than the affluent [did]."[22] Because the urban poor have no space to call their own, they have no reason to be enthusiastic about civic consciousness and public cleanup campaigns. The public space is not their space; they are barely citizens. The waste of a nation is hardly something they care for.

Population, Poverty, and Prosperity

For purposes of understanding the magnitude of public sanitation in India, even small improvements in the living standards of urban people have large, cumulative consequences. Between 2001 and 2011, the population of urban India rose by about 90 million people (Table 2.2 and Figure 2.2). The number of urbanites grew, and the proportion living below the official poverty line fell from about one person out of every four to about one in seven (Table 2.3). We should not make too much of this. The methodology for calculation of poverty lines in India is dis-

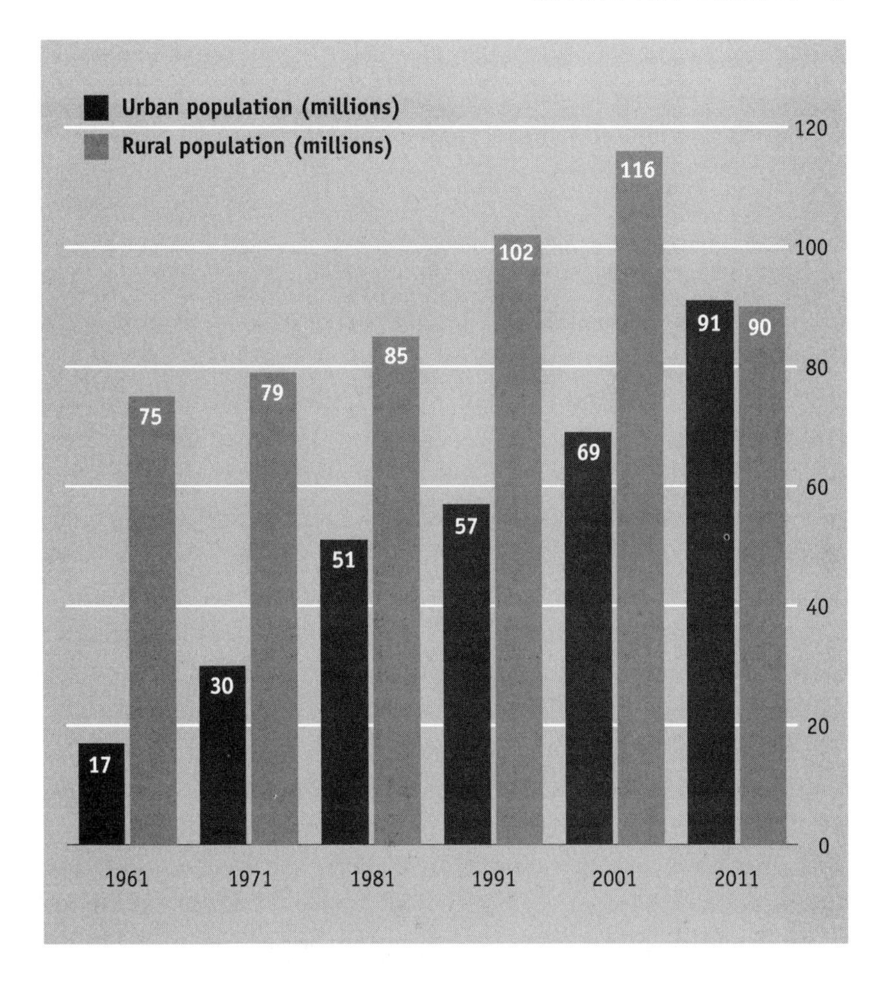

Fig. 2.2 **Growth in each decade: urban and rural population, 1951–2011**

puted, and no matter what the methodology, the poverty line is desperately low.[23] But even allowing for these qualifications, the number of urbanites living at a standard where they had acquired things to throw away grew significantly.

In the 1990s, the characteristics of what Indians threw away began to change. For growing numbers of people, middle-class consumerism became possible, respectable, and desirable. The Gulf War of 1991, which dried up foreign-exchange remittances from Indians working in West

Table 2.3 Population Below the Poverty Line (BPL), 2004–2005 to 2011–2012

	2004–2005	2009–2010	2011–2012
Rural BPL (millions)	325.8	278.2	216.7
Rural BPL (%)	42	34	26
Urban BPL (millions)	81.4	76.5	53.1
Urban BPL (%)	26	21	14

Source: Reserve Bank of India, "Number and Percentage of Population Below the Poverty Line (BPL), 2004–05 to 2011–12," https://goo.gl/HfxD8n.

Asia, helped trigger liberalization of the Indian economy. Foreign-exchange reserves, already low, were depleted further, and the country borrowed from the International Monetary Fund to pay for oil and petroleum imports. In July 1991, a newly elected minority Congress Party government with Manmohan Singh as finance minister introduced a budget that reduced regulation of domestic business and opened sections of the economy to foreign investment.[24] Controls on the products and ceilings on the quantities that could be produced were removed. By the mid-1990s, Japanese and Korean car companies were competing with the arthritic Ambassador cars that had been India's signature automobile from the 1950s.[25]

The process by which India's throwing-away habits changed was not unique to India. Europe, North America, and Japan had similar experiences. "An urban and industrial material culture had come into being," writes Charles Rosenberg about the United States in the nineteenth century, "in a society whose habits of thought and patterns of collective action had been those of a simpler, largely rural world."[26] The description fitted India beginning in the 1990s, but it omitted, as we shall see, a social ingredient that made India's throwing-away and picking-up habits uniquely Indian: caste.

In the 1960s, simple consumer goods had been middle-class treasures. Razor blades and trustworthy shoelaces were welcome gifts in Chandigarh in 1968. Durable flashlight batteries and simple plastic bags to hold wet laundry or provide waterproofing during the monsoon were carefully husbanded in the 1970s. As late as the 1980s, visitors would be especially welcome if they brought watches, pocket calculators, robust ballpoint pens, or good chocolate. For Jeffrey, a realization of change came in the spring of 1993. Doing interviews in Thiruvananthapuram, he knocked his small tape recorder off a table. It smashed on the cement floor. He sighed. Without a tape recorder, future work would be more difficult. Someone, however, assured him, "You'll be able to buy a new one in Mumbai." He thought, impossible, except in a back-lane black market? But it was true. Harboring memories of nursing the batteries of his pocket flashlight in Kerala in 1974, he was amazed to be able to buy a new Japanese tape recorder and sturdy batteries in Dadabhai Naoroji Road within a few hours of arrival in Mumbai. But what to do with the smashed tape recorder and the dead batteries that powered it? Jeffrey put them in the waste basket at his hotel, and they disappeared. India's "urban and industrial material culture" was in liftoff.

Bite-Sized Waste

One of the most common consumer items in the cupboards of urban households in the West for the past hundred years or more has been the toothbrush and some sort of toothpaste or tooth powder. In India, this had not been so, and the topic of toothpaste helps us understand the magnitude of India's collision with hard waste (plastic, glass, paper, medical, electrical). The toothpaste tube, popularized in the United States and Britain in the 1890s, exemplifies a hard-to-get-rid-of artifact of modern urban life. Throughout the nineteenth century, tooth powders, which were sold in glass jars, became popular in industrializing countries. Toothpaste was an innovation of the 1870s, and glass jars of toothpaste were arriving in India in the 1880s.[27] It was expensive at nearly a rupee "per pot" and intended for a tiny European market.[28] By the 1920s, however, the Chicago-based Pepsodent Company was promoting Pepsodent in India by offering a "10-Day Tube Free."[29]

Toothpaste tubes were originally made of tin and lead, but they were transformed into an aluminum-tin-and-plastic amalgam during World War II. They became purely plastic or plastic-and-metal laminate in the 1990s.[30] Although toothpaste tubes can be recycled, "the small size, blended material and leftover toothpaste inside toothpaste tubes . . . make recycling almost impossible."[31] Unlike the glass jars in which toothpaste was originally sold, they cannot be reused.[32] Toothpaste tubes are a packaging innovation that animals and the elements cannot deal with. Tubes go to rubbish dumps or lie in the open until swept into drains and bodies of water.

In India, the tool for cleaning teeth and gums had long been a twig usually taken from a neem tree (*Azadirachta indica*), which can be plucked each morning, chewed into a teeth-cleaning brush, and then thrown away. Neem also has medicinal properties.[33] Tooth powders gained popularity in towns and cities in preindependence times, but in smaller towns as late as the 1960s shops that sold toothpaste had to be searched for. Consumption of toothpaste was meager. India's toothpaste industry in the mid-1970s was estimated to produce about 1,200 metric tons a year for a population of more than 600 million.[34] An Australian population of 16 million consumed 5,000 metric tons of toothpaste.[35] By the late 1980s, the Indian market was said to be growing rapidly, but the industry estimated that only 15 percent of the population used toothpaste and that per capita consumption was only 30 grams a year.[36]

As for toothbrushes, between 70 and 85 percent of the population was estimated not to use them, thus presenting a delicious potential market for manufacturers newly freed by the economic liberalization of 1991.[37] As marketers were well aware, oral hygiene was time-honored bait to tempt simple-living people to join the mass-consumer world. Katherine Ashenburg recounts that the profits of the company that made the mouthwash Listerine rose by a factor of seventy in seven years in the 1920s when its advertising campaign persuaded Americans of the hazards of halitosis.[38] A widely circulated 2003 survey found that the toothbrush was the device that Americans believed they could least live without, more important even than their cars.[39] But toothbrushes also pose problems. They are hard to recycle because they require the labor-intensive and unrewarding task of separating the bristles from the handle.

Doron observed some of the effects of toothbrush marketing in Varanasi. As the sun rose one morning in 2016 near the steps leading down to the river, he watched the daughter of a boatman brush her teeth for ten minutes with toothpaste and a toothbrush. Her father, on the other

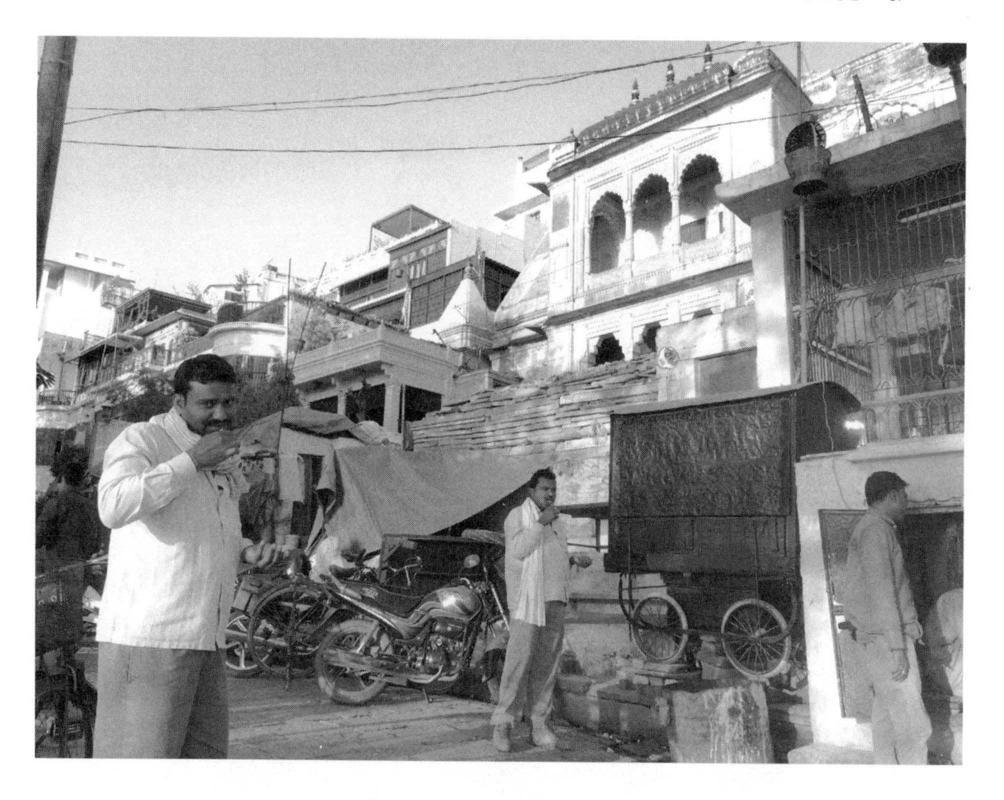

Fig. 2.3 **Brushing with *daatuun*, a neem twig, on the ghats in Varanasi.** Photo © Assa Doron, 2015.

hand, held his *daatuun* (neem twig) and chewed it well to turn it into an effective brush. He explained that he used the *daatuun* regularly and that it was better than a toothbrush. His daughter laughed with approval. She told Doron how she and her sister first began using a brush at the age of eight and were now used to brushing. "It's fresh," she said. She also had a tongue cleaner, a strip of metal used to scrape the tongue. She and her sister used the same tongue cleaner. But she also said that it is *juutha*, or "touched," and thereby polluted, just as the used-every-day toothbrush. "We use and reuse it. It's dirty. That's not as good as the *daatuun* [which is thrown away each day]." During festivals, "like Durga puja and others, before we worship we always use the *daatuun*, because *daatuun* is pure, not like the toothbrush, and you need to be pure before worship." Doron then talked to a woman who sold *daatuun* on

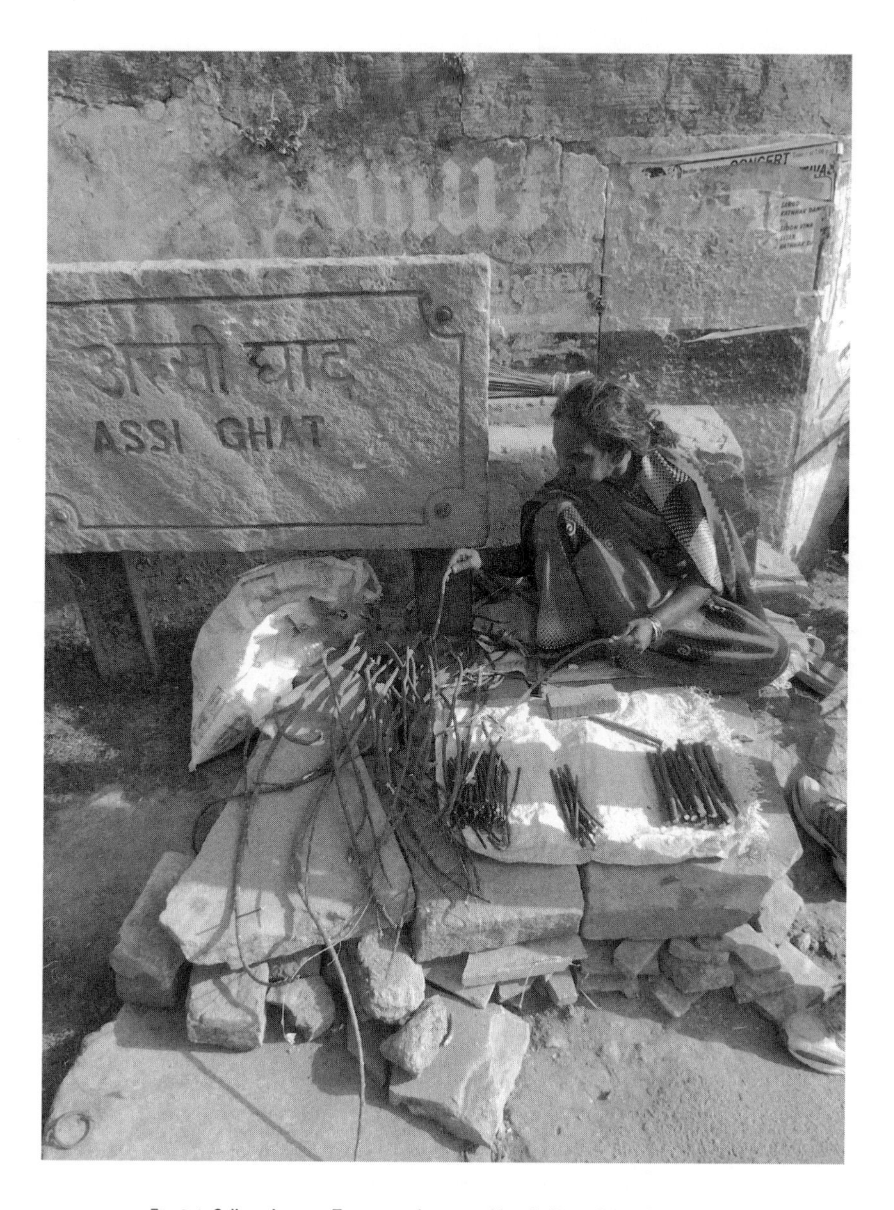

Fig. 2.4 **Selling *daatuun.* Two rupees buy a toothbrush.** Photo © Assa Doron, 2014.

the ghat. She bought one hundred twigs for Rs 100 and sold them for Rs 200. Business, she said, was steady, but the *daatuun's* future seemed to lie increasingly in ceremonial use as a ritually appropriate tool during religious festivals.

The uses of the toothbrush marked the gradual adoption of various new hygiene practices by boatmen. *Daatuun* was generally used at dawn, when boatmen arrived for work. It was part of a series of public displays of cleanliness and purification, including washing in the river, gurgling Ganga water, and spitting and hoicking on the ghats. Increasingly, however, boatmen used a toothbrush and bathed at home. Indeed, the gradual abandoning of the neem twig signified a broader move toward a hygienic mode of conduct, which was inseparable from changing living arrangements, access to electricity and water supply, and ideas about work and leisure.[40]

The use of toothpaste provides a guide to the growth of solid waste in India. By 2014, a single new factory set up in Gujarat by Colgate-Palmolive was capable of making 15,000 metric tons of toothpaste a year, more than ten times the quantity produced in all of India two generations earlier.[41] Marketers estimated that 70 percent of urban India and 40 percent of rural India used toothpaste out of a tube. Even though annual consumption was estimated at less than 150 grams per person a year, India by 2015 consumed more than 80,000 metric tons of toothpaste, or more than 800 million 100-gram tubes a year.[42] Their manufacture was estimated to grow rapidly as the 60 percent of rural nonusers, and Doron's friends, the boatmen on the Ganga at Varanasi, were made aware by their daughters of the virtues of toothpaste from a tube (not to mention the joys of a brush with a plastic handle).

Waste on Wheels

America's second-most-needed item, after the toothbrush, the automobile, is also a major contributor to industrial and hazardous waste. To anyone negotiating Delhi traffic in 2017, India might have appeared to have too many cars. Relative to urbanized countries, however, India's love affair with the automobile has been sedate. In the United States, there were estimated to be 802 motor vehicles for every 1,000 people; in

Table 2.4 Registered Motor Vehicles, 1951–2011 (in thousands)

	1951	1961	1971	1981	1991	2001	2006	2011
Buses	34	57	94	162	333	634	992	1,604
Goods vehicles	82	168	343	554	1,411	2,715	4,436	7064
Cars, 4 wheelers	159	310	682	1,160	3,013	7,058	11,626	19,231
Two wheelers	27	88	576	2,618	14,047	38,556	64,743	101,865
Others	4	42	170	897	2,506	5,795	7,921	12,102
Total	306	665	1,865	5,391	21,310	54,758	89,618	141,866

Source: "Total Number of Registered Motor Vehicles in India during 1951–2012," https://data.gov.in/catalog/total-number-registered-motor-vehicles-india.

India, the estimate was 18 per 1,000.[43] By 2011, India had an estimated 142 million motor vehicles, 70 percent of them scooters and motorcycles (Table 2.4 and Figure 2.5), and this grew to 174 million by 2015.[44] Acute air pollution in Delhi, the country's most motorized city, led to attempts to improve emission standards and limit motor traffic. Because many vehicles were old, the government had an interest in replacing them with less polluting models. A program in 2016 offered benefits to 10 million owners of old vehicles if they scrapped them and switched to newer, less polluting and more fuel-efficient transport.[45]

In dealing with the wastefulness arising from humanity's love affair with automobiles, India had advantages. The United States, for example, junked an average of 13 million vehicles a year in 2002–2014.[46] India, on the other hand, recycled relentlessly, partly out of habit, partly out of necessity. Habit stemmed from the frugality that prevailed in much of India until the 1990s, a frugality resulting from limited wealth and opportunity. In the car industry, especially when there were only two or three manufacturers and models, small shops and artisans were spread across the country, each one able to take cars apart, store the pieces, and use them to repair other cars. Little was left to go to landfills or the vast car graveyards that characterize other parts of the world. (The United States was said to have 25,000 car junkyards in 1951.) Most Indian cars stay on the road until they fall apart. "Cars do not perish," journalist Binoy

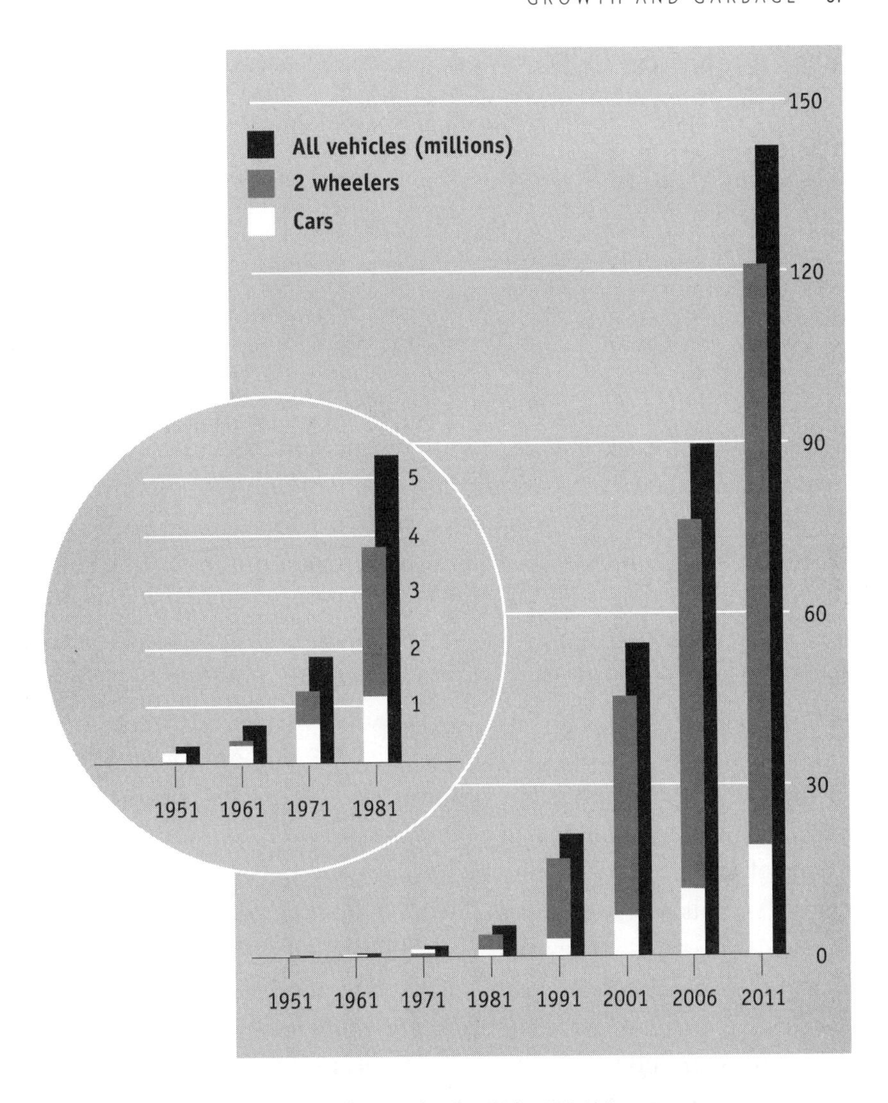

Fig. 2.5 **Registered motor vehicles, 1951–2011**

Prabhakar said after a visit to Soti Ganj, the car rebirthing center in Meerut, northeast of Delhi, in 2011. "They come back to life coated in fresh paint, fitted with shiny alloy wheels and often, powered by new engines."[47] Critics claimed that Soti Ganj was also a haven for sellers of car parts from dismantled stolen cars.[48] The first car shredder, an industrial plant that destroys and recycles old vehicles, was not due to open until

2018.[49] However, as India's car population rises, it will not be able to follow the twentieth-century strategy of the United States where, by 1970, it was estimated up to 30 million cars had been dumped in fields, lakes, and rivers.[50] India's density of population leaves no room for such extravagance.

Switched-On Waste

Television further underlines a relentless growth of consumer capitalism. In 1959 All India Radio in Delhi began "broadcasting television programs every Tuesday and Friday from 7 P.M. for about 90 minutes each day." Twenty community TV sets were distributed in the neighborhoods within the 12-kilometer (7.5-mile) range of the signal.[51] By 1980, the country had seven broadcast centers and 1.5 million TV sets, but Bengaluru, today's high-tech center, still eagerly awaited the opening of its station.[52] In 1973, the central government pondered the introduction of color television, but until 1982 that was dismissed as a needless frippery.

By 2011, however, the census recorded 116 million households—47 percent of all households—with televisions.[53] A color television became an object of achievable desire. In Tamil Nadu, the crafty old leader of the Dravida Munnetra Kazhagam promised poor voters a color TV if his party was elected in 2006. It was. During the next five years, 16 million color televisions were distributed by the government.[54] (It did the Dravida Munnetra Kazhagam no good; it was soundly defeated in 2011.) Many of the old black-and-white sets appear to have finished up in landfills. India's capacity to deal with electronic waste is limited to colonies of specialized waste workers and creative, exploitative entrepreneurs. The methods of dismantling are often crude and dangerous.[55]

The model of the throwaway society, with its planned obsolescence, a feature of consumer capitalism in the West for many years, assumes that Indian modernity must follow the same path.[56] India's local economy tells a different story. First, the sheer magnitude of population and the quantities of waste an all-consuming India could generate make the prospect physically impossible. India would choke. Second, and more optimistically, India's recycling economy has long existed; it is innovative and subversive; and although it is constrained by its cottage-industry structure, it is propelled by flexibility. It can deal with changing inputs and cater to local needs. But it relies on an underclass constantly grappling with social, economic, and health risks.

The mobile phone is the global necessity of the twenty-first century, and this book began when Doron visited Seelampur, a suburb of Delhi, noted for its rough-and-ready recycling of electronic waste. Seelampur stamped a lasting impression on Doron about waste. Phones were stripped bare, circuit boards pried open to enable nimble fingers to strip them for the recycling pile.[57]A report in 2011 estimated India was dealing with 400,000 metric tons of e-waste a year, with annual growth estimated at 10 to 15 percent. By 2014, e-waste was estimated at between 1.5 and 1.7 million metric tons.[58] Ninety percent of e-waste is recycled in the lanes of cities and towns. The risks are great, because recycling concentrates on salvaging precious metals, such as platinum and gold, and the required techniques involve solder-stripping (a segregation method) and acid baths (see Chapter 4).

What Kind of Waste?

The sanitary engineers and recycling industries that deal with waste have well-defined categories. So far, we have been referring to solid waste, emanating from homes and businesses, and liquid waste—sewage and storm water. But as Elizabeth Royte points out in *Garbage Land,* "municipal solid waste constitutes just 2 percent" of waste in the United States.[59] Most waste comes from mining, industry, and agriculture. Tucked away within these categories are specialties like hazardous waste, medical waste, and C&D—construction and demolition waste. All these require extra effort to minimize their harm and to reuse what's valuable.

"Hazardous waste management is a new concept for most of the Asian countries," said a report on India's new rules for managing and handling hazardous waste in 1990.[60] Before economic liberalization began in 1991, hazardous waste in India, including chemicals, industrial sludge, and contaminated metals, amounted to a modest 4 million or 5 million metric tons a year. The United States at that time generated 275 million metric tons.[61] Even by 2015, India's hazardous waste was estimated at less than 8 million metric tons a year.[62] The capacity to deal with hazardous waste was limited. Only twenty-two plants in all of India were accredited to deal with it in 2009, and seven of those were in one state, Gujarat.[63] In 2015, a single plant at Haldia near Kolkata was the lone center for West Bengal and Sikkim.[64] The plant did not receive enough waste to operate at full capacity and ran its high-combustion incinerator for only about two weeks each month, as we discuss in Chapter 7.[65] The relatively small quantity of hazardous waste processed in a region populated by more than 130 million people highlights two features of waste and growth in India. First, large amounts of hazardous waste were being dumped illegally wherever the producers could find a spot. Second, hazardous waste was bound to increase as India's economy grew, and recognition of its dangers and the capacity to handle it was severely limited.

Medical waste, which also requires specialized disposal, posed similar problems. The high-quality steel in disposable needles—"sharps"—can be reused, but the process requires appropriate equipment, and needles, once used, carry infection.[66] The same applies to bandages, plastics, bed linen, and other hospital equipment. A national study in 2009 emphasized that "expansion of health care facilities as well as the recent trend in using disposables has led to an unprecedented burden of health care related waste. . . . Unregulated handling of biomedical waste is emerging as a serious threat to human health and safety." The study concluded that biomedical waste management was "grossly deficient" at all levels—from primary care to secondary and tertiary care.[67] More than 80 percent of the 150,000 subcenters for providing basic care in rural areas had little understanding of safe ways to handle used needles and other medical waste. Even at higher levels, 54 percent of community health centers had no "credible [biomedical waste management] system."[68]

A lesson lies in the story of biomedical waste. To make its recycling, reuse, and safe disposal effective, people have to profit in some way. India in 2008 had only 177 biomedical waste treatment facilities with high-combustion incinerators and equipment for cleaning plastics and dealing with steel instruments.[69] These facilities, many of which are public-private partnerships, charge for their services, and hospital operators and government health centers sometimes lack the will or capacity to pay.[70] The state of Kerala, with a relatively well-developed health care system and 35 million people, had a single such center. IMAGE, a project of Kerala members of the Indian Medical Association, claimed to be the largest "Biomedical Waste Management project in the country." An effective transport system, IMAGE claimed, enabled it to collect three-quarters of the biomedical waste of the entire state, totaling close to 5,000 metric tons a day in 2013. This volume made the plant economically viable.[71]

Population growth and medical developments present further challenges to waste management. Antibiotics, readily available over the counter in India, are a widely used first remedy for ailments. Indiscriminate use for prevalent illnesses such as diarrhea and respiratory diseases increases the stock of antimicrobial organisms in the environment and leads to development of organisms that can resist antibiotics.[72] Antibiotics are also used for non-therapeutic purposes "such as growth promotion and mass disease prevention . . . in intensive farming of food-producing animals such as poultry and fish."[73] India is a major producer of drugs in cities such as Hyderabad and Bengaluru. Some of the production plants send untreated pharmaceutical waste into water bodies. Studies have consistently found high levels of antimicrobial drugs in soil and water bodies close to such plants and to other sites where antibiotics are commonly used.[74] These circumstances contribute to the growth of "superbugs," an immense threat in India but also throughout the world. "Our children and grandchildren may well die of resistant infections," Britain's chief medical officer warned in 2017.[75] The Government of India began to recognize antimicrobial resistance in 2016 with the publication of a National Action Plan calling for increased awareness, improved hygiene, and stricter regulations on industry.[76] Control of liquid waste and sewage thus emerges as one of those insidious perils that confront a growing India.

Since 1947 India's generation of these distinctive categories of waste had been slow but accelerated markedly in the 1990s. Generation will continue to increase as the economy grows. To deal with these materials safely and economically requires investment, broad-based participation, and relentless regulation and management, a theme we return to in Chapter 7.

Measuring Magnitude

The volume and steady growth of rejected things—waste, garbage, rubbish, refuse, sewage—pose immense challenges to India. But how do we measure these challenges in ways we can grasp? Estimating quantities of waste is a crude exercise unless one is sitting at the weighbridge of a modern waste transfer station where the contents of every vehicle are carefully weighed and recorded. For our purposes, we need only general indicators of India's advantages and handicaps.

When Indian governments began to analyze waste, the Central Pollution Control Board surveyed fifty-nine cities to calculate the volume. That exercise suggested that in 2004 these cities generated about 50,000 metric tons of waste a day, or less than 20 million metric tons a year.[77] Over the next ten years, various measurements and informed (and not so informed) guesses estimated annual waste collection in towns and cities at somewhere between 50 million and 90 million metric tons annually.[78] Table 2.5 emphasizes the difficulty of measuring waste. Most all-India estimates are based on taking census figures for the number of households in an area and imputing to them a certain daily production of waste. About 0.5 kilogram (1.1 pounds) per household per day is often used as a rule of thumb for India. Only in places with sanitary landfills, where trucks pass over weighbridges, do we begin to get more accurate measurements. Such landfills were rare in 2017.

Ranjith Annepu, in a pioneering effort to provide an overview of India's waste, laments that "lack of data and inconsistency in existing data" are "a major hurdle" in understanding waste's magnitude and consequences. He surmises that waste volume increased by 50 percent between 2001 and 2011 and speculates that India will generate 230 million metric tons of urban waste annually by 2041.[79]

For a picture of these growing numbers, think of the world's most popular car, the Toyota Corolla. A Corolla weighs about 1.7 metric tons. Imagine a gigantic set of scales. Put 65 million metric tons of India's annual waste on one side. On the other side, you will need 38 million Corollas to make the scales balance. That's about the same number of Corollas that Toyota has sold in the past fifty years. And to park 38 million Corollas would require about 350 square kilometers (135 square

Table 2.5 Estimates of Annual Urban Waste Generation in India

Estimate (millions of metric tons)	Year	Source
49	2008	Ravi Kant, Ramky Enviro Engineers, "Financial Analysis and Risk Allocation in PPPs: Public Private Partnership for Sustainable Growth," Department of Economic Affairs, 2008, http://pppinindia.com/ppp-nodal-officer-round-table.php.
90	2008	Mufeed Sharholy, et al., "Municipal Solid Waste Management in India Cities," *Waste Management,* no. 28 (2008): 460. The calculation includes "industrial, mining, municipal, agricultural and other processes."
69	2011	Ranjith Kharvel Annepu, "Sustainable Solid Waste Management in India" (master's thesis, Columbia University, 2012), 3, 145.
69	2011	Anjor Bhaskar and Poornima Chikarmane, "The Story of Waste and Its Reclaimers: Organising Waste Collectors for Better Lives and Livelihoods," *Indian Journal of Labour Economics* 55, no. 4 (2012): 595.
65	2013	*Times of India,* 25 September 2013, quoting A. R. Rajeev, principal secretary (environment), Maharashtra, at a Confederation of Indian Industry seminar on waste management. He put the daily collection at 178,000 metric tons.
47	2014	*Indian Express,* 22 January 2014, speech by Dr. Amiya Sahu, president, National Solid Waste Association of India. He put the daily collection at 127,486.
53	2014	Almitra H. Patel vs. Union of India, Original Application No. 199 of 2014, National Green Tribunal, annex 6, citing 144,000 metric tons a day.
52	2016	Central Pollution Control Board, cited in Sunita Narain and Swati Singh Sambyal, *Not in My Backyard: Solid Waste Management in Indian Cities* (New Delhi: Centre for Science and Environment, 2016), 5. Narain and Sambyal emphasize the weaknesses of the estimates and cite figures ranging from 47 million to 62 million metric tons.

Table 2.6 Population Densities of Selected Countries, 2017

Country	Density / sq. km	Total pop. (millions)
Bangladesh	1,134	163
South Korea	514	51
Netherlands	413	17
INDIA	402	1,322
Philippines	349	105
Japan	335	127
Vietnam	283	94
United Kingdom	271	67
Pakistan	260	209
Germany	232	83
Nigeria	208	192
China	144	1,387
Indonesia	138	262

Source: "List of Countries and Territories by Population Density," Wikipedia, accessed 11 October 2017, https://goo.gl/8FT9Pz.

miles). That's nearly double the area of Washington, DC, and three times the area of the Union Territory of Chandigarh in India. And waste doesn't go away; it accumulates. At a steady pace of 65 million additional metric tons a year, India in ten years would need an area as big as the state of Goa for its landfill—or a parking lot for 380 million Corollas.[80]

The magnitude of India's encounter with consumer capitalism and urbanization presents unique problems. Of the world's major countries, only a handful surpass India in population density—Bangladesh, South Korea, and the Netherlands. Bangladesh stands out for its combination of a huge population and a small size. But Bangladesh has yet to generate the industrial expansion and exploitation of natural resources that India has.

India's population will continue to grow. Whether at 1.2 percent a year or slightly less, this still entails an additional 15 or 20 million people a year. National governments aim for annual economic growth of at least 7 or 8 percent. And "there is no escape from urbanization," wrote the Sivaramakrishnan. "It is a demographic, economic, and social reality. India has to come to terms with it."[81] India faces unique problems of magnitude and density.

3

SEWAGE AND SOCIETY

Of all the things that humans want to dispose of, the wish to be rid of their own excreta is common to all peoples and all times. Today, we often measure health and comfort by the quality of plumbing, sewers (the pipes), and sewerage (the system) and by wastewater management. Ancient peoples, once they came together in towns and cities, were similarly keen to put feces and urine at a distance. The ancients of Dholavira in today's Gujarat, part of the Mohenjo Daro civilization and predating the Romans by 1,900 years, built toilets that emptied into drains carrying much-needed water to the fields of a dry region. And Rome's Cloaca Maxima, which might have begun as an open drain, became a giant sewer that carried water and human waste into the River Tiber and away from the nostrils of Romans.[1] Urban sewerage, however, made little progress until relatively recent times.[2] An Oxford scholar in the twentieth century despaired that his college "denied him the everyday sanitary conveniences of Minoan Crete," Rose George tells us in her admirable book about sewers and toilets, *The Big Necessity*.[3]

To understand India's challenges in coping with waste in the twenty-first century, the management of liquid waste is fundamental because it throws up inescapable questions that relate to caste, health, and infrastructure. Some of these questions are unique to India.

Caste

On the day we began to write this chapter, January 19, 2016, Indian media crackled with accounts of the suicide of a Dalit graduate student at the University of Hyderabad. He and his Dalit student organization had clashed with a Hindu-chauvinist student organization aligned with the Bharatiya Janata Party (BJP) over screening of a film that the BJP-affiliated organization wanted banned.[4] The university administration had supported the ban and punished the five Dalit students who had protested the ban on the university campus. The young man then wrote a poignant note and hanged himself.

On the same day, the online edition of the *Hindu,* one of India's most respected daily newspapers, based in Chennai, carried a four-paragraph item in its web edition: "Four die of asphyxiation as they enter septic tank at Chennai hotel."[5] To give the *Hindu* its due, the Chennai edition of the print version of the newspaper on January 20 gave the deaths of the four sewage workers a two-column headline at the bottom of the front page. But the top story of the day, with a five-column headline, was the suicide in Hyderabad.

Both these stories of appalling, avoidable deaths relate to problems of sewage, public sanitation, and ideas about purity in India. At first, such a statement may seem hard to justify. The connection is clear in the deaths of the four men attempting to deal with a poorly built cesspit. But where is the connection with the death of the PhD candidate in Hyderabad? The answer lies in caste prejudice and ethno-religious tension being inescapably part of the politics of public sanitation in India and in all five of the men who died having suffered from the stigma of being Dalit. Even those who join the minuscule elite of scholars with doctorates encounter the slurs of deep-rooted prejudice. The full and equal citizenship for all guaranteed in the constitution sits uncomfortably with a sanitary infrastructure that continues to rely on enduring forms of inequality and oppression. The young scholar who took his own life in Hyderabad was on his way to becoming part of a tiny Dalit middle class, and his death, which had heavy political implications, was a major national story. The deaths of the four cleaners in the cesspit were an everyday reality, imbued with a stifling inevitability.

In 2006, a group of India-based researchers published *Untouchability in Rural India,* an exceptional book based on five years of interviews and fieldwork by several teams of researchers working across rural India.[6] To be a Dalit in rural India, Ghanshyam Shah and his colleagues conclude, "involves internalizing a repressive regime of self-control and servility in everyday life."[7] The Dalit laborer is typically paid less and forced into the worst jobs. Even opportunity in construction work is limited, because many higher-caste villagers fear being polluted by Dalits:

> Beliefs regarding purity and pollution are strong constraints while hiring persons for constructing houses—it was seen in about one-third of the sample villages that Dalits are considered unacceptable for this kind of labour. . . . Moreover, in Bihar we found that Dalit women were rarely employed for cooking and cleaning grains and other eatables, tasks which involve physical contact with food.[8]

Exploitation and humiliation are worse for rural Dalit women, who labor under the "triple oppression" of caste, class, and gender hierarchies. Dalits are trapped in a vicious circle of social discrimination and economic exploitation, validated by religious ideology. "The 'impurity' of the task and of those who perform it," Shah and his colleagues write, "are mutually reinforcing . . . ; in the circular logic of untouchability, the tasks are 'impure' because they are performed by Dalits, and Dalits are impure because they perform these tasks."[9]

The practice of untouchability has been illegal since the constitution of 1950. But law is different from practice, and in practice, cruel and glaring prejudice still exists. In town and countryside, it manifests itself in whispered sneers and sniggers, in lamentations of higher-caste Hindus about the ill effects of reservation (affirmative action to foster Dalit social mobility) on academic and professional standards, and in coercion and violence against Dalits who assert their rights or display signs of prosperity.

Dalits, however, are not a single, unified entity. Within the official category of Scheduled Castes (the administrative term for Dalits) are scores of subcastes, or *jatis,* and a *jati* is exclusive to a single language (see also the Introduction). Members of, for example, Tamil-speaking *jatis* do not have caste fellows who speak a different language. *Jatis* also tend to rank themselves in hierarchies, with some claiming superiority over others.[10] Not all Dalits take up manual scavenging or work in urban sewers, but many are born to it. "The [Dalit] mother-in-law feels very proud in giving a scavenging basket and broom," writes Bezwada Wilson, "as the first gift to her daughter-in-law, as part of her legacy. I have seen innumerable such instances with my own eyes."[11] One of Bhasha Singh's informants tells her, "In my parents' home we didn't do this work. The first time I did it was in my in-laws' place. . . . My mother-in-law took me with her and made me begin this work."[12] The practice of a family owning the right to collect human waste from particular localities has a long history. The *Scavenging Conditions Enquiry Committee* report of 1960, one of those magisterial documents produced by Indian governments, identified jealous possession of such "rights" by many—but by no means all—Dalit families as an obstacle to improvement in dealing with human waste.[13]

Bezwada Wilson, who won a Magsaysay Award in 2016 for his work to eliminate manual scavenging, is a Dalit born in 1966 into a family that lived by manual scavenging. He grew up in the Kolar Gold Fields east of Bengaluru in Karnataka. He became a full-time organizer of the Safai Karmachari Andolan, "a movement to eradicate manual scavenging in India," in the 1990s.[14] Wilson describes the degradation, stigma, and alcoholism that he saw around him as he grew up. His family protected him from manual scavenging, and he was able to complete the tenth standard (grade ten) at school. His transformation into an activist came, as he tells it, one day when he went on rounds with manual scavengers he knew. They were emptying a cesspit, transferring the excrement to a tanker to carry away. A bucket fell into the cesspit. The man who dropped it "just leapt into the pit, and he started searching for the bucket. . . . I started shouting, 'What are you doing? Stop! Stop!' They said, 'We can't do the work without the bucket and you are coming and disturbing us.'"[15] Others began scooping feces from the cesspit with bare hands. The experience led the teenage Wilson, who had been relatively sheltered by his higher education, to become a full-time organizer, letter writer, data gatherer, and thorn in the side of politicians, officials, and any organization that allowed manual scavenging.

In legal terms, Safai Karmachari Andolan might have claimed success in 1993 when the national Parliament passed the Employment of Manual Scavengers and Construction of Dry Latrines (Prohibition) Act. But legislation alone does not change practice. Twenty years later Parliament wrung its hands, recognized that little had changed, and passed the Prohibition of Employment as Manual Scavengers and Their Rehabilitation Act of 2013.[16]

Disagreement over definitions clouds discussion of manual scavenging. An official definition treats only those people who remove excrement from dry latrines as "manual scavengers." These are mostly women. This definition omits thousands of men who enter sewers and cesspits—as the four did who died in Chennai in 2014. Mumbai alone was estimated to have 38,000 such workers.[17] Throughout India, as many as 2.3 million people were involved in manual scavenging according to an estimate by the national executive of the ruling BJP in 2015.[18] Wilson's organization, founded in 1995, had itself recorded 1,327 "sewer and septic tank deaths" in less than twenty years.[19]

Despite their illegality, dry latrines still exist, notwithstanding denials by various governments and organizations. The census of 2011 calculated that 0.32 percent of India's 260 million households—more than 800,000 households—had latrines cleaned by human hands.[20] As we discuss in Chapter 1, other estimates range from 600,000 to 2.6 million. The point is that although they are illegal, no one denies there are still a lot of them. Indian Railways, the country's largest employer, itself works through subcontractors to hire people to clean the excrement that falls onto the rails from thousands of passenger carriages every day. But only household dry latrines qualify officially as manual scavenging.

Caste complicates efforts to deal with human waste. It imparts a ritual power to excrement that exceeds the distaste felt by people in other parts of the world. From early childhood, millions of people are presented with the idea that groups designated by their birth are the appropriate people to carry away human waste and other repugnant material. For the orthodox, such ideas are justified by religious doctrines of merit, duty, and rebirth; for the less orthodox, widespread practice is passed on routinely from one generation to the next.

Desperate poverty adds a further ingredient. Because the tasks of maintaining antiquated and inadequate sewerage are so unpleasant, they provide a sure source of permanent employment. The people who perform these tasks don't like doing them, but many value their certainty, because they know that other people live still more precariously than they. Bhasha Singh explains: "The thought of leaving manual scavenging fills them with dread because this entails giving up something that, for centuries, has been associated with a source of economic security and prestige."[21] The prestige comes from the right to clean the latrines of a group of families in small towns and villages, a right possibly being held by a single Dalit family, usually through a female member who does the work. It is a *jagir*—an inherited right. "What property do we have except this?" a woman asks Bhasha Singh. Manual scavengers, says Bhasha Singh, "are made to believe they have a lot to gain from manual scavenging—caste-based security, clothes and sometimes loans."[22] It may be loathsome work, but because it must be done and no one else will do it, it is guaranteed work.[23]

"Through eradicating manual scavenging," Safai Karmachari Andolan's website states, "we will break the link imposed by the caste system between birth and dehumanizing occupations."[24] One of the key factors in creating a cleaner India lies in undermining belief that removal of tainted things, of which human waste is the most tainted, is the responsibility of people who are born to the task.

Infrastructure

Humans can deal with urine and feces in limited ways. The most basic is the one still widely prevalent in India: to deposit the offending matter as far from the creator as convenient and let nature, in the form of sun, wind, rain, and animals, take its course. The dangers to public health of this method have been accepted by scientists and civic leaders since the 1850s and widely known since the 1890s.

In rural India, liquid waste—runoff water and excreta—ends up in surrounding fields, or in the case of cow and buffalo dung, is collected and used for fuel. Rural India resisted the British system of concentrating excreta in cesspools. People went to the fields, as they still do in many places. In the 1940s, the anthropologist M. N. Srinivas reported the awkwardness of needing to relieve himself outdoors during his fieldwork in a south Indian village:

> Within a day or two of my arrival, Rame Gowda the headman's eldest son told me quite casually and before a few people, that there was a big tree, a *Ficus Indica,* about two hundred yards behind the house where I should answer calls of nature, under its protective shade. Incidentally, he commented on the virtues of the tree and the spot he had recommended. I knew that the land and the tree belonged to the headman. But I was astonished that Rame Gowda could so matter of factly discuss such a personal matter with a relative stranger like me. Two hundred yards to the ficus tree were not always easy, especially when it was hot or raining. There was also the chance of meeting someone on the way with the certain prospect that the exchange of pleasantries would take several minutes.[25]

Srinivas was a highly educated Brahmin, and the social and physical discomfort he described was negligible compared to the dangers faced by disadvantaged groups, especially women, when they venture to the fields to relieve themselves. A Dalit woman who worked as a laborer for powerful Jat farmers told researchers, "There is no daily wage labor here, people are forced to go outside to earn money and they come back here to defecate. And Jats even benefit when we defecate in their fields, because some time later it turns into fertilizer!"[26] Not only was Dalit labor extracted, but their bodily excretions benefited their landlords. Open defecation and human waste were not seen as a problem to be solved but rather a resource to exploit.

Towns and cities, however, do not permit going to the fields. Similarly, in towns and cities, vegetable waste—fertilizer for fields or feed for animals in the village—needs to be disposed of in other ways. What are the other ways? Simply dumping refuse into the nearest gutter or onto the nearest piece of vacant ground is one, widely practiced not just in India but in the cities of Europe, North America, and Australia throughout the nineteenth century.

In towns and cities, slums and shanty colonies might have cesspools where human waste was allowed to collect and that eventually leached their contents into the ground. Open drains, led by gravity toward rivers, lakes, or the sea, could carry away waste when there was enough water to make them flow. And for the better off, daily visits from manual scavengers removed waste. An Australian city such as Melbourne, built in the 1870s and 1880s, had back lanes to all properties so that workers could collect excrement from the dry latrines at the back of houses. Their cart then carried its contents to sewage farms in the countryside—or quietly dumped the contents into a secluded drain. Such door-to-door collection had the advantage of requiring neither expensive infrastructure nor large quantities of water. It had the humiliating drawback of stigmatizing the people who did the daily collection—"nightmen" in Australian terms, Bhangi in the Hindi of north India.[27]

In the 1870s, as Britain itself woke up to the attractions of flush-and-forget, water-driven sewers, efforts were made in a few of the major cities and cantonments in India to build sewerage, primarily to serve the European population. But to build sewers and connect them to households is disruptive and expensive. Sewerage, wrote a Kolkata-based British official in 1881, "involves an enormous expenditure, and requires the existence of three main features, viz., a complete system of underground sewers, a sufficient and efficient water supply, and a convenient and unobjectionable outfall for the contents of the sewers. Where all these conditions do not exist, . . . the hand-system . . . must be adopted."[28] Unsurprisingly, when the British left in 1947, few places beyond Mumbai, Kolkata, Delhi, and Chennai had enclaves with sewerage. The committee that reported on manual scavenging in 1960 concluded that "it is a story of the far distant future to think of all the towns having underground sewers."[29]

In 2017, most urban households do not have connections to sewers, and most towns and cities do not have sewerage. "The country actually treats," a report to the national Planning Commission stated in 2011, "30 per cent of the human excreta it generates."[30] The census of 2011 counted 67.2 million urban households; 24.1 million were connected to sewers. In major centers of more than 100,000 people, less than half of households (47 percent) had sewage connections. In small towns,

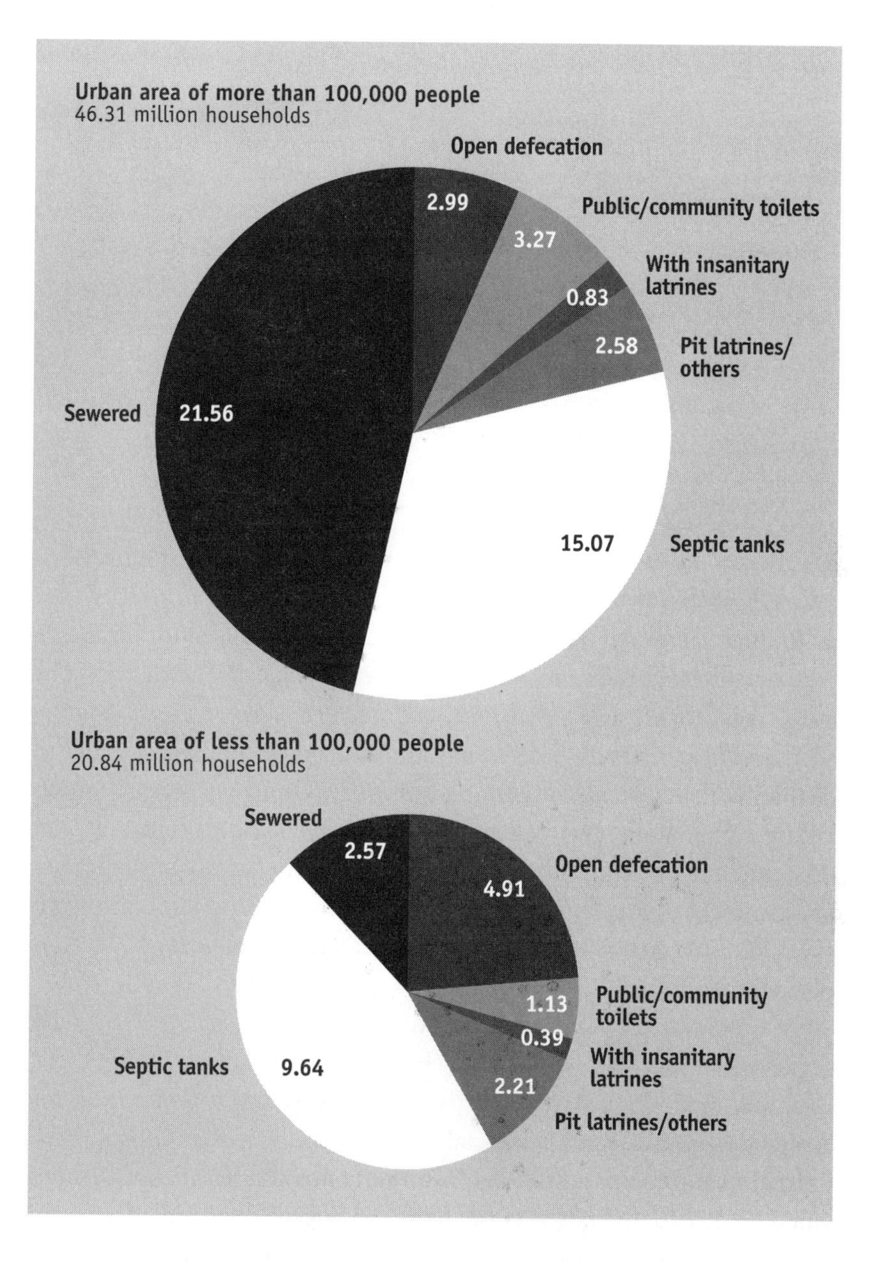

Fig. 3.1 Urban Households connected to sewerage (in millions), 2011

Table 3.1 Urban Households Connected to Sewerage, 2011

City size	No. of towns	Households (millions)	Households connected to sewerage (millions)	Households connected to sewerage (%)
More than 100,000 people	476	46.31	21.56	47
Fewer than 100,000 people	3,565	20.84	2.57	12
Total	4,041	67.15	24.13	36

Source: Ministry of Urban Development, *Annual Report, 2014–15*, 82, accessed 4 January 2016, http://moud.gov.in/pdf/582d962fe1282English%20Annual%20Report.pdf.

more than 85 percent of households were not connected to sewers. (See Tables 3.1 and 3.2.)

In the twenty-first century, as the government focused on the country's irresistible urbanization, sewerage expanded slowly. In 2005, the 892 largest towns and cities were estimated to generate twenty-nine thousand megaliters of sewage a day and had treatment plants capable of dealing with about one-fifth of this volume.[31] (One megaliter is 265,000 U.S. gallons; about twelve thousand Olympic swimming pools can hold twenty-nine thousand megaliters.) Ten years later, a similar rule-of-thumb exercise calculated that urban India was producing sixty-two thousand megaliters of sewage a day and had the capacity to treat 37 percent of it.[32]

Of the fast-growing small towns of fewer than 100,000 people, only 12 percent of nearly 21 million households were connected to sewers. The most frequent alternatives were septic tanks—often a polite term for cesspits. (See Table 3.2.) The social consequence of septic tanks was the periodic need for people to remove the contents and dump it somewhere. That usually meant Dalits to do the removal and a contractor to organize the dumping, almost certainly not at a sewage treatment plant.

A sewer system has two features. First, it uses water to carry human waste out of homes. Having done that, however, a system must dispose of the excrement it accumulates. The time-honored way, going back to prehistory, ancient Rome, and nineteenth-century Europe, was to use

Table 3.2 Urban Households Not Connected to Sewerage, 2011 (millions of households)

Size	No. of towns	Households	Households using septic tanks	Households using pit latrines / others	Households with insanitary latrines	Households using public / community toilets	Households using open defecation
More than 100,000 people	476	46.31	15.07	2.58	0.83	3.27	2.99
Fewer than 100,000 people	3,565	20.84	9.64	2.21	0.39	1.13	4.91
Total	4,041	67.15	24.71	4.79	1.22	4.40	7.90

Source: Ministry of Urban Development, *Annual Report, 2014–15,* 82, accessed 4 January 2016, http://moud.gov.in/pdf/582d962fe1282English%20Annual%20Report.pdf.

creeks and rivers to carry waste downstream from the urban center that produced it. When populations were relatively small, and the downstream inhabitants were inferior in power to town elites, such techniques could work, and flowing water can purify itself over a distance. Today, the Ganga, Yamuna, and other Indian rivers receive sewage and carry it downstream. However, as populations and their volumes of excrement increase, not only does opposition grow from others who need the river but so do inescapable consequences for environment and public health. (See Map 3.1.)

In modern urban history, London's Great Stink of 1858 is a landmark. In the year that the Great Revolt was suppressed in India, the summer in England was unusually hot—an "Indian heat," as it was described. The Thames, into which London's cesspools and drains had emptied for hundreds of years, was now carrying more effluent than imaginable in the past, and the river stank so strongly and pervasively that people no longer would travel on its steamboats. Conditions were right for a binding crisis, similar to Surat's plague of 1994. As a catalyst for change, the Great Stink had another advantage: it was at its worst at Westminster, the seat of Parliament. "In the burning heat of 1858," Lee Jackson, the author of *Dirty Old London,* writes, "the building was filled with the reeking stench of sewage—'pregnant with disease and perhaps with death.'"[33] Just the sort of thing to concentrate the minds of the powerful.

Binding crises affect the poor and the powerful, not equally but inescapably. By August 1858, as the hot weather continued, the short-lived Conservative government authorized the London Metropolitan Board of Works to raise funds and go ahead with a long-discussed program of sewer building. The government and the ruling classes had other pressing problems to consider: passage of the Government of India Act, which replaced the East India Company with the British Crown as ruler of India. The *Times,* as Jackson points out, linked public sanitation in Britain with revolt in India: "That hot fortnight did for the sanitary administration of the metropolis what the Bengal mutinies did for the administration of India. It showed us more clearly and forcibly than before on what a volcano we were reposing."[34] Within seven years, London's new sewer system, although far from complete, was officially opened by the Prince of Wales, the later Edward VII, Emperor of India.[35]

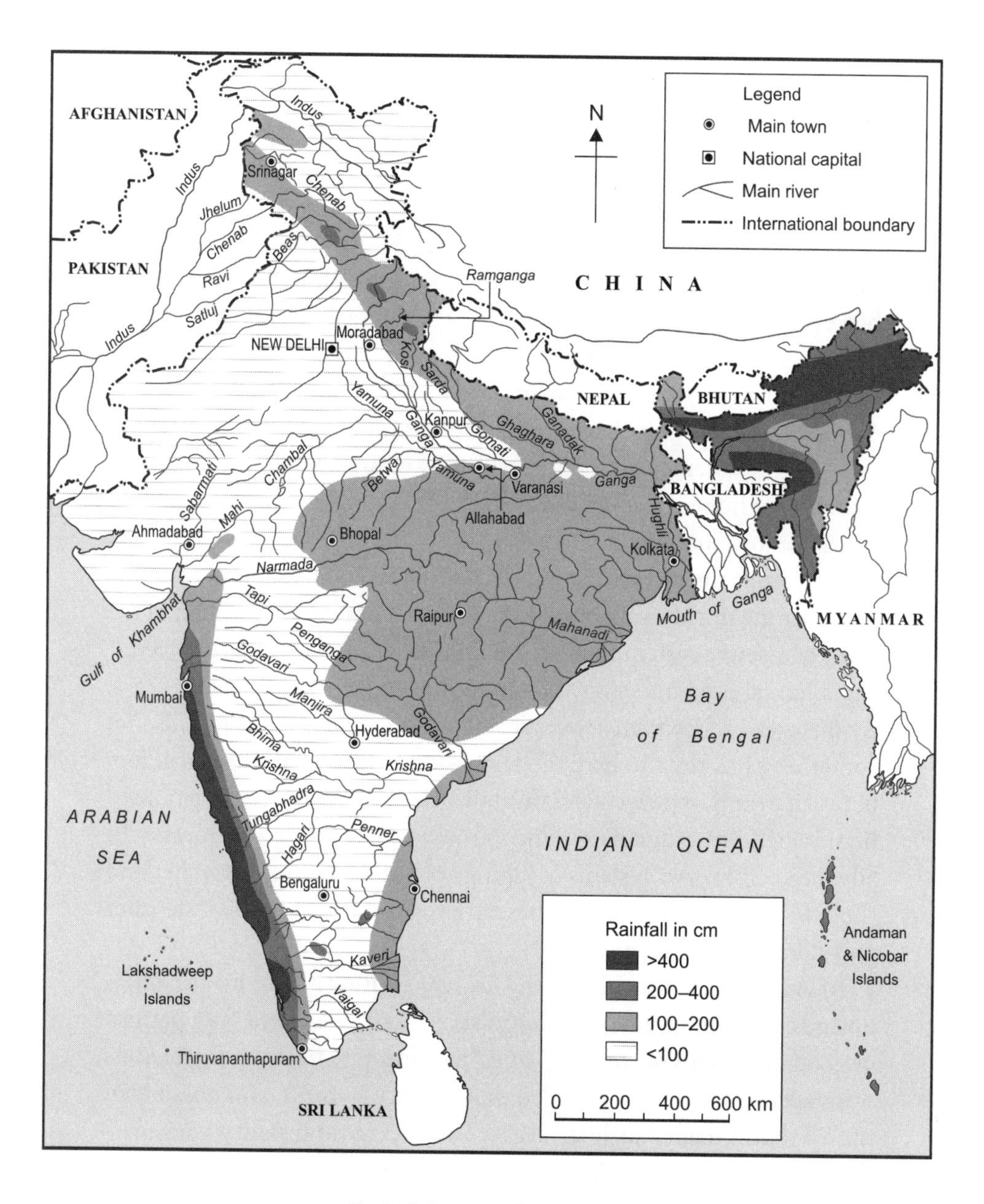

Map 3.1 India: rivers and annual rainfall

New Delhi in the twenty-first century has something in common with London in the nineteenth: a befouled river. The National Capital Territory of Delhi straddles the River Yamuna. When it is in spate during the monsoon, the Yamuna used to flow strongly across a vast floodplain, and when Delhi was a city of 1.7 million as it was in 1951, the Yamuna could keep itself and Delhi relatively refreshed. In 2011, however, Delhi had a population of more than 16 million. In contrast to the Thames, however, the Yamuna does not flow at the doorstep of the Indian Parliament. A smelly Yamuna is five kilometers (3.1 miles) from the noses of the country's leaders. Parliamentarians at Westminster were among the first to know when the Thames stank or turned yellow.

London's sewerage helped make the city cleaner, but it simply shifted dumping of human excreta down the river and made the North Sea responsible for purifying it. The grandeur of the engineering—"a perfect shrine of machinery," the correspondent of the *Times* reported from the gala opening in 1865—supported the idea that once a technical fix in the form of a sewer system had been engineered, problems were solved.[36] India has labored under such assumptions for more than thirty years. By themselves, however, sewers solve nothing. They collect liquids, but something has then to be done with them. There is a difference, too, between drains, which collect rainfall, and sewers, which carry tainted liquids including human excrement from households and businesses. In advanced cities, two systems of piping are built, one for wastewater and the other for rainfall. Today, these are often referred to as wastewater and storm-water systems.

In 1906, C. C. James, one of the drainage authorities of his time, was optimistic about Bombay. The city "stands out," he wrote "as a pattern of good local self-government" and "has now practically completed its sewerage works."[37] He concluded that "no city in India, and possibly in the East" had made "such strides . . . in sewerage and sanitation generally." As recently as the 1880s, urban sanitation had little scientific basis and "the system of 'trial and error' had inevitably to be resorted to."[38] However, "the ignorance and indifference of former times in sanitary matters are now happily well nigh things of the past" and civic leaders were taking "a keen, helpful and most intelligent interest in sanitation." He alluded to the result of a binding crisis, the plague of the 1890s: "The last nine years of plague have taught many lessons, not the least valuable . . . of which is the appreciation of cleanliness and sanitation, which seems to be now becoming general even among the humblest."[39] Bombay in 1906 had a population of just over 800,000.

By 2011, the population of Mumbai had grown to 18.4 million, and authorities and citizens were less cheery than James had been in 1906. "Discharge of untreated sewage is the single most important cause for pollution of surface and ground water," the Maharashtra Pollution Control Board reported in 2013. "There is a large gap between generation and treatment of domestic waste water," which was "responsible for about eighty percent of water pollution." As a whole, the state of Maharashtra had 26 cities with populations greater than 300,000, but only 18 had treatment plants for domestic sewage. Of 230 smaller urban centers, only 10 had plants for sewage treatment.[40]

Many of James's observations in 1906 remained relevant in the twenty-first century. "The genuine religious sentiments of the people" often obstructed innovations in public sanitation, "far too few conveniences [toilets] are provided," there was a need for "educating the lower classes to the necessity for sanitation," public fixtures of all kinds "were constantly being jerked off and stolen," and "authorities of many Indian towns . . . make no attempt to purify the sewage before it is discharged" into rivers and other water bodies.[41] The remarks remain strikingly appropriate more than a hundred years later.

The period before World War I proved the pinnacle (although not a very high one) of public sanitation in India during British rule, as James's optimism indicated. Germ theory had become widely understood and accepted, and as a result, engineers, scientists, and officials now found common ground. At the same time, the pressure on Britain to clean up its empire that came from other imperial powers made British officials less reluctant to finance public sanitation projects in merchant centers, such as Mumbai. The plague outbreaks of the 1890s had served that purpose. To avoid bans imposed by other imperial powers on contaminated British ships, the empire needed to present a cleaner face to the world.

The moment did not last. World War I drained finances and administrative energy. Indian sanitation became a low priority for British officials. A militant nationalist movement, galvanized by British wartime repression, meant European officials and Indian-led local governments were invariably adversaries. There were more urgent causes than sewers and water supplies, and urban infrastructure developed sporadically. "Before 1947," a government publication recorded in 1953, "not much progress was made in . . . public health."[42] After independence, national and state governments focused on building what promised to be the great institutions of modern states—industrial capacity and higher education—while paying lip service to a vague Gandhian ideal about the virtues of village life. The latter inclination aimed to discourage people from migrating to urban areas and downplayed the needs of towns and cities. Although one might have expected urbanization to be a key part of a program of modernization, it seldom was. New cities were started—Chandigarh and Bhubaneshwar—and New Delhi received a masterplan,[43] but it was the 1980s before urbanization gained wide acceptance among politicians as an unstoppable process that needed to be adapted to, not resisted.

In the 1960s, officials who sensed the need for urban investment generated inquiries that pointed to huge deficiencies in public sanitation. But drains and sewers had little appeal to politicians. "The income of local authorities," a 1966 inquiry concludes, "is hardly adequate for normal maintenance of civic services and facilities." Anything beyond that was "impossible." Urban sanitation since 1947 "appears to have improved, though only marginally." In most small towns, "the shift to wheel barrows has only been partial with sweepers continuing to carry it [excrement and other refuse] on head loads [*sic*] or in buckets."[44]

By 2013, the Government of India believed that less than 20 percent of wastewater, including human waste, was captured by sewerage, even in towns and cities.[45] Mumbai was one of the few with a highly developed system of underground sewers. More than 90 percent of the greater Mumbai area was claimed to have such access.[46] But to have households and businesses connected to extensive sewerage means little if the raw effluent is discharged into lakes, rivers, and seas. As one of the country's wealthiest states and with Mumbai as its capital, Maharashtra probably managed sewage better than most. But its Pollution Control Board regretted that local governments had not been able to build enough sewage treatment plants. Those that were operating "generally neglected . . . sludge removement & its treatment." Unreliable power supply disrupted treatment of sewage, and plants suffered from "poor operation and maintenance" as a result of "deputation of unqualified . . . staff."[47] Cities like Kochi in Kerala with a metropolitan population approaching three million had no sewerage at all. In the past, the backwaters surrounding Kochi dealt with storm water; households used pit latrines and septic tanks.[48] Most towns and cities still rely heavily on open drains (*naalas*) and natural water channels. During rainy seasons, storm water sweeps up the refuse in its path—from plastic bags and industrial chemicals to dead rats, dogs, and other animals—and carries it into water bodies.

What happens to sewage from households that have flush toilets but whose towns have neither sewers nor sewage treatment plants? Residents will often say that their house or housing colony is connected to a septic tank; but not all septic tanks are equal. Effective septic tanks are hardworking but slightly delicate systems. They have carefully placed entry and exit pipes emanating from two sealed chambers; they have a solid cap on top of the tank. In a properly functioning septic tank, bacteria remove impurities from water and reduce solids to nonthreatening sludge. The sludge that accumulates at the bottom of the tank eventually has to be pumped out and deposited somewhere. One estimate suggests that a septic tank designed to serve ten people might need pumping out every five years. If it were serving a hundred people, it would need pumping out every six months.[49]

India had fifty-five million septic tanks and twenty-three million pit latrines, according to the census of 2011.[50] But most septic tanks are simply containers for holding human waste—cesspits, which were a standard way of mitigating liquid waste in the past. Sucking out the contents of septic tanks and the cesspits that impersonate them is a thriving industry as middle classes try to put as much distance as possible between themselves and human waste.[51] Entrepreneurs and nongovernmental organizations in Bengaluru have attempted to turn the contents of cesspits into valuable manure for agriculture. Locally built pumping units installed on trucks clear up to seven cesspits a day. These trucks are known in some parts of India as honey-suckers. The sludge is deposited on suitable land on the outskirts of the city, covered over, and allowed to mature into a rich manure.[52] In ideal conditions, such systems minimize the need for sewage treatment plants and for manual cleaning of cesspits.

But honey-suckers can become outlaws. Kerala's pit latrines control human waste, but they are often not connected to sewerage. In a state of thirty-five million people, hundreds of cesspits need emptying every day, and shady honey-suckers pump out the contents and dump it wherever they can. Households have a functioning latrine that channels human waste and keeps the household and its neighborhood clean; but rivers, backwaters, and the sea receive thousands of liters of illegally dumped, untreated sewage and sludge every day.[53] The tankers, writes M. Suchitra, a correspondent of the environmental magazine *Down to Earth,*

> come close to midnight along with . . . suction pumps and hoses. . . . Nobody, not even the neighbours, get to know of it. Residents are cautious not to ask the cleaners where the sludge goes. . . . When the streets are clear of cops, it [the tanker] moves to the city's periphery and slyly dumps the waste at any convenient place—an open field or one of the numerous streams, canals and rivulets.[54]

The contrast was striking between Kerala and Bengaluru. In Bengaluru in 2016, there were said to be close to five hundred honey-suckers doing a fairly well-regulated and manure-producing traffic.[55]

One of the attractions of the honey-sucker concept as envisaged in Bengaluru was captured in the headline of an enthusiastic website: "Eliminating Manual Scavenging—The Honey-Sucker Approach."[56] Cesspits and septic tanks cleaned regularly by honey-suckers place a layer of technology between human waste and the human beings responsible for dealing with it. In the Bengaluru model, the sludge is turned into productive manure. More important, the people who clean out cesspits control a substantial piece of machinery, and that gives them a certain standing and importance. One might deal contemptuously with a manual scavenger carrying a bucket and a scraper, but someone driving a truck and operating an outsize suction pump commands some respect. And because work related to contact with human excrement is invariably done by Dalits, the conferral of respect is an essential element in improving public sanitation by undermining caste prejudices. To be sure, the owner of a honey-sucker may not be a Dalit, but even to put a Dalit in the driver's seat marks a small social advance. Waste management will improve as the conditions and dignity of the people who handle waste improve—when they have suitable uniforms and premises, acknowledged civic rights, and the responsibility and the skills to operate the equipment. When that becomes widespread practice, it will be evidence that attitudes to ritual pollution and caste are shifting slightly.

For the urban middle class, arrangements that remove excrement from their vicinity are what matters, especially if those arrangements appear to be cheap. In everyday life, people seldom think about polluted and shrinking water supplies and public health and nutrition. Change is expensive and disruptive. It takes the enhanced awareness generated by the crisis of a Surat plague to provoke change. To build, maintain, and extend sewerage, streets have to be dug up, pipes laid, and households and businesses connected. And there must be water—plenty of water—to flush effluent through the system. An old-fashioned toilet requires up to twelve liters for every flush. If every one of India's 260 million households had a flush toilet and used it six times a day, toilet use alone would require a reservoir the size of Sydney Harbor once a month.[57]

Flushing human excrement out of sight and smell of a household or a community is only the beginning. To expel untreated effluent into water bodies simply moves pollution from one place to another and carries potential infections farther afield. Sewers need treatment plants. Treatment plants need space; they are costly to build and demanding to maintain. The city of Pune, one of the country's most prosperous cities in the richest state, manages to treat about three-quarters of its daily sewage before pumping it and the untreated 25 percent into its rivers. "There are treatment plants on paper," the chair of the Maharashtra Pollution Control Board told a conference in 2015, "but the final disposal is either in open drains or we don't know where the sewage goes."[58]

Ahmedabad, the capital of Gujarat on the Sabarmati River with a population of about six million, illustrates the limitations of sewage treatment plants. In 2013, Ahmedabad had seven working sewage treatment plants treating 1,100 million liters of effluent and producing 20 metric tons of sludge a day. Once treated and made benign, the water was released into the Sabarmati. The newest of these plants—"India's . . . largest" plant of its kind, a brochure declared—cost Rs 55 crores, or about $14 million, when it was completed in 2009. As Ahmedabad sprawled, new housing and industries on its outskirts were not integrated into the sewerage network, and 300 million liters of untreated effluent went straight into streams flowing into the Sabarmati.[59] Sewerage—the trenches, the pipes, the individual connections, the maintenance, and the treatment plants—entails planning, disruption, and substantial investment, which India's local governments do not have the capacity to initiate, as we discuss in Chapter 6.

It proves easier to leave things as they are. Local governments call on workers, who are mostly Dalits, to do the dirty, dangerous work of maintaining primitive systems for removing human waste. They do the work because they have few other ways to earn a living. The gated communities of the urban middle class call on honey-suckers to pump out cesspits and septic tanks and dump the contents out of sight and smell.

By 2017, more than a third of India, close to 450 million people, lived in towns and cities where 60 percent of the feces and urine generated each day found its way, uncontrolled, into water channels and onto open ground. At a low estimate, an adult produces more than 100 grams of excrement and a liter of urine a day. That adds up to 270 metric tons of excrement and 270 million liters of urine released untreated in towns and cities daily.[60] The health hazards are one thing, but the lost energy is another. Feces can produce energy and, having done so, leave behind rich, benign fertilizer. Urine is heavy with nitrogen, and India uses more than 10 million metric tons of nitrogenous fertilizer a year, second only to China. With suitable technology and immense change in attitudes and practices, India's waste problem could become an asset.

Health

Rural India suffers from a silent crisis documented in Diane Coffey and Dean Spears's pathbreaking book, *Where India Goes*.[61] If widely understood, this silent crisis might become a binding crisis for transforming attitudes and practices.

Rural India's silent crisis lacks the drama of Surat's plague of 1994, but it appears to affect both the poor and the better off, as diseases like typhoid and cholera once did. Childhood stunting is the invisible calamity and in 2015 was estimated to affect 39 percent of Indian children under the age of five. A child whose height is significantly below the median for its age is stunted according to standards established by World Health Organization research in 2006.[62] Public health specialists widely agree that the World Health Organization methodology is sound and that "there is no genetic reason for cross-country differences in child stunting prevalence."[63] Children who are stunted fail to "attain full developmental potential," and the consequences—including "poorer cognitive ability," hampered physical growth, and "more anxiety and depression"—"have a profound impact on the developmental capacity of entire societies."[64]

Stunting does not result solely from a lack of food. Beginning in the 1990s, researchers into nutrition and public health concluded that intestinal parasites and bacteria contribute to stunting in young children. Parasites compete for food in the child's gut, and bacteria lead to diarrhea, which prevents children from absorbing nutrition from the food they ingest.[65] The most common way for bacteria to get into babies is through "contamination of drinking water, soil, utensils, food and flies."[66] Open defecation, which is higher in India than in sub-Saharan Africa, greatly increases the risks of contamination.[67]

Studies that compare India to its neighbors and to states within India confirm that problems of childhood nutrition are strikingly affected by open defecation and the resulting contamination. "A large fraction of the difference in average child heights between Africa and India," one researcher argues, "can be explained by the prevalence of open defecation."[68] Various factors explain why some babies are stunted. These include the health, height, and education of the mother; the wealth of the family; access to health care; and whether open defecation is widespread in the neighborhood. In most of these categories, north India appears more favorably positioned than countries of sub-Saharan Africa or Bangladesh. Yet rates of stunting in north India are higher.[69] Open defecation stands out as a key factor. In Uttar Pradesh, India's largest state, with more than 200 million people and the highest rate of stunting, more than 50 percent of people defecated in the open, and 56 percent of children under five were estimated to be stunted. In Bangladesh, 36 percent of children were stunted, and 8 percent of the population defecated in the open.[70] In the state of Kerala, child stunting was 21 percent, and open defecation 5 percent.[71]

Perhaps the most intriguing comparison is with Bangladesh, the most densely populated major country in the world and one of the poorest. Bangladesh, however, has lower rates of stunting than most of India—*and* Bangladesh has a higher proportion of households having access to a toilet. "Unlike its South Asian neighbours India and Pakistan," Bangladesh's leading English newspaper gloated in 2015, "Bangladesh is on track to meet the global targets for reducing stunting among children under five."[72]

The story of stunting attracted wide attention. The *International New York Times* carried a front-page account—"starving, but not from the lack of food"—by an award-winning science reporter, Gardiner Harris, in July 2014.[73] Nicholas Kristof, the *New York Times* columnist, devoted a column to the topic: "Stunting," he wrote, "is worse in India than in Burkina Faso or Haiti, worse than in Bangladesh or North Korea."[74]

In the distressing story of stunting, there may be a glimmer of promise. Because a large proportion of the children of better-off rural families are also stunted, not merely the children of the poor, stunting is becoming a little more widely understood as an affliction endangering everyone. Stunting affects "a third of children from [India's] richest families," according to one survey.[75] This is because flies and bacteria are democratic and blind to caste and social class. The preference for open defecation in rural areas leads to widespread contamination of water, vegetable gardens, courtyards, household utensils, and human hands. Even the children of well-off rural families ingest contaminants and have their development impaired. Better-off children play in the same dust as poor children, drink tainted milk and water, eat food insufficiently cleansed, and are fed and cared for by relatives who have dirty fingers and have not been exposed to ideas about germs. Childhood stunting and its causes could constitute a binding crisis.

If it were widely known that well-off children were in almost as great danger as the children of the poor, building and using toilets might become desirable, even fashionable. If village leaders do it, others will emulate it. If germ theory becomes well understood, awareness grows of a threat that can be mitigated by enlisting everyone—rich and poor—in a system of hygienic treatment of human waste. In France in the 1880s, as Louis Pasteur's theory of germs became widely understood, awareness grew that "shared life . . . makes us all interdependent one on another. These organisms [microbes] . . . penetrate everywhere, . . . into our drink, into our food. . . . The hygiene of a town can never be ensured so long as it continues to be neglected in its poorer districts."[76]

The lingering problem in rural north India is not so much building toilets as it is inducing people to use them. Infrastructure is more than simply about money and mechanics; it is equally about the practice of government and access to resources.[77] It is also about social relations, people, and ideas, as we detail throughout the book.[78] A recent study of rural Tamil Nadu shows continued preference for open defecation across caste groups, despite targeted financing and technological interventions. Increased access to subsidies for building toilets provided little incentive for ongoing latrine usage. Rather, people expressed concern about the pollution—ritual and otherwise—generated by latrines built inside the household. When perfectly functioning community latrines were installed, they too were rarely used, largely because of their location near Dalit neighborhoods.[79] Cultural schemas and ideas do matter when trying to stimulate infrastructure and effect behavioral change. Equally important is basic sanitary education of the kind that an adequate primary school education imparts. In Kerala, where such primary schooling has been universal for three generations, more than 90 percent of households have access to toilets. These may not be toilets that lead to satisfactory processing of excrement, but they restrict it and lessen the exposure of children to excrement-derived pathogens. And a solid primary education teaches about germs, the need to wash hands, and the need to purify water. In Kerala, the infant mortality rate in 2012 was twelve deaths per thousand live births. In Uttar Pradesh, it was fifty-three.[80]

For habits to change, health education and follow-up are essential and go hand in hand with making affordable toilets available. A survey of campaigns to eliminate open defecation in India, Indonesia, Mali, and Tanzania found that Mali showed the best results. After being introduced to the program, villages were visited every month for a year to encourage commitment and resolve problems. Mali offered almost no subsidies or material incentives for toilet building, but it was the only country where there was an improvement in the height of children, a measure of nutrition and stunting. In India, although there were subsidies to build toilets, only a single introductory visit supported the campaign, which did little overall to improve the health of children.[81]

Other countries have attempted to spread the message that germs lead to sick babies. An emotion-driven campaign in Ghana in 2003 brought significant results, particularly from a television advertisement "aimed at mothers [that] depicted a woman leaving the toilet with a strange digitized red stain on her hands, which she transferred to the *fufu* (popular staple food) she was preparing, which the child then ate."[82] Follow-up surveys suggested that more than 70 percent of the audience remembered the advertisement, 13 percent began washing hands with soap after using the toilet, and 41 percent began washing hands with soap before eating.[83] Even before the Modi government's Clean India campaign began in 2014, there were patchy examples that the "toilets are good for everyone" message was being picked up and propagated. One of the perverse results of the previous government's Total Sanitation Campaign, begun in 1999, was reported from Maharashtra: "High-caste villagers were motivated to build latrines for the entire village with the observation that otherwise flies would carry particles of low-caste people's feces into high-caste people's food."[84] Such motivation adds a uniquely Indian caste prejudice to the attitudes of nineteenth-century European and North American middle classes that sought to protect themselves from the infections of the poor.

The crisis of managing liquid waste in India is quiet and insidious. Conscientious primary education and clever advertising can support suitable toilet technology and well-targeted policy. In the first year of the Swachh Bharat campaign, the government of Prime Minister Narendra Modi spent Rs 94 crores (about $20 million) on advertisements; however, the messages were aimed at the urban middle class.[85] More than two-thirds of India still lives in the countryside, where improvement in public sanitation can benefit the health of all classes.

One way of conveying a sense of urgency is by generating sanitation chatter in the media. Jairam Ramesh, then the Rural Development minister in the national government, provoked controversy in 2012 by saying that "toilets are more important than temples. No matter how many temples we go [to], we are not going to get salvation. We need to give priority to the toilets and cleanliness."[86] Ramesh was criticized from all sides for daring to fuse the sacred and profane. But the message "toilets first, temples later" got renewed currency from Modi in the run-up to the 2014 elections.

Gender

Jairam Ramesh's sanitation campaigns continued a series of programs that began in 1999. In television advertisements, Vidya Balan, a Mumbai film star, appeared as a kind and reasoning woman visiting rural India to impart sanitation gospel.[87] One ad had Balan in a village, marveling at a little girl's mathematical skills. The little girl, called Munni, hints to her mother that she needs to go to the field to relieve herself. Her mother tells her to go. Balan then takes out several strips of pills and hands them to the mother. "Keep these [pills], Munni is about to get sick." "Sick?!" replies the mother. Balan then explains that when relieving yourself in the open (*khule mein shauch karegi*), flies will gather around the excreta and "then the same flies pollute the food and hence make Munni sick." The concluding message was commanding: "Get a toilet in the house and use it!" (*Ghar mein shauchaalaya banva, aur istemaal kar!*). Similar ads spoke of the need to provide a daughter-in-law with a toilet in her new home to safeguard her from the dishonor and risk involved in going outside to defecate. In another ad, Balan praised a woman who for the "sake of her honor and cleanliness" (*izzat* and *swachhta*) left her in-laws because they failed to provide a toilet. Similarly, the film *Toilet: Ek Prem Katha* (Toilet: A Love Story), made international headlines for helping spread the message using the tried and tested Bollywood formula, and for promoting the Clean India campaign. The film describes the struggle of a newly married couple in rural India to introduce secure toilets for women in their homes. It was released to coincide with Independence Day celebrations on August 15, 2017, and was an instant box office hit, widely endorsed across social and traditional media outlets.[88]

Such advertising campaigns and films highlight gender-related issues. The lack of clean, secure toilets reinforces gender inequalities and confronts women with huge disadvantages. Girls drop out of school when there are no toilets. Women suffer from urinary and genital infections because they don't drink during the day because they don't want to have to urinate. They relieve themselves and change menstrual cloths after dark in unsanitary conditions.

The sanitation needs of women differ between urban and rural India. In urban India, the sociologists Shilpa Phadke, Sameera Khan, and Shilpa Ranade write, "if we had to pick one tangible symbol of male privilege in the city, the winner hands-down would be the Public Toilet."[89] In towns and cities, the lack of usable public toilets reinforces gender oppression and hampers women's mobility.[90] In the countryside, the lack of household toilets exposes women to sexual harassment when they go to the fields. This is especially so for those who do not have land of their own and are therefore forced to defecate on the property of others, often from higher castes and classes. This was the case in a widely reported rape and murder of two girls from Badaun District in Uttar Pradesh in 2014.[91] The risks involved in open defecation are both physical and social.[92] They include harsh weather, snakes, scorpions, and other hidden dangers. Equally threatening are social relations and ritual hierarchies that make women, especially of low status, a target for sexual assault and police harassment.

The concluding refrain of the advertisements involving Vidya Balan was unequivocal: "Get a toilet in the house and use it!" When toilets are built in rural India, they are often unused. According to one official, this is for practical reasons, because cleaning the toilet is considered a task for lower castes or is another task for women, who have to bring extra water, often a scare resource, to keep the toilet clean. Studies also point to mistrust that some rural people feel toward nongovernmental organizations and government institutions that promote sanitation. Rural people question the design and viability of toilets and complain about unreliable support and limited financial assistance to build them.[93] Another common explanation for unused toilets is that rural people enjoy the experience of defecating in the open air and find a closed toilet unpalatable and slightly frightening. Or that many rural women appreciate an opportunity to be able to meet other women and escape the confines of a household dominated by elders. Whatever the reason for their preferences, the assumption that a private toilet will be instantly embraced by village women is often belied by their actions.[94]

Any intervention in sanitary practices must consider gender roles, power relations, and preferences.[95] To assume that a private toilet keeps women safe from predatory men who prowl the streets and fields reinforces the patriarchal claim that a woman's place—and safety—is in the home. Homes are not necessarily safe from violence. Studies in many countries, including India, have documented the varieties of physical and psychological violence that women can face at home every day. In these circumstances, being able to leave the house to go to the fields can be a welcome respite. Convenient toilets are desirable in their own right. But it is important to draw attention to the unstated assumptions of some of these campaigns, which take for granted that public spaces belong to men. In efforts to get toilets built, such campaigns, films, and advertising, and some nongovernmental-organization-led interventions seldom question women's roles as housewives and the premise that keeping women at home is the best way of keeping them and their honor safe.[96]

Rivers

India's river systems are also its sewers. (See Map 3.1.) The Government of India accepted a statement in Parliament in 2015 that "nearly 37,000 million litres [i.e., 37 gigaliters] per day of untreated sewage water flows into rivers across the country."[97] If that is so, it represents a Sydney Harbor's worth of raw sewage—never mind industrial pollutants—every two weeks.

Costly programs to clean the Ganga, the most famous and revered of India's rivers, have been going on for more than thirty years.[98] In its progress from the Himalayas to the Bay of Bengal, the Ganga flows past cities, twenty-nine of which have a population of more than a million.

When the Yamuna joins the Ganga at Allahabad, the Yamuna adds the pollutants of New Delhi and those of towns and villages along a nearly thousand-kilometer (620-mile) stretch between New Delhi and Allahabad. "Most rivers in the country today are just fetid sewers," writes Raghu Dayal in an excellent analysis of the failures of Ganga cleanups. Dayal calculates that 75 percent of Ganga pollution comes from "municipal sewage from the cities, towns and villages located along its banks."[99]

Varanasi, the most revered city on the Ganga and the constituency of Prime Minister Modi, illustrates the difficulties in keeping rivers clean. More than 80 percent of the city has no sewers, and the sewerage that exists is antiquated.[100] The city's four sewage treatment plants face maintenance problems and frequent power failures with the result that raw sewage from the plants often flows directly into the river. Faulty sewerage can present more problems than no sewerage at all. "Water pipelines, the main source of water in the city, are broken at many places," writes B. D. Tripathi, chair of the Ganga Research Program, "and sewer lines are built next to them. During the day, due to water pressure sewage does not mix with clean water but at night when the pump is switched off, pressure goes down and sewer water enters treated water pipelines."[101]

Migrants and pilgrims drift in and out of Varanasi. Like the urban poor, they have few options except to defecate in open spaces, such as the railway tracks or along *naalas* flowing into the river.[102] Women of the boatmen community, whose association with the city is as old as the city itself, wake up before dawn to relieve themselves at the Ganga's edge. More than thirty thousand bodies are cremated on the ghats annually, and three hundred metric tons of ash is immersed in the river. An estimated two hundred metric tons of half-burned human flesh and three thousand unburned human bodies are found in the river every year.[103]

As Varanasi's new member of Parliament in 2014, Narendra Modi aimed to succeed where others had failed. Citing his experience in cleaning up the Sabarmati River at Ahmedabad when he was chief minister of Gujarat, he spelled out his vision:

> When I took over as [chief minister] in 2001, the condition of Sabarmati was similar [to the Ganga's]. Switch to 2014 and

> things are very different! We have brought water from the Narmada and now water flows through the Sabarmati. A world class Sabarmati River Front was created, which has emerged as a popular recreation and cultural spot in Ahmedabad . . . this is what we intend to replicate in Varanasi. . . . Once we are able to give the required impetus to tourism, it will not only bring more tourists but also enhance the livelihood of the poorest of the poor. More tourists mean more income for those associated with temples, those who are living on the ghats, those who ride the ferries on the Ganga . . . [and] the entire town and surrounding areas will receive a much needed facelift.[104]

Dangers, however, lie in expectations that technology alone can overcome India's problems with sewage. The Ganga Action Plan, Rajiv Gandhi's grand scheme to clean the river in the mid-1980s, adopted the Thames Water Authority as one of its models. The Thames Water Authority transformed the Thames in the 1970s, but the model for the European river does not translate to India's climate, geography, and ecosystem.[105] The Thames is no Ganga, and the Chiltern Hills are no Himalayas. Technology is vital to improving India's treatment of sewage, a theme we return to in Chapter 5. But the technology must suit the social and physical diversity of where it's applied.

4

RECYCLING AND VALUE

THERE WAS A TIME NOT SO long ago, on sleepy afternoons in small towns in north India, when you would hear the cry "Kuh-baa-DEE! Kuh-baa-DEE!"—Rubbish-man coming! Rubbish-man coming! A creaking black bicycle with sacks over the rear wheel like saddlebags would bring a rider to your door to offer a small payment for your old newspapers or a broken saucepan or anything else you might care to haggle over.[1] The *kabaadiwala*—the rag-and-bone man—was a feature of Indian life. In those days, the man on the bicycle might have had a patch of ground somewhere that he had managed to cordon off, or even a tiny shop, where he could sort his collections and receive drop-offs before selling the carefully segregated items to specialists who dealt in glass, paper, metal, or rags.

Most middle-class families have a *kabaadi* story—probably about a family member carefully husbanding objects to pass on to the *kabaadiwala*. A girlhood experience in western Tamil Nadu in the 1980s illustrates the keen frugality that was part of life:

> Plastic items were relatively rare—and valuable, even if discarded, in those days, and poor people—like my so-called "servant"-cum-best-friend—would hoard small items like combs with teeth missing, rubber bands, old bookmarks, odd plastic thong-straps and so on, from our waste-baskets as well

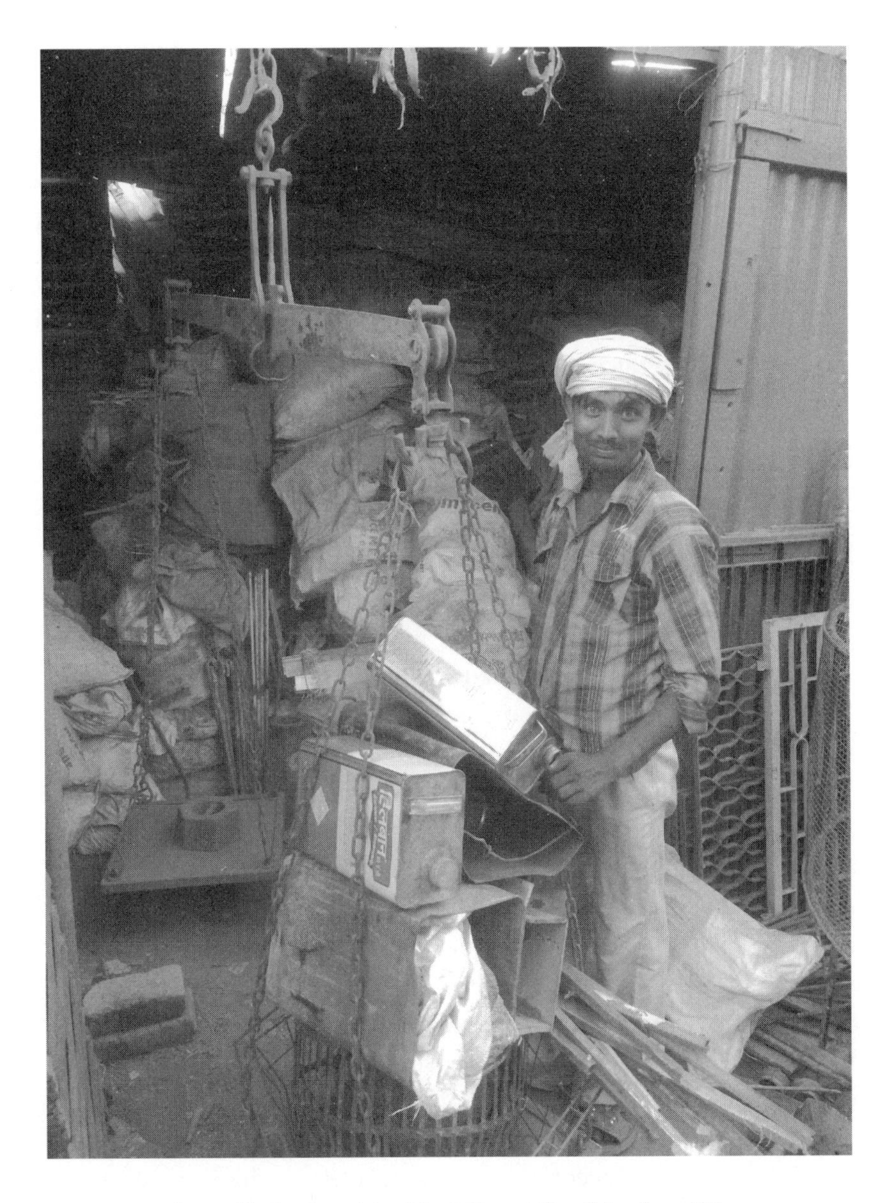

Fig. 4.1 **Weighing in at a *kabaadi* shop in Varanasi.** Photo © Assa Doron, 2014.

> as from the public dump spots at the . . . corners of streets. . . . Every few weeks our friend would walk optimistically into town with a shopping bag full of an extraordinary variety to be exchanged. . . . Our friend argued about the price of her loot long and patiently with the old man in charge. This was one of life's miraculous bonuses.[2]

A symbol of such miraculous transformations lies in the city Chandigarh, built from scratch after 1947 as a capital for the state of Punjab. The Rock Garden in Chandigarh is a make-believe village of statues and tableaus, built out of broken bangles, smashed ceramics, and any inspiring waste that came to the hand of the founder, Nek Chand (1925–2015). Today, the Rock Garden is probably Chandigarh's most popular attraction, surpassing the celebrated buildings of the city's famous designer, Le Corbusier. The Rock Garden captures the old spirit of letting nothing go to waste.[3] Vestiges of old-style frugality survive. These customs, however, are being steadily supplanted as a growing middle class devours a dizzying variety of products and embraces throwaway practices of the developed world.

Up to this point, we have been trying to do two things. The first is to persuade readers of the magnitude of India's task in dealing with an immense urbanizing population that consumes growing volumes of stuff that eventually it wants to discard—from toothpaste tubes to cars and construction debris. The second concern has been to put India's circumstances into historical and geographical perspective. India today confronts experiences that industrializing, urbanizing countries have faced for two hundred years and that are similar to those that many other countries are facing. India's size, however, means its challenges are unprecedented; and although some of its customs have helped lessen the distress that has accompanied full-throttle modernity elsewhere, the cultural politics of caste and class present particular challenges.

The chain of people and activities involved in existing arrangements to turn thrown-away things into commodities of value—recycling—is complex. These arrangements are still largely haphazard. India has a long tradition of people making livelihoods out of other people's discards, but the country is not particularly successful in comprehensively capturing discarded objects. At the same time, its vast labor force, eager for work, has led to the dumping of some varieties of Western waste in India, where Indian workers process it to extract value for astute middlemen. If experience and bountiful labor can be organized effectively, India has the potential to recycle with great thoroughness and to benefit the lives of large numbers of workers. Pockets of such achievements exist, but local examples prove difficult to expand to cover great cities. Scaling up is hard.

People who seek to understand public sanitation—government officials, nongovernmental organizations, and private industry—calculate that India discards a larger proportion of food scraps and by-products (wet waste) than industrial countries. That is because Indian consumption of packaged goods and throwaway manufactures has not reached the scale of the West. In the United States in the 1980s, about 20 percent of waste was wet. In India today, the figure is closer to 50 percent.[4] For waste-pickers, wet waste is something smelly and decaying that camouflages items, such as plastic, paper, glass, and metal, that have recognizable value. For local governments, NGOs, and private enterprise, however, wet waste can supply electric power and good fertilizer and can be dealt with locally, thereby greatly reducing the cost of transport to a landfill. But even small-scale centers that turn wet waste into community benefit require persistent supply and maintenance.

The characteristics of thrown-away things are the keys to unlocking new value. In the countryside until recently, most waste was biodegradable and reclaimed by the soil through natural decay or eaten by domestic animals. In urbanizing India in the twenty-first century, the mix in most towns and cities is reckoned to be almost half biodegradable, 30 percent inert material (dust, gravel, street sweepings), 10 percent plastic, 10 percent paper, 5 percent rags, and 2 or 3 percent glass and metal.[5] But these proportions vary regionally, and as William Rathje and Cullen Murphy sagely observe in their book about garbage in the United States, no one "really knows how much garbage Americans produce."[6] We can say the same about India, and we can also say that the volume of discarded things is growing rapidly.

A complex chain of relationships takes the humblest of things—a single strand of discarded hair, for example—and transforms it into

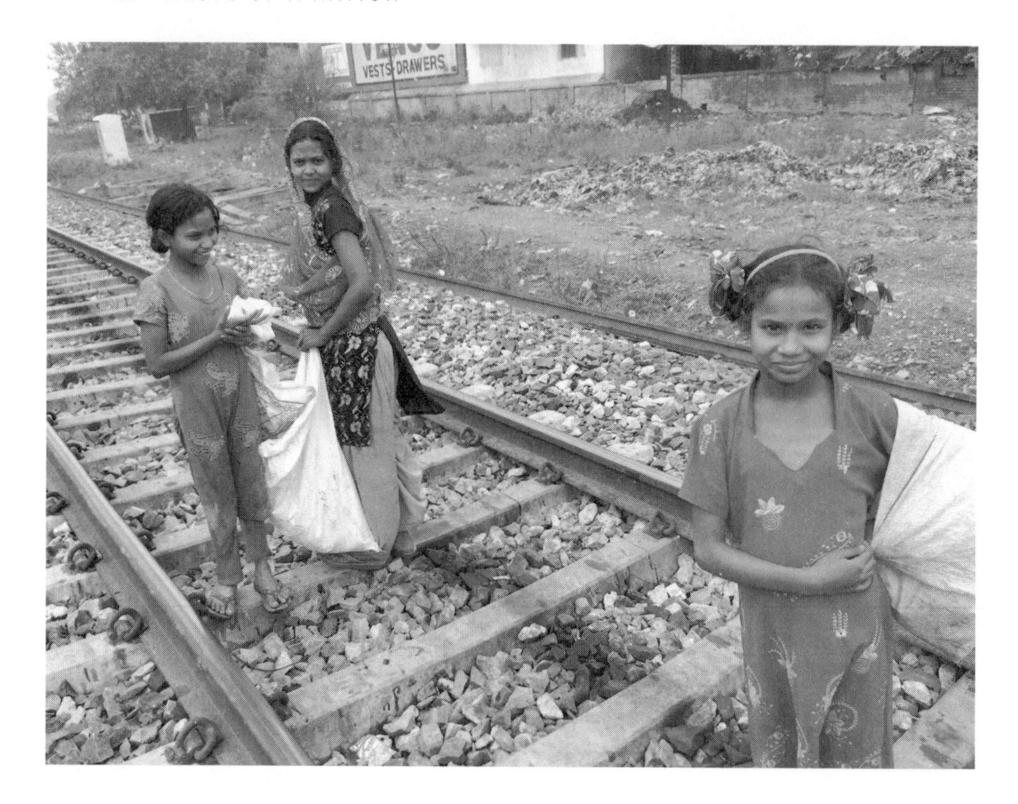

Fig. 4.2 **Helping the family by collecting recyclables in Varanasi.** Photo © Assa Doron, 2015.

something of value, and the way recycling—although it was never called that in the past—is carried on in India today has remarkable strengths as well as weaknesses. One of the strengths is the enormous pool of workers hungry for employment under almost any conditions. This gives India the potential to collect, sort, and process waste in meticulous ways that would be difficult to replicate in other places. But it is also a weakness, because cheap labor becomes a magnet for discards from elsewhere in the world. Seagoing ships and electronic waste are notable examples. To extract valuable components from such commodities is dangerous to workers and polluting to the environment unless conditions are carefully controlled and regulations enforced, which they seldom are. Because price is everything and varies on the basis of international circumstances, care and safety are seen as costs to be minimized. Nevertheless, there are small-scale examples from around the

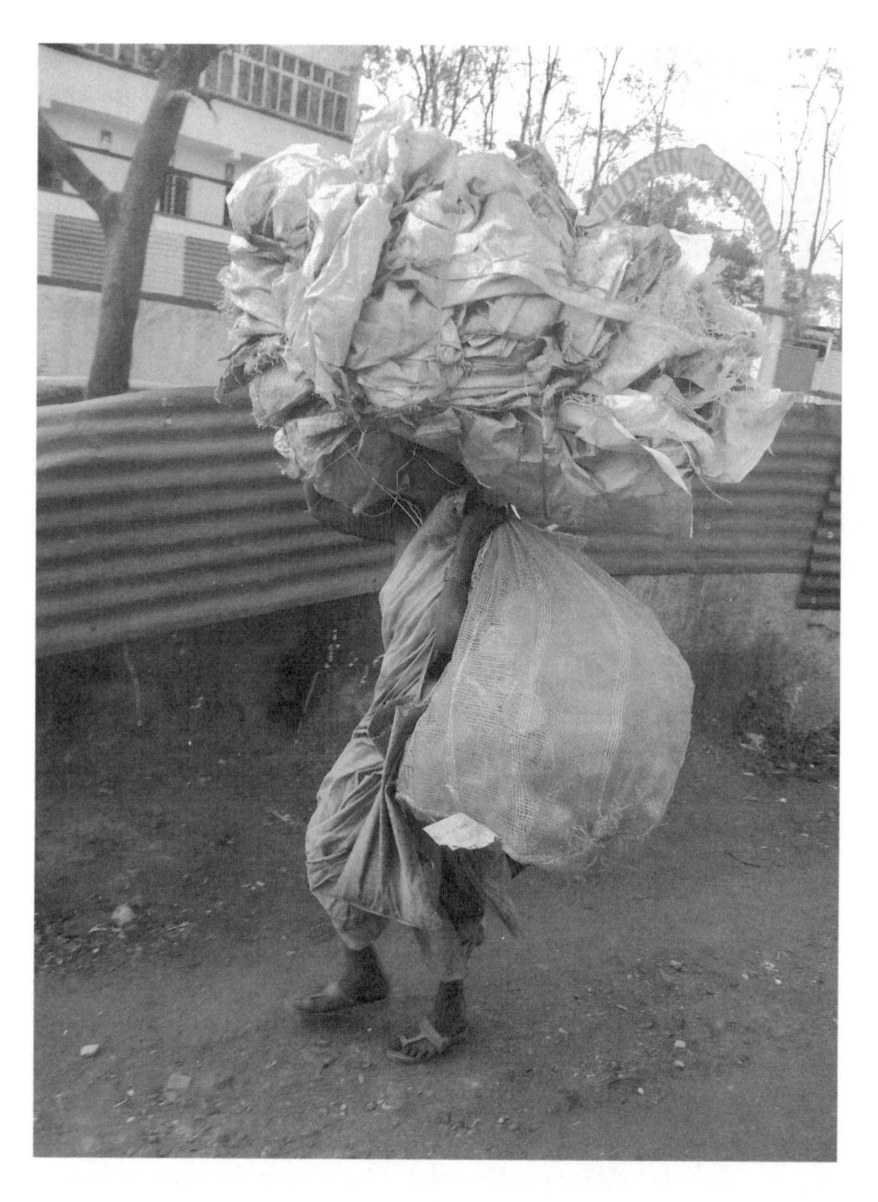

Fig. 4.3 **Harvest of waste. Woman on her way to a *kabaadi* in Pune.** Photo © Assa Doron, 2014.

country where thrown-away things are collected methodically, where there is space to maximize their value by sorting them carefully, and where the people who do the dirty work at the bottom of the chain improve both their income and their sense of dignity. These people are invariably from lower castes, and in the twenty-first century, recognition, which they rarely receive, is as important to them as it is to the proudest high-caste person.

Ships

Why would India import other people's waste? In the right conditions, there is profit to be made. India has the cheap labor to perform tasks that elsewhere would require expensive infrastructure. In a few regions, and the western state of Gujarat is a prime example, some castes have trading traditions and overseas connections built on hundreds of years of experience. Indeed, Gujarat's prehistoric centers of Lothal and Dholavira traded around the Arabian Sea more than four thousand years ago, and in modern times, Gujaratis have been perhaps the most mobile people in India. Gandhi himself was a Gujarati whose formative first twenty years were spent in South Africa before World War I.

Beginning in the 1980s, geography, history, and cheap labor made Gujarat one of the world's largest centers for the demolition of seagoing ships. "Ship-breaking" critics call it. But it is "ship recycling" according to the proprietors of the companies that buy unwanted ships from all over the world. The ships are beached and dismantled, and the components, especially the steel, are sold for profit, if prices are right.[7]

With more than fifty thousand merchant ships on the sea worldwide, the need for demolition and renewal of ships is constant, although fluctuating.[8] The town of Alang is the center of India's ship-breaking industry, which extends for eighteen kilometers (eleven miles) along the western shore of the Gulf of Khambhat (Cambay), thirty kilometers (19 miles) south of the city of Bhavnagar. At its peak, ship-breaking at Alang encompassed 140 spaces on the shoreline where ships could be beached and torn apart. More than 140 companies were involved in the business.[9] The advantage of the location lies in the great tidal variations in

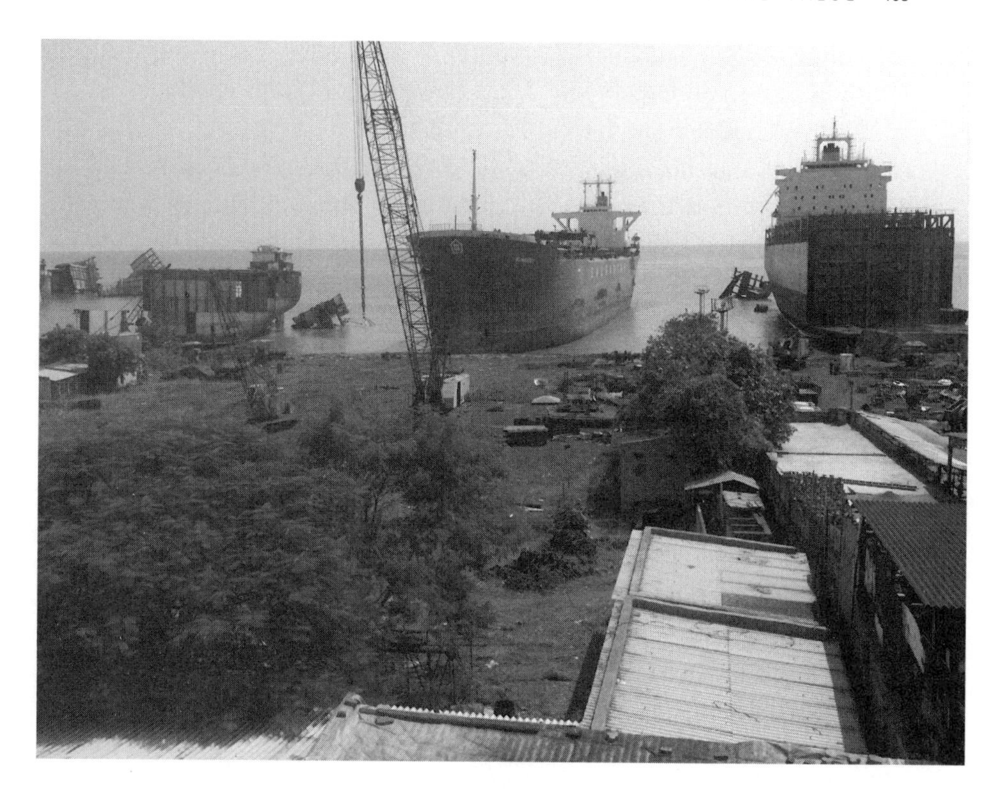

Fig. 4.4 **Ships beached for destruction at Alang, Gujarat.** Photo © Robin Jeffrey, 2013.

the Gulf of Khambhat—a difference of ten meters (33 feet) between high and low tides on some occasions. A ship can be driven far up the shore at high tide until it is firmly beached, and at low tide workers attach steel cables to keep it there. Gangs of workers cut up the ship by hand to recycle the steel and extract everything from lifeboats to kitchen crockery and bathroom fixtures for resale.

Alang's low-tech ship-breaking drew international attention in the 1990s. Investigating the scrapping of U.S. Navy ships in 1997, reporters from the *Baltimore Sun* followed a trail that took them to Alang and a Pulitzer Prize for their reporting. India's environmental magazine *Down to Earth* conducted its own investigation, and Greenpeace, the European environmental group, focused on Alang beginning in 1998.[10] A memorable article in the *Atlantic* brought the agonies of small-scale ship-breaking to international prominence.[11] Photographs of inferno-like conditions accompanied written reports. Worker safety was scant, and the mess of oil and toxic waste in the bowels of old ships endangered workers and polluted the Gulf of Khambhat.

Owners of ship-breaking businesses defended their practices. When Jeffrey met three of them in 2013, they were at pains to reiterate what the *Atlantic* article had reported in 2000: their business did not deal in waste. It was not ship-breaking; it was ship recycling. Less than 1 percent of a ship ended up, they said, as waste.[12] The magazine of the ship-breakers' association spelled out the message: "The ship recycling yard Alang-Sosiya is not the graveyard of ageing ships, but it is . . . the Re-incarnation of these vessels."[13] The owners were aggrieved, defensive, and anxious. A great deal was written about Alang, they contended, without people seeing for themselves. Pictures from Bangladesh, where conditions indeed were bad, were published purporting to be from Alang. At Alang, since 2007, strict rules, imposed by the Supreme Court of India, applied to workers' conditions and even provided for insurance. Margins, they emphasized, were slim. Price was everything. Ship-breakers bid for ships in U.S. dollars, and if the price of steel fell between buying the ship and dismantling it, the ship-breaker lost money.

In the boom year of 2011–2012, Alang's companies cut up more than 400 ships and had a turnover estimated at Rs 10,000 crore (close to $2 billion). By 2015, cheap Chinese steel had become readily available in India, profits fell, and Alang dismantled only 275 ships.[14] As with most dealings in which one person's waste becomes another person's recycling, price was everything. For people who trade in waste and recycling, the summation of Adam Minter, author of *Junkyard Planet*, is basic: "The goal is always the same: take something that costs $0.55—like a pound of Christmas tree lights—and turn it into something that costs $3.12—the London price for a pound of pure copper."[15] Such labor-intensive processes require cheap labor and minimization of expenditure on health, safety, and conditions for workers.[16] At the top of the labor pyramid, the rare worker who lasted twenty years and became a vital, on-the-job supervisor and a worker-aristocrat could earn Rs 80,000 a month (about $1,500). Lowly helpers started at Rs 200 a day (about $3.00).[17]

The ship-breakers of Alang rarely break up Indian ships. They are in a global trade, and the ships that come to Alang arrive because of the cheapness of Indian labor and the favorable tides of the Gulf of

Khambhat. They exemplify how Europe and North America have often dumped their problems on poorer places, just as their own wealthy suburbs send their garbage to poorer regions.[18]

Hair

The ship-breakers of Alang deal with the gargantuan—ships as big as fifty thousand metric tons.[19] The people who do the breaking are lonely men who usually come from eastern India, attracted by better wages than they would get at home—if there were any work at home at all. They have no personal attachment to or cultural beliefs about the ships they take apart.

All this stands in tantalizing contrast with India's recycling enterprise that deals with the tiniest of items—strands of human hair. The collection and processing of human hair is a complex and lucrative business for those at the top. When you break up a ship, the dismantled components acquire value. When you collect hair, the combining of millions of individual strands creates value. Collect enough hair and you can feed your family—or become, in rare cases, a millionaire. Ship-breaking brings the world's waste to India; hair collecting carries India's discards to the world.

Doron first encountered the hair business when he met a group of young boys scavenging for recyclables on the outskirts of Varanasi, Uttar Pradesh. Carrying white polypropylene sacks full of stuff collected through the morning, the boys were happy to unload the day's catch for inspection. The contents looked like rubbish: disordered, moist, and sordid. But as Mary Douglas writes, order is established by acts of elimination and discretion—identification of specific items and judgment about their potential.[20]

The boys sorted and separated their collection on the muddy ground. They picked out strands of hair and separated them carefully from the rest of the refuse, which included a fluorescent-green flip-flop sandal, empty henna bottles, a gray wristwatch, a green soda can, a white cassette tape, and various other items, all of which were put back into the bag. But the clumps of hair were gathered carefully into a plastic container where they formed a substantial black mass, which appeared to

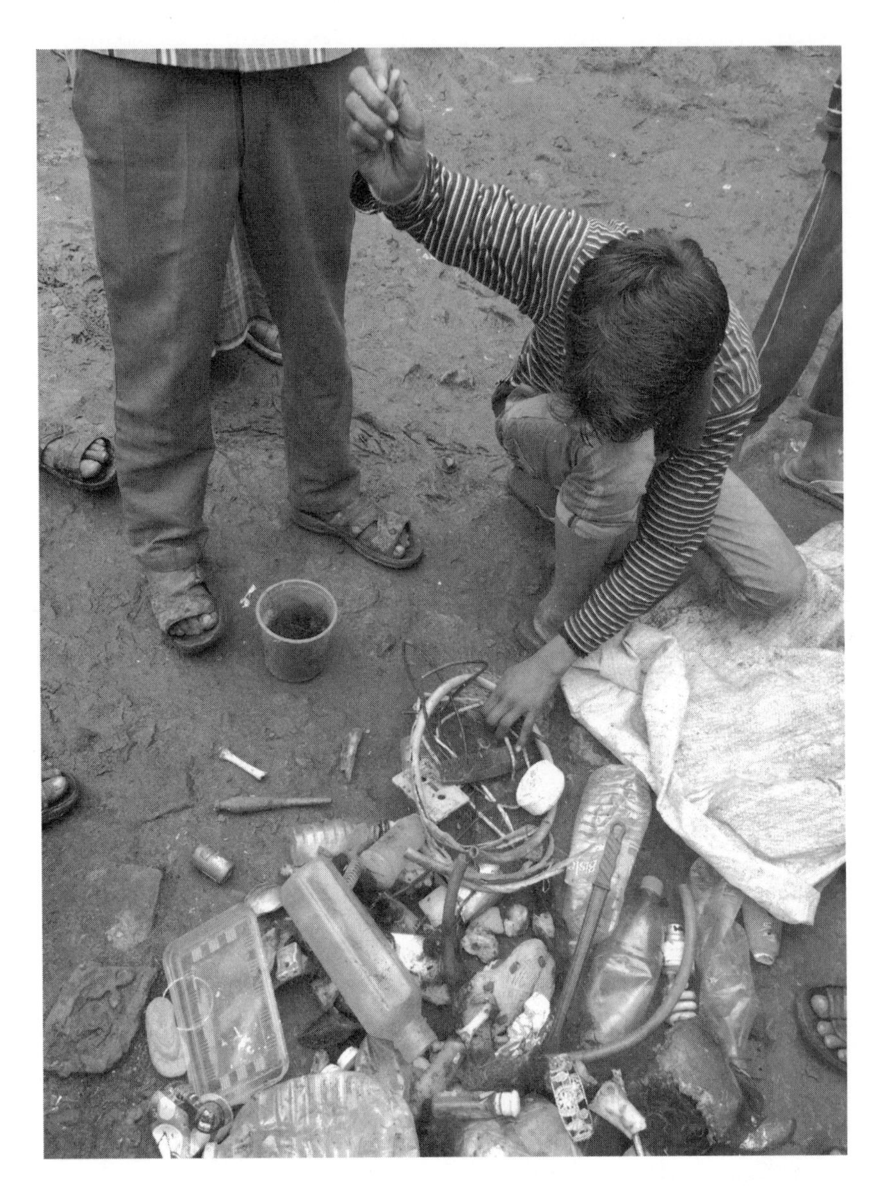

Fig. 4.5 **Separating strands of hair from a street collection in Varanasi.** Photo © Assa Doron, 2014.

be valuable. When Doron inquired about the hair (*baal*), one boy replied, "We just pick it up along the way, anywhere, on the road and drains. Sometimes it just attaches to things and later we separate it."

"But what do you do with it?" Doron asked. The boys explained that they sold it to a Bengali hair trader who lived nearby. The slum where the boys lived housed a community of poor migrants, mostly Muslims. The huts were made of salvaged materials: gunnysacks and tarpaulins stitched together to form walls, held in place with bamboo and metal poles. The roofs were a puzzle of corrugated iron and colored plastic sheets weighed down with automobile tires. Most of the inhabitants relied on waste work for income. Children regularly scoured the nearby streets and rubbish heaps and brought back their finds to be sorted into categories—plastic, metal, glass, paper. These were sold to specialized traders, recognizable by the metal scales at the entrance to their huts.

A few of the children described the scavenging routes they followed throughout the day. Specific rubbish heaps were guarded as the prized territory of particular families. Foraging on larger, more formal rubbish sites near roadside bins was tricky, because such sites were often under the jurisdiction of municipal cleaners (*safai karmachari*) who had first pick of whatever came to the site. What was especially intriguing in this encounter in Varanasi was that the waste-pickers of this slum specialized in something different: hair. Human hair was everywhere.

Outside the huts lay bundles of hair drying on plastic sheets. "The hair is washed and gathered until we have a large enough quantity, and then we sell it to Mr. Khan," explained one of the boys. Water was essential for cleaning the hair, and unlike other slum communities, this one had ready access to water. Throughout the day, women and children armed with buckets waited their turn at a well.

Mr. Khan, the hair trader, was a specialist, a necessary link in any chain that processes waste to give it new value. He had many more connections and higher social status than the hair collectors who sold him their harvest. Mr. Khan's humble office was across an alley opposite the slum, located in a small compound that served migrant rickshaw pullers from Bihar. Most of the hair, stored in two rented rooms, was collected by workers living in the adjacent slum. During Doron's visit,

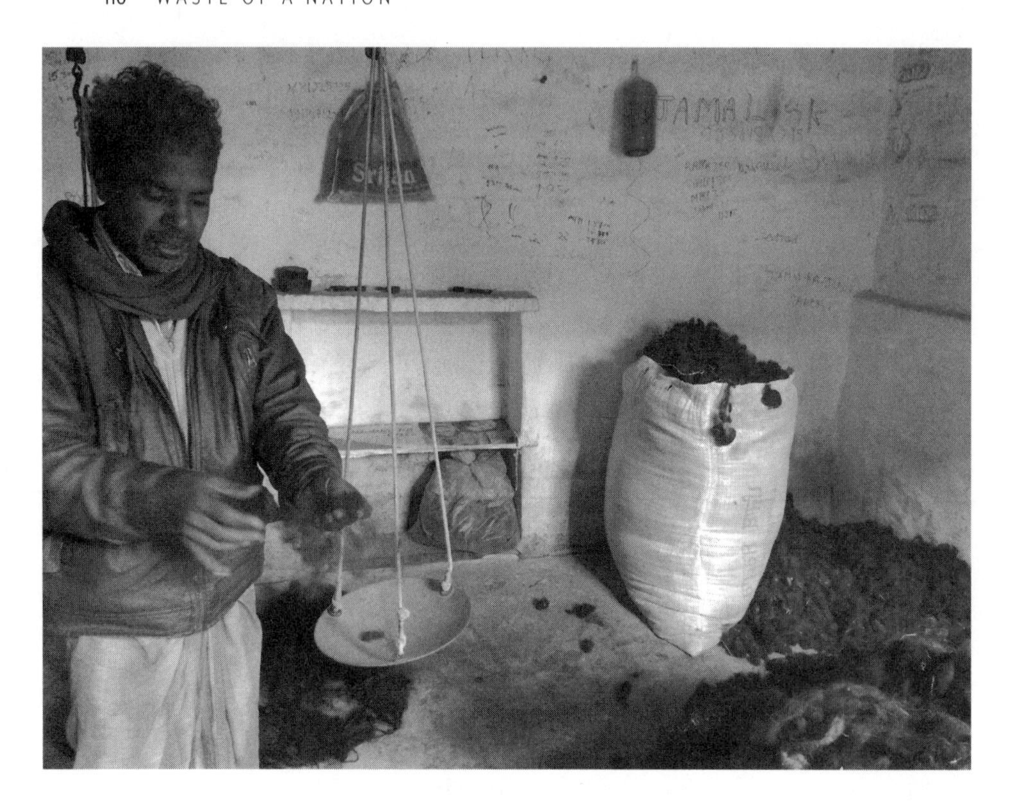

Fig. 4.6 **Weighing and bagging by waste-hair *kabaadi* in Varanasi.** Photo © Assa Doron, 2015.

a boy brought in a bag of hair, which was weighed on large mechanical scales hanging from the ceiling. The boy was given Rs 600 (about $9) for five hundred grams of hair. The quick transaction represented the fruits of a few weeks of hair collecting.

The wad of hair was added to one of the large gunnysacks lying against the wall, each stuffed with hair. Mr. Khan described this as black, *kaccha* hair—raw hair. It fetched a better price than gray hair from the elderly, which was described as *pakka,* or matured, hair.

There were, he said, four general grades of hair, classified according to color, length, and quality (damaged, broken, or dyed). The most prized bags contained women's long black hair, probably shaved for ritual purposes. Varanasi is a leading pilgrimage center, and head-shaving rituals to mark key milestones of life are common.

Emma Tarlo's fascinating book *Entanglement* examines the global hair industry.[21] One perennial source of hair is south Indian temples, famous for prized and pristine hair of pilgrims who shave their heads before worship. Commonly known as temple hair, in professional circles it is called *Remi,* or virgin, hair and is regarded as the purest quality of hair. This black gold sustains a multimillion-dollar global industry of wigs and hair extensions.[22] Indian women's hair is coveted because it is usually unadulterated by dyeing, bleaching, or streaking, and temple hair enjoys its reputation because much of it comes from devout rural women who have carefully groomed and oiled their hair for decades. Tarlo traces the commodity chain—whether comb waste or temple tresses—as it travels along unanticipated routes, from Myanmar hair-processing villages to Chinese factories and to an international hair expo in Jackson, Mississippi. Entangled in social and cultural considerations, the global hair trade is anything but a straightforward commodity chain.

Human hair has long been an object of fascination and reverence in India.[23] For Hindus especially, "the removal of hair is seen as an act of purification and, at a metaphysical level, represents the abandonment of ego (*ahamkara*), the extinction of individuality, which is a prerequisite of achieving the soul's release, *nirvana,* or 'perfect bliss.'"[24] In practice, of course, such lofty ambitions are often much more worldly. Hair figures, for instance, in various life-cycle rituals and pilgrimage rites. Hindus mostly speak of pilgrimage and sacrifice as a form of gratitude to god for granting good fortune, health, or economic success. At Tirupati, the most famous pilgrimage center in south India, thousands of pilgrims line up every day to have their heads shaved in purpose-built tonsuring halls, where barbers employed by the temple authorities do nothing but shave heads. Once shaved, pilgrims go to receive the blessing of the Tirupati deity.

Temple employees collect, clean, and store the hair until it is auctioned to dozens of hair dealers eager to bid for premium material.[25] At an auction in 2016, the Tirupati authorities reported a return of Rs 50.7 million rupees (about $800,000). A year earlier, the starting bid for "first variety" hair, which was black and eighty centimeters (about thirty-one inches) or longer, was Rs 25,500 (about $375) a kilogram. The temple had only 1.3 metric tons of "first variety" to auction, but it had 194 metric tons of "fifth variety," less than five inches long, with an opening-bid requirement of a mere Rs 35 (about 65¢) a kilogram.[26]

The large sums of money derived from selling hair from the temples of south India were a far cry from the small-business venture of Mr. Khan in Varanasi. The majority of the hair that came to him was not temple hair but miscellaneous discards collected by scavengers. If he was lucky, Mr. Khan occasionally received high-quality long hair. It usually came from widows who shaved their heads to mark their new social status after arrival in Varanasi, seeking refuge in the sacred city.[27] "This kind of lengthy hair," Mr. Khan explained, "could fetch up to 1,500 rupees per kg—but it is rare to get." Most of the hair came from pavement barbers and the daily brushing of women. Another source for hair, added Mr. Khan, was the countryside, where roving traders (*pheriwalas*) collected strands of hair that village women gathered from their combs and brushes.[28]

Mr. Khan began as a roving hair trader. His occupation highlights that there are many links in the remarkable chain of people who earn livings by finding, acquiring, moving, and processing waste and thereby turning it into something of value. The harvesting of waste hair was seasonal. According to one waste-picker, winter is an especially good time to forage for hair, because women's scalps become dry and more hair comes out when they brush it. Mr. Khan traveled the countryside of West Bengal:

> I used to come into a village with my bicycle and *damru* [two-headed drum], which drew the attention of children who would gather round asking what I was selling. At the beginning I'd explain that I was after hair, especially of the village women. While they were initially surprised, it wasn't long until I began getting small bundles of hair for which I paid in talcum powder, *bindis* [ornamental dots, placed on the forehead by Hindu women], and sweets. On repeat visits, the hair was already waiting for me, with the kids and women anticipating the [monetary] returns.[29]

Mr. Khan sold the hair to a wholesaler, whose role in the hair business was similar to Mr. Khan's at the time Doron met him. In a substantial apprenticeship the wholesaler had learned the ins and outs of the trade (*jaankaari*) and established his own connections with dealers higher up the chain. He was operating his modest business with the help of his son, son-in-law, and one regular employee. They sourced hair from neighborhood scavengers and a network of hair traders. To manage his business, Mr. Khan had a mobile phone that held two SIM cards, one for Uttar Pradesh and the other to manage business at the West Bengal end, where parceled hair was sent by railway. Although he was less familiar with the details of how the hair was processed in Kolkata, in West Bengal, Mr. Khan was sure that another stage of refinement and classification took place before it was sent overseas.

So far, Doron had found four broad groups of participants in the chain that captures and gives new value to thrown-away things. There were the small boys who first caught his eye in Varanasi. They were connected indirectly to the women who discarded strands of hair. There were the *pheriwalas,* the traveling traders who collect hair on their rounds of small towns and villages, and there was Mr. Khan, who aggregated what had been collected. In south India, there were the great temples, devotees, barbers, and the authorities who organized the auctions. But to find out what happened after hair left Mr. Khan's premises, Doron was directed to Delhi and Mr. Ashok.

Mr. Ashok's export business was located on the top floor of a nondescript building near Delhi's Paschim Vihar metro station. Several women worked in a large room processing hair. Some used large purpose-built combs called hackles to refine and measure the hair. Others packed bundles of hair. A couple of men worked on sewing machines that stitched wefts (loose hair sewn together to make a lock of hair). Outside, on a small veranda, black hair soaked in buckets of chemicals, and treated hair dried on the balcony. The adjacent room functioned as a front office where Mr. Ashok, his wife, and his brother conducted the business. The room had a large desk and brown leather sofas and was decorated with specimens of hair hanging on the walls—Brazilian, curly, raw, single, double-drawn, and colored. Everything was neat and clean.

Mr. Ashok was the son of a farmer in a village near Agra. Like many youths of his generation, he found little appeal in continuing to farm. He completed vocational training at Ambedkar University, and in 2009 he received a master's degree in business administration in 2011 from

Galgotia University in Greater Noida on the outskirts of New Delhi. "I then began working in B2B [business to business] in a job in sales as a marketing manager for three years. This way I could repay my [school] debt."[30]

It was during his MBA studies that Mr. Ashok discovered the world of hair. "I began to research the hair business in detail and traveled across India looking for hair." He managed to trace the commodity chain: from sources of raw material to the processing technologies and marketing strategies at the consumer end. He entered the hair industry as a trader, a middleman selling hair to larger wholesalers, but soon realized there was more potential for profit if he could control most of the transactions along the hair chain. He invested in the technology for processing hair and hired laborers to do the work. "I will not tell you what is involved in the processing," he said. "These are secrets of the trade, but I'll just say that it cost me several lakhs [hundreds of thousands of rupees] to purchase the machinery and learn the know-how." To ensure a superior product, Mr. Ashok had to familiarize himself with the finer details: "I studied even the molecular structure of the hair, the follicles, cuticles and the type of alkaline / acidic aspects of the processing, which takes time and knowledge to understand and apply."[31]

Business grew, and his brother joined him. In 2015, Mr. Ashok bought hair from various sources, including waste hair from *pheriwalas* and temples. He employed around fifty workers and had another factory in Agra where most of the hair was processed and prepared for export. Wholesale prices ranged between $100 and $250 per kilogram depending on the type of hair and the quantity purchased. He exported about 500 kilograms (1,100 pounds) of hair a month to more than thirty countries across Africa and Europe.

Mr. Ashok was a newcomer to the hair trade. Another dealer of comparable size was Mr. Sonu, whose trajectory illustrated the deep roots of waste traders. Expanding a family enterprise that originated with his grandfather, Mr. Sonu took the family waste-hair business to a new level. Based in Delhi and the neighboring state of Haryana, the business had been very local until a few years ago. Mr. Sonu's grandfather, a Khatiik farmer from Haryana, came to the hair trade by chance in the 1970s.[32] "My grandfather," Mr. Sonu said,

> told me how in the late 1970s he visited Bombay and saw people selling balls of hair [*goli*]. Surprised, he decided to get some and took it back with him to Haryana. He told me that when he arrived back home with the hair, he shut all the windows and doors of the house and began to unravel the balls of hair. Hair is dirty you know, but also because he wanted to try this business himself. Then he secretly managed to collect some four to five kilograms [9 to 11 pounds]. He kept the whole thing to himself until he found reliable suppliers from the countryside [*pheriwalas*] and established connections in Bombay to sell the hair he collected. Those days, he just moved the hair from one place to another. But these days we also clean and process the hair after getting it from countryside *kabaadis* and even from some small temples.[33]

Most of the hair his grandfather procured ended up in Mumbai, intended for wigs and the entertainment business. Poor-quality hair was sold for stuffing mattresses. But Mr. Sonu had bigger ideas for the business and looked beyond the domestic market. After some extensive Web-based research, he decided to travel to Brazil, his first-ever overseas trip. His parents disapproved of his frivolous adventure. "Why go to Brazil? Business is just here," they told him. Eventually, he convinced them and set off for Brazil with a new passport and bundles of waste-hair in a couple of suitcases. He said, "It was amazing how fast I managed to sell the hair, and the money covered my flight tickets and accommodation, and I even had some money left; I could not believe it."

Several fruitful trips followed, and Mr. Sonu began to travel regularly to Brazil, carrying suitcases full of hair. But smuggling hair in suitcases had its limits, as he discovered during the soccer World Cup of 2014. Airport security was beefed up, and the kilograms of hair in his luggage were confiscated. "I lost everything. The custom officials even gave me a receipt. That's when I realized I must do things differently."

Mr. Sonu decided to formalize his export business, and over the next few months he acquired the right documentation and licenses and "lubricated the right people, otherwise nothing gets done here." In 2015,

Mr. Sonu exported between fifty and one hundred kilograms a month to his Brazilian partner. "Business is getting better every day," he said as he showed off recent text messages from clients in France, Angola, and Spain. "Next month I am off to Norway. Have you been there?"[34]

At this point, Doron reflected on the people he had met since talking to the small boys collecting strands of hair in the gutters of Varanasi. Mr. Khan aggregated Varanasi hair. Mr. Ashok had discovered the hair trade and created a network of suppliers. Mr. Sonu had taken a family business and found international markets. There was, however, still another level in the hair business, represented by a national award winner, sometimes referred to as "the king of hair."

The hair trade earned its moment in the national limelight in 2015 when the president of India presented an award from the Federation of Indian Export Organizations to the self-styled king of waste hair for his company's stellar export performance. A pioneer of the industry, D. C. Solanki and his company claimed to be exporting an astonishing sixty metric tons of waste hair a month.[35] "Last year," he said, "my business was named the top export business in India. We are the largest traders in raw, waste hair in India, which is used for wigs, hair extensions and many different products." A wall-size poster of India's president with Mr. Solanki and his family adorns the entrance to the company's factory in north Delhi. "I don't deal with temple hair, it's too expensive; here we only use waste hair," Mr. Solanki said. "I have lakhs [100,000s] of workers all over India," he said, referring to the armies of freelance waste-pickers whose collections reached his factory through a chain of middlemen like Mr. Khan in Varanasi.[36]

The Solanki factory spanned a whole block. At one end, a roofed bay contained hundreds of large polypropylene bags stuffed with hair. Once unpacked, the hair was processed in several large halls. The sacks of hair were piled at one end, with brown boxes, ready for export, stacked at the other. Workers combed, cut, measured, classified, and weighed bundles of hair before packing and loading them onto trucks, destined mainly for China, Africa, and Europe. The factory floor was a typical production line, but instead of producing automobiles or grading apples, workers used specialized tools to ensure quality, standardization, and uniformity—of waste hair.

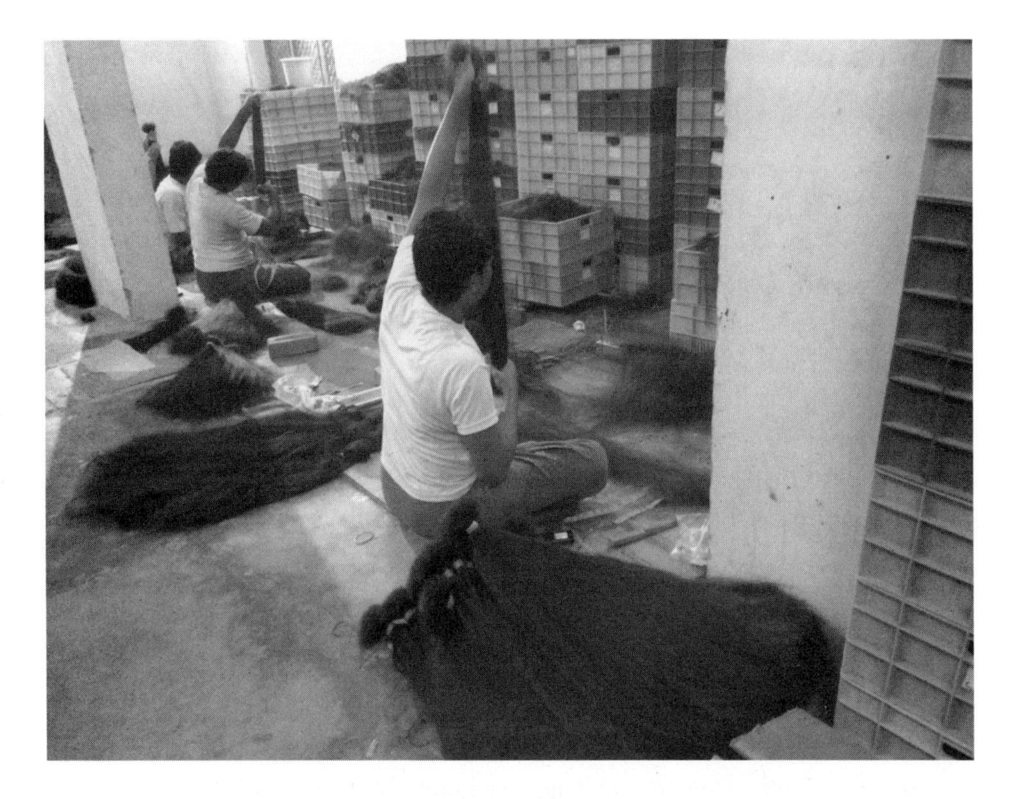

Fig. 4.7 **Adding value: processing long, black waste hair in New Delhi.** Photo © Assa Doron, 2015.

The male employees were dressed in dhotis and color-coded T-shirts (yellow, orange, and pink) that indicated their role in the factory. The yellow shirts operated in a hall that housed dozens of large plastic crates piled high with waste hair. Young men sat cross-legged on the concrete floor, combing the product on hackles, machines that looked like miniature fakir beds—long rectangular planks of wood fitted with nails pointing upward. These hackles were designed for refining large bundles of hair, after which the hair was measured for length and quality. The now-smooth hair was divided into small, silky bundles, wrapped with different colored ribbons, and placed in one of the plastic crates according to its grade and length.

This repetitive work continued in another large hall. The classified and color-coded hair was measured again, trimmed to size, and gently laid in cardboard boxes. Like glassware, luxurious hair has to be handled with care. The boxes were weighed and an information slip placed on top, noting the amount, type, and length of hair. Once sealed, the boxes were moved to another large hall before being loaded onto trucks.

The trucks that took Mr. Solanki's processed hair to the airport might appear to be the end of the waste-transforming chain. The waste hair was purged of its former life, transformed into a commodity, and subjected to the forces of the market. However, as a commodity in a global market, Indian hair—as with other recycled objects—is subject to further surprises in the form of unexpected price fluctuations. In 2004, the hair industry received a setback from the actions of a Jewish community in Brooklyn, New York.

In many Orthodox Jewish communities, women must cover their hair after marriage as a mark of modesty (*tziniut*). They wear head coverings (*sheitel*) such as hats, scarves, or wigs. Wigs have become increasingly fashionable among Orthodox women, some investing thousands of dollars in wigs made of human hair. Such stylish wigs were often made of the best-quality hair in the market—Indian hair. But in 2004, an Israeli rabbi who discovered that most human-hair wigs came from Indian temples deemed such wigs to be idolatrous and issued a ban. A crisis followed:

> Synthetic wigs flew off the shelves yesterday at Yaffa's Quality Wigs in the Borough Park section of Brooklyn. On the crowded streets of the neighborhood, an increasing number of Orthodox Jewish women were seen wearing cloth head coverings, having left their wigs at home. Sarah Klein, a neighborhood resident, said that until the confusion was cleared up, she would leave the house only if she wore a baglike snood.[37]

As Emma Tarlo observes, the tainted wigs were seen as too vile and dangerous for anything other than destruction by fire.[38] By 2016, Orthodox Jewish women were unlikely to wear wigs made of Indian temple hair, and the Indian hair industry had recovered from the shock of losing a section of the Jewish market.

This globalization story is instructive in two ways. The most obvious is the complexity of the chain of waste reuse—of recycling—in global capitalism. The boundaries between the informal and formal sector are blurred, entwined, and interdependent. Strands of hair like those that first attracted Doron's attention when he saw the boys pulling them out of the gutter in Varanasi can cause a minor religious panic in New York City and a temporary collapse in the demand for waste hair in the back lanes of north India.

These stories also highlight less obvious qualities that inhere in waste and recycling. Material things have histories arising from everyday personal rituals, such as combing hair. Waste can become highly symbolic and produce strong reactions, and discarded hair can acquire abstract qualities in which it becomes idolatrous. More concretely, the transformation of waste produces chemical reactions, many of them injurious.[39] The processes involved in reusing waste tend to obscure the practices, ethics, and unequal power relations of waste and recycling industries. In the case of the ship-breakers of Alang, their labor in creating new value out of unwanted objects exposes them to both immediate and later danger, such as the barely visible asbestos fibers released from some of the ships they dismantle.[40]

Gold

Ship-breaking and hair collecting highlight the variety of value-extracting industries and the many links in the chains of reuse. The recovery of precious metals from electronic waste underlines another aspect: the painstaking invention and evolution that characterize generations of frugality and husbanding in India.

As with hair, salvaging gold from electronic waste requires knowledge and skill. Unlike hair, gold does not decay; it is more likely to gain value than lose it. Gold symbolizes class, value, and wealth, and the salvaging of gold waste has a history that some have dated back to the Mughals.[41] In one of their efforts at cataloguing and recording, the British described the people who recycled gold. *Tribes and Castes of the Central Provinces,* published in 1916, explains the word *niaria:* "An occupational term applied to persons who take the refuse and sweepings from a Sunar's [goldsmith's] shop and wash out the particles of gold and silver."[42] Such practices and occupations still exist. India is said to be the world's largest consumer and importer of gold, and gold bullion and jewelry remain the preferred gifts for Indian weddings and other festivities. With years of government restrictions on the import of gold, jewelers have had to rely on recycled gold to cater to booming domestic demand. The scale of the industry is measured in hundreds of tons: "Kumar Jain, who runs a gold retail business in Mumbai's Zaveri Bazaar, a bee-hive of gold traders, expects about 400 tonnes of recycled gold to enter the market this financial year to March 2014. Normally, about 130 tonnes of old gold gets recycled."[43] There are various sources for old gold. Some jewelers melt heirlooms, and others use gold recovered from the same markets and jewelry shops in which gold is sold and processed.

Goldsmiths have a symbiotic relationship with *niarewalas*. The latter pay goldsmiths a fee to be allowed to "clean their shops after nightfall and the streets alongside."[44] The collected dust and dirt are washed and sieved to extract the tiny flakes of gold that fall from a jeweler's bench. Less well-connected *niarewalas* rely on the sweepings and sludge they collect around the jewelers' shops. Armed with brooms and dust pans, young boys scour the gutters, and others wake up at dawn to filter gold specks from drain water that flows as a goldsmith takes his bath. Once filtered and accumulated, the specks of gold are melted into ingots that are sold back to the goldsmith.[45]

Jewelry shops are especially protective and discreet about their waste. One long-time jeweler and goldsmith in Varanasi was willing to elaborate on the different types of waste found in his modest shop:

> First there is our regular rubbish, so the paper we burn and plastic we throw. Then there is the normal dust, which comes from the files we use when polishing the gold and metals. This dust accumulates on the workshop table, and we carefully collect it daily in paper bags so I can then melt it back to gold or silver. But then there is the shop-making dust, because even when we are very careful to file and collect, we will always lose some. You see, there is the fan, wind, etc., and people coming and going in the shop, so we never get out of 10 grams the full 10 of gold, but more like 9.5. Where does the half gram go? It goes in the shop, in my house, wherever I go, in my clothes and

> even sticks to my hands. And that's why all my workers clean and wash hands in one tub only, we don't wash everywhere. These leftovers in my shop are called *niara*.[46]

This jeweler collects around ten kilograms of mixed dust and sand during the year, which he then sells during the festive season of Diwali to the *niarewalas*. According to him, this ten kilograms of mixed waste, which contains mostly sand, with some metal dust (*niara*) mixed in, fetched around €1,000 in 2015. This was one of his most significant single transactions of the year. Value hides in a nondescript bucket containing gray floor sweepings. Yet this value can be realized only through a range of social relations and the use of technologies to identify, extract, and measure what would otherwise be waste.

Electronics

Deriving value from waste relies on extensive networks of collectors and the various middlemen, subcontractors, and contractors who add a little value at every link in the chain. The informal labor force involves whole families and communities, including women and children. They collect, carry, and sort discarded things that harbor value. These processes are vividly seen in the electronic waste that began to grow with the arrival of mass television in the 1990s and became an avalanche after the spread of mobile phones beginning in the twenty-first century.[47]

Gaffar Market in New Delhi is a hub for electronic repairing. After discarded phones or other devices have been cannibalized for spare parts, they move from repair desks to containers awaiting pickup for the final journey to the place where dead phones go. Two or three times a week, Doron was told, a man would arrive with a large bag and collect the discards. In 2013, prices varied from Rs 15 for a mobile device to Rs 300 for a computer monitor or Rs 150 for a keyboard. Gaffar Market was the start of an e-waste trail, marked by defunct mobile phones.

The majority of collectors of e-waste in Gaffar Market amassed their goods in the neighborhood of the Jama Masjid, one of India's largest mosques. The area served as a port, and its godowns (sheds) stored different types of e-waste waiting for dispatch across north India. Space was critical. The Jama Masjid area was packed, land values high, and processing e-waste there was illegal. Waste workers knew this and aimed to ensure an efficient flow of materials. Once rudimentary segregation was completed, the goods were quickly loaded onto trucks. The accumulation of e-waste grew every day, and fast processing and movement of goods were essential.

Delhi was becoming a global magnet for electronic waste, and Gaffar Market was only one source for a stream of electronic discards feeding a huge sector. The Associated Chambers of Commerce and Industry of India (ASSOCHAM) reported in 2014 that "Delhi-NCR is emerging as the world's dumping yard for e-waste and is likely to generate to an extent of 95,000 metric tonnes (MT) per annum by 2017 from the current level of 55,000 MT per annum growing at a compound annual growth rate of about 25 percent."[48] This was despite the dismantling and processing of e-waste in the informal market being illegal. With such clandestine practices drawing the attention of global media, authorities were keen to minimize public activity.

Established slums, such as Dharavi in Mumbai, were recognized as recycling hubs for certain commodities, and this was legal. But the neighborhoods around the Jama Masjid were not similarly recognized; they were unlicensed and increasingly scrutinized by the authorities. Patronage and bribery lubricated the movement of waste. This differed starkly from Dharavi, where the plastic and metal recycling establishments had licenses, often framed on the office wall. Many paid an annual fee to formal associations that represented their interests with the authorities and helped them source laborers from Bihar and Uttar Pradesh. But unlike the Jama Masjid area of Delhi, Dharavi did not process electronic waste.[49] Waste processing was regulated in Dharavi, but dealing in e-waste was illegal.[50]

In Delhi, the waste processed discreetly near Jama Masjid needed legal and political protection, and moving goods efficiently and quietly was imperative. Some e-waste was sent to Gujarat and Uttar Pradesh, but Seelampur, a predominantly Muslim settlement on the eastern side of the Yamuna River, in Delhi, was a center for e-waste processing—tearing items apart and separating them into their component materials.

In 2014, it was known for the many scrap-metal dealers who operated there. From the embankment at Seelampur, the Yamuna was a pitiful stream, iridescent green and gray, meandering among islets of sludge and blotches of foul-smelling foam.

Beyond the embankment, a semisealed road was crowded with vehicles churning dust. Auto and cycle rickshaws, small trucks, and improvised vehicles loaded with scrap cargo brought in mounds of electronic goods, already sorted and classified. A cycle rickshaw, remodeled as pedal-driven truck, carried hundreds of gray and black keyboards. On the side of the road, men unloaded computer monitors off a small truck, while a recycling vendor using a locally fitted-out wheelbarrow waited to unload.

Beyond this road lay Seelampur's lanes, with rows of apartment blocks casting shadows over the narrow streets. Only cycle rickshaws could enter. At ground level, the streets were lined with concrete shop fronts, and scales at the door indicated the presence of recycling vendors. Inside the rooms lay an array of discarded goods, piled up according to type. Computers, printers, fax machines, and monitors lined the walls alongside sacks filled with CPUs, TVs, mobile phones, keyboards, TV remotes, and more—a cornucopia of electronic discards. Some scrap dealers specialized in larger items, such as refrigerators and washing machines, but most dealt in everything.

The activities were mundane. Children and adults stripped plastic coating from wires to recover the copper. The rhythmic beating of keyboards and computers to extract their parts provided background noise. Workers segregated piles of metal and plastic. Classification and sorting was key to extracting value. Basic physical segregation—banging and tearing—could be heard all around, but the succeeding processes, which required more sophisticated techniques, remained hidden. The alchemy of the e-waste industry, where high-value materials were reclaimed, was not visible. When Doron inquired about gold, silver, and copper being extracted through grinding, burning, pulverizing, and chemical extraction, he was told that such things happened elsewhere. Much of this extraction took place outside New Delhi.

The politics of waste raises concerns about the dumping of toxic materials in third-world countries, but it also has a distinctly local character. At the ground level, waste workers are part of a social order anchored in long-standing prejudices and inequalities. As Ghazla Jamil, a longtime observer of Delhi's Muslim communities, showed in her study of Seelampur, localities that began as slum resettlements decades ago could not avoid the social and economic marginalization of the increasingly capitalist setup of recent years. For Muslims, such marginality was different from Hindu strictures of caste, but the stigma and prejudice were similar. The lack of political networks and reliable infrastructure combined with their religious identity constrained the opportunities of those involved in the scrap trade. It was hard to "move beyond being a limited part of the supply chain in any industry."[51] The risks involved in this unregulated sector also meant that much of the alchemy of waste took place in distant towns away from the gaze of the media and from the law.

Moradabad in western Uttar Pradesh was once celebrated as the Brass Capital of India, but it is now notorious as a center for e-waste processing. The industry was built on the declining fortunes of its famed brassware sector. According to a report from the Centre for Science and Environment, the brass industry suffered a severe blow from the global recession of 2008. Dwindling demand led people practiced in metalwork to make the "natural" move into the e-waste industry, and streams of electronic goods began arriving from across the country and beyond.[52] The figures, according to one estimate, were staggering: "50 per cent of the PCBs [printed circuit boards] used in appliances in India end up in Moradabad."[53] With more than nine metric tons of waste arriving daily, the industry was said to employ tens of thousands workers, most of whom earned between Rs 100 and Rs 300 a day.[54]

Like other industries in the informal economy, e-waste is a family affair, with women and children often assigned the task of breaking apart and segregating printed circuit board components. Dismantling electronic goods entails prying open the object and separating the gold-, silver-, and copper-plated components and the plastics and aluminum. How this art of recycling is performed has been shrouded in mystery. Yet locals in Moradabad were happy to describe the process, explaining that once the basic dismantling and separation were achieved, different methods of extraction followed. Typically, these were burning, grinding, washing, and bathing in acid. Such processing was heavily guarded, with policemen standing at the entrance to the slum area on the outskirts of the town where much of this illicit work took place.

This protected area, known as a major e-waste processing site, was situated beside the bridge over Moradabad's Ramganga River. It was a predominantly Muslim neighborhood near the Jama Masjid Bridge Road, and from the road one could see locals washing the ash from burned e-waste and using sieves to recover fragments of metal. The policemen were positioned at the entry to the slum at an improvised gate. Men managing the flow of goods were visible from the bridge, as rickshaws carrying electronic discards made their way through the gate and disappeared into the alleys. Rhythmic hammering echoed up to the bridge. The role of the police presence was hard to gauge, but according to one local there was an arrangement between the police and various parties.

Presumably, the police presence intended to demonstrate that strict regulations on e-waste processing were in force. In fact, however, the gate-keeping function was to exclude outsiders. Local people believed that the police received money and goods from e-waste dealers who wished to protect their businesses and that benefits flowed up and down the chain of command. The lowly police on the gate relied on small gratuities, but locals suggested that bigger favors went to more senior officials. The e-waste industry required protection from busybodies who might want to enforce the law or from potential competitors who might pry into their business and steal clients.

On a subsequent visit to the town, Doron and an Indian friend took an unexpected opportunity to enter the slum during the Muharram observance in November 2012. There was little activity that day, and no police at their posts. Shop fronts were mostly shut, the usual hammering had fallen silent, and a peacefulness prevailed. Several children, curious about a Hindi-speaking foreigner, explained that no one was around on this holiday. One boy, however, pointed to a large room facing an alley.

Sacks, brimming with segregated components, were stacked up—connectors, integrated circuits, diodes, resistors, capacitators, and computer microprocessors. Inside a dimly lit house, a fire was burning in a pit furnace built into a cavity in the clay floor. A crystallized golden substance had accumulated on the rim of the furnace. Because of the deafening sound, the person who lay beside the wall was unaware of the arrival of Doron and his companion, but another soon noticed and demanded they leave immediately.

Moradabad's old specialty of brass manufacture simplified the shift to recycling electronic waste. Brass making requires high heat to melt and combine copper and zinc. Pit furnaces, used to turn the recovered metals into ingots, were available and well understood. Once the circuit boards from phones and computers were burned to dislodge metals from plastics, they were turned into powder by ball mills of the kind used in brass manufacturing. The powder from the dissolved circuit boards was separated by sieves or by washing in water. The pit furnaces finished the task of melting metal into ingots. Copper was by far the largest proportion of metal recovered in this extraction process, and much of the copper was sold back to the brass industry in the city.[55] The recovery of much smaller quantities of platinum, gold, and other precious metals was worthwhile because of their high market value.

Later on that Muharram day, the same children were flying kites on the river bank. Below them, a herd of buffaloes drowsed under a hot sun, and a few men washed clothes. But it was not a picture-postcard river scene. A visual cacophony littered the banks—plastic bags of all colors, plastic cups and plates, and an array of shimmering sachets used for shampoos, hair oils, washing powder, sweets, toiletries, and above all, *paan masala* (mouth freshener with added tobacco). The fast-moving consumer goods revolution had taken India by storm. Millions of Indian consumers can afford to buy only tiny quantities at a time, and the revolution was said to be about "sachetisation in capital letters."[56] But sachets, along with plastic bags, left a waste trail across India and led to blocked drains in towns and cities and blocked intestines in grazing animals like the buffaloes lounging on the river bank below. From the bridge in Moradabad, the bags and sachets were a flashing sign of the country's growing confrontation with consumerist waste and a daily annoyance to middle-class citizens. But beneath this everyday eyesore, the mud of the river concealed a more insidious detritus that was a consequence of the e-waste industry.

High levels of heavy metals, such as zinc, copper, arsenic, chromium, lead, and nickel, are present in the river bed and river bank, according to analysis carried out by the Centre for Science and Environment. The river water itself showed "the presence of heavy metals such as arsenic and mercury above permissible limits."[57] These toxic elements resulted from e-waste processing. All the liquid waste of the settlement poured into drains and then flowed directly into the river and seeped into its banks. The continuities with the brassware industry were clear, as a Centre for Science and Environment report observed:

> There is a strong linkage between the e-waste recycling and the existing brass industry in Moradabad. Metals such as copper, iron and aluminum extracted from PCBs of e-waste are fed into the brass-making units. A lot of the brass work carried out informally in Moradabad is pollution-intensive and employs child labour. It is done mostly in small houses in narrow streets but also in well-furnished large units. In household units, the work is carried out within houses, creating noise beyond the decibel counts permissible for the human ear. Metallic dust, chemical fumes and smoke emanate from various processes and affect the respiratory systems of workers. In larger units, many workers work together in over-congested conditions.[58]

E-waste will continue to plague the subcontinent. The increase in electronic discards from a more affluent population compounds the problem of waste dumping from developed countries. Lax regulations and a cheap labor force make India an attractive place for disposal and processing. This e-waste industry relies on what anthropologist Anna Tsing calls "salvage capitalism," in which value is gained with little capitalist control and regulation.[59] Indeed, many of the transactions and restrictions characterizing the Moradabad slum depended on a local, noncapitalist economy that has its own value system. Families work in dismal conditions to sustain an elaborate network of exchange. But this informal economy creates value for capitalist enterprises that benefit from the semiclandestine activity. The police presence in the slum was meant to demonstrate the authority of a modern state governed by the rule of law. However, this was a performative stance, part of the "translation mechanisms for getting access to value procured through violence."[60]

The offshoring of industrial hazardous waste from first-world countries to the third world is notoriously difficult to track, identify, and quantify.[61] But there is evidence to suggests that illegal dumping continues unabated.[62] In the absence of an international standard coding that clearly defines what constitutes hazardous or toxic waste, it becomes relatively easy to smuggle across borders with impunity. This is further facilitated by a host of actors and institutions that populate the waste trade and handle transnational waste flows with entrepreneurial innovation.[63] Along the commodity chains we find a range of people at different stages of the process.[64] Some collect raw materials, some distribute, repair, or manufacture new things, and others conduct the exchanges and relationships that exploit market opportunities.[65] Such recycling chains, including these illegal ones, have their own dynamics—often emerging from the product itself, whether it is ships, hair, e-waste, or plastic.

Plastic

For the millions of poor people who derive a little of their income from foraging in waste, some items bring obvious and ready return. Plastic is one. Because plastic is visible and lightweight and can be reengineered even at the level of a cottage industry, in India plastic gets recycled more completely than any other product and more completely than in many places in the world. When the Government of India issued new Plastic Waste Management Rules in 2016, it estimated that the country recycled 60 percent of the 5.6 million metric tons of plastic thrown away every year.[66] In 2012, the United States was estimated to recycle only about 9 percent of 31.8 million metric tons of plastic it discarded annually.[67]

"The Indian plastics industry made a promising beginning in 1957," according to the Plastics Promotions Council.[68] However, it took more than thirty years for plastic to pervade Indian life as it was doing elsewhere. In 1979, "the market for plastics" was "just being 'seeded' by the . . . state-owned Indian Petro-Chemicals," and it was 1994 before plastic soft drink bottles became a visible annoyance.[69] "In the wake of plague scare" in Surat in 1994, citizens in other cities decried the state of public sanitation and urged governments to "ban the production, distribution and use of plastic bags."[70]

Since the mid-1990s, plastic has pervaded Indian life. Mumbai was said to be using five million new plastic bags a day by 1996.[71] Plastic waste became a mainstay for the humblest waste-pickers, especially women trying to scrape together livelihoods in any way available. For waste-pickers, plastic waste has advantages. Its chemical composition means it can be reprocessed in small-scale operations, not far from where it is collected. It is light and easy to handle, and a kilogram of plastic is usually worth more than a kilogram of glass. "Plastic came along," a lower-caste trader told Kaveri Gill, "and with it came more earnings. In plastic, we are becoming landlords, so we much prefer it."[72]

Plastic comes in half a dozen varieties that have to be segregated if they are to be broken up successfully and made into something else. If you look carefully at a plastic container, you see a triangle with a number from one to seven stamped in it. These resin identification codes proclaim the chemical makeup of the object. Soft drink bottles, for example, are number one, which is PET (polyethylene terephthalate).[73] When waste-pickers collect plastic, they improve their returns if they separate their collection into its various categories before selling it to intermediaries, who may send truckloads of crushed plastic long distances to more industrial-style reprocessing industries. A survey of plastic waste in Bengaluru in 2011 reckoned that 80 percent was "exported out of Bangalore" to Delhi, Mumbai, and Gujarat. The rest was dealt with by three hundred or four hundred "reprocessing units . . . operated as a micro enterprise, in an informal way."[74]

Such micro enterprises can be very micro indeed, and they flourish in any town or city large enough to generate quantities of plastic waste. Doron visited such businesses in Tirunelveli in Tamil Nadu and elsewhere (see Chapter 7). Jeffrey saw similar units at work in Kolkata. There, in rooms no bigger than a badminton court, plastic waste was sorted and chopped into pellets before being heated and transformed into sturdy black window brackets. Other forms of plastic waste were extruded

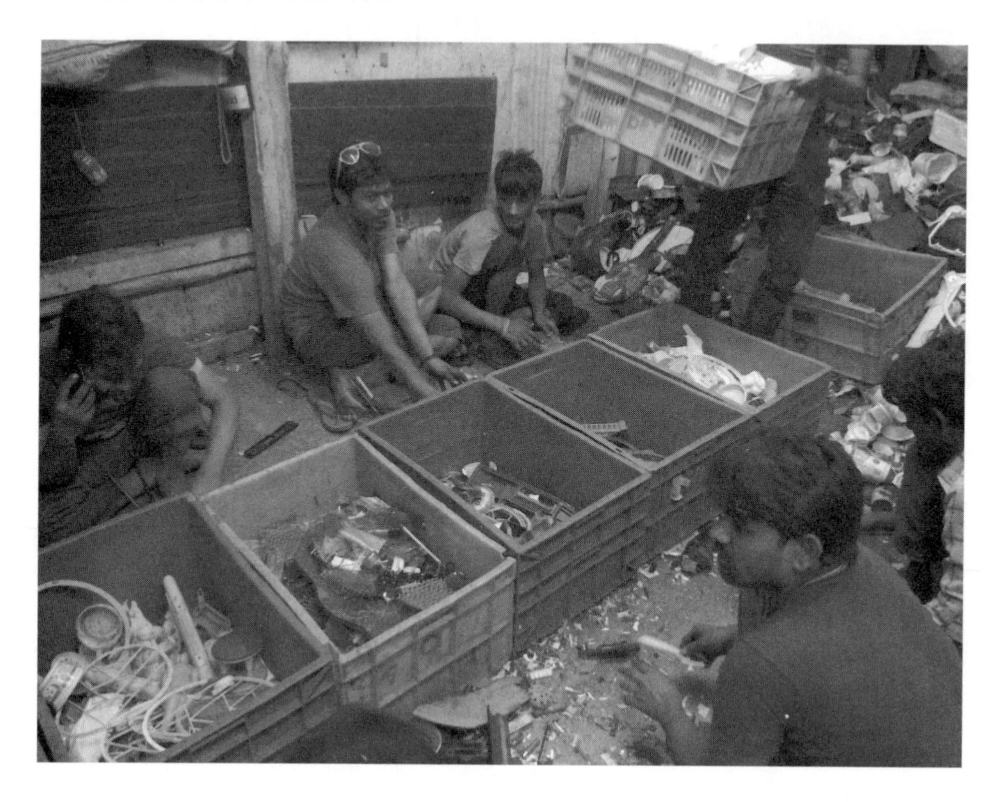

Fig. 4.8 **Sorting and separating plastic and metal waste in Dharavi, Mumbai.** Photo © Assa Doron, 2016.

into sheeting. The proprietors of these establishments do not welcome visitors, domestic or international; there are no factory tours. Such operations often exist outside regulations, and some steal their electricity, siphoning it from public supply lines.[75] Some units make only pellets, which they sell to manufacturers; others make pellets and manufacture basic products; others are simply buyers of pellets for the manufacturing of more elaborate items.[76] In a splendid essay, Vinay Gidwani describes Mundka, an area of eastern New Delhi that claimed to be "Asia's largest plastic recycling market" with five thousand businesses—"small and large, licit and illicit"—"devoted to finding an afterlife for Delhi's discarded plastics."[77]

All plastics are not equal. Different plastics when mixed together corrupt each other, and to reuse plastic effectively, it must be segregated. Therefore, at some point in the waste chain, plastics have to be separated, and this requires space and skill.[78] Waste-pickers often have neither, so additional links appear in the chain. A *kabaadi* who has a shop with a courtyard employs people to sort plastic. He knows where to sell these value-added products and closely follows the fluctuating prices for different kinds of waste.

Paper, Glass, Cloth, and the World

Paper was once a *kabaadi*'s staple. Householders hoarded their newspapers and relished a regular haggle with the *kabaadi* over the price per kilogram that he was willing to pay. Wastepaper often ended up in shops and roadside stalls as packaging. In Mumbai, old copies of the *Times of India* were "considered the best wrap for fish that people bought at Crawford Market or Colaba," writes Kamla Mankekar, one of India's first women to be a full-time journalist.[79]

Consumption of paper increased steadily after economic liberalization began in 1991, but the ability to recycle paper did not keep pace. Cheap plastic competed with paper as a packaging material. The old *kabaadi* collected mostly newsprint and household paper, but much of the growth in consumption was from paper used in offices. By 2015, India was disposing of perhaps twelve million metric tons of paper a year, of which more than half was going to landfills. To fuel its paper mills and meet demand, India imported more than two million metric tons of finished paper and four million metric tons of wastepaper.[80]

For the poorest waste-pickers, paper has always been a challenge. It is heavy and hard to carry, and substantial quantities are needed to earn even small sums. You also need to know where to sell it. And when bundled paper is dumped in a landfill, it doesn't degrade. Air cannot get into tightly packed bundles, chemical breakdown doesn't happen, and the bundles sit in lumpy masses taking up space for decades.[81]

The price of paper, especially newsprint, fluctuates with global demand and supply. A metric ton of newsprint cost about $1,000 in the mid-1990s; it cost $500–$600 in 2016.[82] The potential for capturing much more of India's wastepaper is great, but the need for volume means it requires greater organization than waste-pickers and the traditional *kabaadi* can supply on their own. Big businesses, such as ITC, see opportunities, as we touch on in Chapter 7.

The contrast between the value of plastic and glass was underlined on a British website in 2016 that quoted a base price of £35 a metric ton for mixed plastic waste; but for mixed glass, the website indicated that there might be no buyers at all, and the very best a seller could expect was £35 a metric ton.[83] In her remarkable book *Behind the Beautiful Forevers*, Katherine Boo explains what fluctuating prices, resulting from the global financial crisis of 2007, meant for the waste collectors of Annawadi, a Mumbai slum: "A kilo of empty water bottles once worth twenty-five rupees was now worth ten, and a kilo of newspaper once worth five rupees was now worth two: This was how the global crisis was understood."[84]

Cloth and old clothes were another commodity that the *kabaadi* on a bicycle used to deal in. He sold them either to be cut up and used to patch and mend or to be ripped apart for their fiber. But in those days, clothing was never a staple of the *kabaadi*'s trade, partly because clothing was rarely thrown away. In the past thirty years, however, old clothes from the West have been a globally traded commodity, as Lucy Norris, an authority on these matters, has described in books and articles.[85] They come to India for two purposes: either to be ripped apart for the fiber and turned into cheap blankets and shawls, or to be sold in secondhand markets.[86] Neither of these activities produces the kind of waste that contributes to an unclean India. But the trade in old clothing illustrates, as Norris makes clear, "the complexity of the market as vertical hierarchies of dealers negotiate and expand the multiple spaces between legal and illegal commodity flows, and formal and informal economies."[87] Similar complexity prevails in all areas of recycling.[88]

In campaigns to raise global awareness of uncontrolled waste and wastefulness, plastic often features as a kind of nuclear weapon—an agent of mass destruction. The Great Pacific Garbage Patch afflicts and kills marine life across thousands of kilometers of the Pacific Ocean. Plastic microbeads in toothpastes and cosmetics pass into the environment and invade the bodies of living creatures. And trillions of runaway plastic bags are bemoaned as an eyesore and condemned as a hazard.[89]

Plastic is not inherently evil. Its light weight and adaptability have made it an essential aspect of everyday life, and discarded plastic can be used for other purposes. In a few respects, some of India's waste handlers, and their buyers farther up the waste chain, provide examples of what can be done on a small scale.

Plastic changed ragpicking in India once it arrived in a major way in the 1990s. Small-scale manufacturing units that had once worked with metal turned to remaking plastic, and others followed. Waste-pickers found a new source of income in the thrown-away plastic that became a big part of the waste stream. The economies of recycling that grew up around plastic now provide income for millions of waste workers. Those economies are characterized by unequal social relations, poor legal frameworks, and oppressive work arrangements. And they do not come close to capturing all the plastic India discards every day. But they suggest what might be done if workers were organized, collection was thorough, methods were regulated, and small-scale inventiveness continued to be rewarded. ("Recycling gets done not because it is a good thing; it gets done if it is a profitable thing," the authors of *Rubbish!* caution).[90] In short, could the inventiveness and abundance of labor be combined in ways that were thorough and profitable yet at the same time protected the environment and workers' lives?

Recipes

Waste was once treated as part of the commons, a resource from which families could eke out livings. The British began to change this perception as early as 1919 when the Madras (now Chennai) City Municipal Corporation Act of 1919 declared that "all things deposited in depots or place[s] provided or appointed . . . shall be the property of the corporation."[91] That meant that informal waste-pickers were breaking the law, although the law was impossible to enforce. However, in the post-1991 era of market reforms, waste becomes a resource for capitalist enterprise to exploit. This process, write Vinay Gidwani and Amita Baviskar "is inevitably accompanied by displacement and deprivation for populations that were sustained by these commons."[92]

Thrown-away things have value if skillfully handled. Food waste, which constitutes at least half of what most Indian households discard, can decompose and go back into the land as compost. So too can the flowers and offerings made at temples every day. Composting is sometimes referred to as managed rotting, in which bad smells, flies, mosquitoes, and vermin are excluded and leachate is contained and enabled to evaporate. Regular management in well-built facilities accelerates these processes, and the methane created by decomposition can be burned to make electric power and mitigate production of carbon. However, if plant and animal matter rots randomly, it is a menace, a magnet for flies that transmit bacteria and potentially creating a breeding space for mosquitoes that carry dengue and malaria. Random rotting clogs drains and brings vermin and stray dogs, which partly explains India's estimated twenty thousand deaths from rabies each year, one-third of such deaths worldwide.[93] Many of these deaths are of children who were foraging around rubbish piles.[94]

India's waste is valuable, even if only fractions of it are currently exploited. Glass containers can be washed and reused, and broken glass has the potential to be remade into new glass. Plastics can be made into other plastic or put into tarmac to improve road surfaces. At worst, they can be burned to generate heat and power in incinerators designed to control the resulting toxic gases. Paper can have multiple lives. But waste must be properly handled and tamed; all the processes entail risks.

India's immense population and its potential for huge increases in waste of all kinds give an urgency to limiting the production of waste and dealing effectively with the things that are ejected. India is sometimes seen as a place where waste is thoroughly scavenged for items of value, but this is not so. Although millions of people derive income from waste, the majority are unorganized, expendable, and almost powerless—ripe for exploitation. Their goal is to survive, not to clean a city thoroughly, organize systematic collections, or recycle its waste.

The challenge lies in achieving comprehensive systems that include most of the people who draw some small income from collecting and selling waste. For the next generation at least, a large population and cheap labor can be an advantage. The arduous collecting and segregating, which maximize the uses of waste, can be tackled in ways that are impossible elsewhere. But to create such systems requires regulation, transparency, and an improvement in the conditions and the dignity of the people who deal with waste. In return for thoroughness, regularity, and discipline, there have to be material and social rewards, a concern we return to in Chapter 7.

Activists, officials, and professionals who work to improve public sanitation understand these needs.[95] Localities scattered around the country have developed working systems that have lessons for everyone, and the updated 2016 Solid Waste Management Rules appear to recognize the informal sector's role in waste management.[96] Human energy and perseverance are essential, whether those qualities come from officials, community groups, or activists. Such people understand the localities where they work, and they tell a persuasive story about the perils and opportunities presented by waste to those who make it and those who deal with it. Such systems provide safe spaces where waste can be sorted and segregated to enable materials to begin the journey to another incarnation. Fair and reliable payments are made to the people who collect, sort, and process the waste, and they experience enhanced dignity and well-being, often in the form of bank accounts, identity cards, uniforms, technical skills, and suitable equipment. Penalties are enforced against people who don't abide by the rules. One can see examples of such practices in Chennai, Pune, Bengaluru, towns in Andhra Pradesh, and elsewhere.

But any change in the makeshift methods by which value is extracted from thrown-away things will affect some of the links in the long, disjointed chain. If valuable incentives are provided for effective collection and processing of recyclable materials, larger financial interests will be increasingly attracted to the recycling business. When large-scale management practices operate over wider geographical areas, there are pressures to reduce wages. Efficiency means profit for investors; investors will also demand to own any item of value. When practices begin to enhance the rewards for an activity, more influential people and organizations may take over. In Uttar Pradesh, when the wages of Dalit waste collectors employed by local governments improved, higher-status people took over the jobs and salaries, employed Dalits for lower wages to do the work, and pocketed the difference.[97]

The principles of effective recycling are understood. But integrating effective localized practices into citywide systems for huge populations presents major difficulties. And recycling processes need to limit the damage they may do to a struggling environment. Technologies offer some possibilities, as we try to show in the next chapter, but technologies must be selected and developed with keen appreciation of the localities in which they are deployed.

5

TECHNOLOGY AND IMPERFECTION

TECHNOLOGY IS ONE OF THE KEYS to improving public sanitation, but it must be appropriate and well understood. Technology with a capital *T* can be a temptation and a trap. In 2012, the Municipal Corporation of Thiruvananthapuram, the capital of Kerala, was under immense pressure to do something about mounting volumes of garbage. Once a coconut-canopied, slow-paced tropical town, Thiruvananthapuram's population quadrupled between 1971 and 2011—from 400,000 to 1.7 million. More important, during those forty years Kerala's people flooded to the Persian Gulf for work, came home relatively prosperous, and adopted a highly consumer-conscious lifestyle. Kerala, too, has always been densely packed—today, more than 800 people per square kilometer (2,080 per square mile). (The U.K. density is about 250; the Netherlands, 500.) Kerala has heavy monsoons, a dozen rivers flowing westward out of the hills into the Arabian Sea, and little room for dumps or landfills. To cope with its waste problems, the Municipal Corporation contracted with a company in Gujarat for a mobile incinerator.[1] It arrived early in November 2012 in the form of a green-painted, forty-two-meter (140-feet)-long body towed by a Tata truck. Expectations were high—and rapidly fell.

"Mobile Stupidity," declared Shibhu Nair, one of Kerala's most committed and knowledgeable advocates of small-scale waste management. He posted a video on YouTube showing the agonies of a technician trying to make the incinerator work.[2] The company contracted to provide the incinerator complained that the city authorities had not provided the diesel fuel needed to run it, had failed to collect the ash and wastewater the incinerator produced, and were not providing it a regular flow of waste. The company claimed it was owed for ten days' worth of diesel. The city authorities refused to pay for the incinerator until its design was modified, including increasing the height of its chimney.[3]

The green incinerator became a white elephant. A year later authorities in Kerala were going to court to force the company to repay Rs 1.5 crores ($160,000). The incinerator had operated for less than two weeks and was moved out of the city to languish in a suburb in July 2013. "The incinerator did not function properly," a municipal official said, "mainly due to the technical faults, besides consuming a huge quantity of fuel. The operators went back to Gujarat after 15 days and they did not return. . . . We could not operate it without expert operators."[4] In following years, the incinerator moved north up the Kerala coast, passed on to other local governments with waste problems. It was at the center of a dispute in the Kochi Municipal Corporation in 2016. A Kochi official said the incinerator was "a failure and the pollution caused by it was found to be high."[5] In Thiruvananthapuram, as management of waste deteriorated, residents often fell back on old-fashioned methods of incineration: they burned waste at the side of the road.

A second vignette comes from north India. On May 1, 2016, Prime Minister Narendra Modi launched several solar-powered boats on the Ganga at Varanasi. It was a media event, and the boats were described as a noise-free, clean alternative to the diesel-engine boats commonly used on the river. The boatmen, who had invested some of their own money in converting their boats into e-boats, soon complained that they were useless (*bekaar*). Of the dozen boats, only a handful now operate occasionally. One boatman maintained that the solar panels were not properly fixed to the boats, even during Modi's visit, and that Modi's boat was actually battery operated: the solar panels were cosmetic. "Solar panels are a problem," said a boatman, "they are dangerous, especially in small boats, because the river has wind and strong currents, and they can shake the boats." His cousin had bought an e-boat on a loan that he was still paying off, but it was hardly worth it. "It is very complicated to charge the batteries," a relative said, "because you need to take it to [distant] Ravindra

Puri for charging. There are no charging points near the river." The heavy batteries had to be carried a considerable distance to charge them, and even then they lasted only six hours. "It has not succeeded," concluded a boatman. "The currents and winds are too strong. It might have worked on a lake, but not on the Ganga."[6] A *Wall Street Journal* reporter similarly observed that boatmen opposed Modi's e-boat initiative on the grounds that "they are unsuitable for strong currents of the Ganges and will affect the livelihood of thousands of boatmen and their families." He quoted a community leader: "If the government really cares about the pollution in the river, then it should first stop the sewage and waste materials that are entering into the river."[7]

The point of focusing on the green incinerator of Thiruvananthapuram and the battery-powered boats of Varanasi is not to ridicule local authorities or innovative attempts to control pollution and waste. Rather, it is to highlight dilemmas. As the responsibilities of local governments increase, they search for rapid solutions to problems that foul the environment, anger voters, and grow every day. But quick fixes from outside seldom solve problems. Improvements in public sanitation and control of pollution require involvement of the people who create, experience, and have to deal with the problem.

Humans have buried, burned, or washed away unwanted materials since prehistoric times, but modern population densities and production capacities pose unprecedented problems. Although superior technologies are essential for the success of the Modi government's Swachh Bharat initiative, they must be accompanied by superior training and conditions for the low-status workers who operate them and widespread change in attitudes toward public sanitation. For officials responsible for achieving Swachh Bharat targets, there is a temptation to adopt uniform methods that appear to offer single, comprehensive answers to truly "wicked problems."[8]

Earth

Dumps are as old as human settlement. Even in the distant past, people found isolated places to discard unsavory and unwanted things. Urban life, however, makes it more difficult to find such spaces, and by the second half of the nineteenth century, rulers and officials of expanding cities in Europe and North America had to make arrangements to deal with the thrown-away things of their residents.[9]

Mumbai grew too rapidly in the 1860s. The American Civil War halted supplies of cotton to British mills, and Indian cotton, exported through Mumbai, was in high demand. With the arrival of the railway in the 1860s, street sweepings from the commercial southern end of Mumbai Island were taken by rail to be dumped on vacant ground at Kurla near today's airport. In 1875, British authorities decided to use these nightly collections to fill in swampland in the areas around Love Grove and Tardeo, today some of Mumbai's prime sites facing west to the Arabian Sea.[10] (See Map 1.1.) By the 1880s, more than 50 hectares (about 120 acres) had been reclaimed. The Bombay Municipal Corporation bought 320 hectares (800 acres) at Chimbur on the eastern side of the island in 1897 and began dumping there.[11] Mumbai's growing population drove dumping farther up the island to Deonar, where today's dump, said to be the largest in India, began in 1927. In the 1860s, Mumbai had a population of about 800,000; it had doubled to 1.2 million by 1932. In 2016, the greater Mumbai area held more than 18 million people and generated more than eight thousand metric tons of waste a day. The Deonar dump grew to cover 130 hectares (321 acres), rising nearly 50 meters (164 feet) above sea level and receiving scores of truckloads of garbage every day.

Independent India inherited these uncontrolled dumps in 1947, and little was done about most of them until the 1990s. The story of Chennai was not very different from Mumbai's. Most of Chennai's waste in 2015 went to overflowing dumps at Kodungaiyur in the north of the city and Perungudi in the south. Each site was said to receive more than two thousand metric tons of garbage a day.[12]

Amendments to India's constitution in 1993 were intended to enhance the importance of local governments. With that enhanced importance came inescapable responsibilities for public sanitation and for the unregulated dumps around every town and city. We come back to the dilemmas of local government in Chapter 6. As local governments struggle to meet the expectations of the Swachh Bharat program, they face decades of accumulated and compacted waste. Mumbai's Deonar, celebrating its ninetieth anniversary in 2017, has thousands of waste-pickers working its heights each week. In 2014, a wall around it attempted to control access, but breaks in the wall made it easy to find a way inside and to climb the heights.[13] Access became more difficult after Deonar gained international attention early in 2016 when its smoldering fires burned with greater intensity than usual and shrouded portions of the city in smoke and haze for weeks.

The "technology" of these uncontrolled dumps is based on hope rather than science. Originally, they were sited at a distance from settlements and began with the wistful belief that nature would take its course. Birds, animals, and very poor people might come to pick through it, and biodegradable materials would lapse back into nature. Everything else would be covered by new layers of waste, and eventually the whole thing might be enclosed and help reclaim swampy land. That was the Mumbai hope in the late nineteenth century. But dumps don't do that, as the University of Arizona's Garbage Project showed.[14] Dumps grow and regurgitate; toxic material buried long ago bubbles up to cause trouble years later.

Growing towns and cities reach a point where the production of waste each day exceeds the capacity of the dump to accommodate it, so what might have begun as a hole or a patch of swampy ground becomes a mound, then a hill, and eventually, as Deonar and Kolkata's Dhapa did, a small mountain.[15] Citizens' complaints about vermin, smells, and the fires from ignited methane gas that the bubbling cocktail produces force local governments to act.

Unregulated dumps violate the Solid Waste Management Rules of 2000 and 2016, which carry the authority of a directive of the Supreme Court. The 2016 rules state that "existing landfill sites . . . shall be improved in accordance of the specifications given in this Schedule." Schedule 3 runs to thirty-three paragraphs and 1,900 words of excellent direction on how to construct a "scientific land fill" and how to dismantle an existing dump. The 2016 rules contain detailed regulations for different categories of waste, including plastic, construction and demolition, medical, and hazardous waste.[16]

The technologies for renovating existing dumps and building scientific, or sanitary, landfills are well known and implemented in various parts of the world. Such landfills begin from the same principle as a dump: they are located at sites as remote as possible from habitations yet as close as possible to the sources from which waste comes. Sites are carefully prepared. They are excavated, surveyed, and divided into cells that are filled one by one. A cell is lined with a layer of hard clay over which is laid a blanket of tough plastic (HDPE) to contain the polluting liquids that leach out of suppurating material.[17] Pipes are installed to capture the leachate, which is poured back over the contents of the cell so that constant evaporation prevents leachate from escaping to contaminate groundwater. Additional piping draws off the methane gas that decomposition produces, and this methane is burned off, sometimes to create electricity. Filters capture toxic emissions from the burning. In the ideal type, the cell into which material is dumped is covered each night to minimize access to birds and rodents and annoyance to neighbors from odors and wind-blown rubbish.

Although the technology is straightforward, implementation is complex and costly, and maintenance requires unremitting, daily attention. And landfills require space, something that in India is in painfully short supply. To establish a new landfill requires painstaking discussion with people living nearby. Examples of failed waste-management projects, such as the site at Vilappilsala on the outskirts of Thiruvananthapuram, reinforce suspicion that proximity to waste will make nearby life unpleasant, degrading, and dangerous. The cost of preparing a sanitary landfill in the United States was calculated in 2005 at roughly $1.5 million a hectare. In India, more recently, estimates suggest that building a sanitary landfill of unspecified size needs about Rs 15 crores ($3 million).[18] Where such landfills have been created, the contract for ownership, operation, and maintenance is a complicated document usually negotiated between a local government and a private corporation but with scrutiny by the state government, nongovernmental organizations, unions of sanitation workers, and wary citizens.

In 2014, India had ninety-four sites that aspired to be sanitary landfills, according to survey answers received by the Central Pollution Control Board.[19] The best of these sites resembled the model that sanitation specialists expect to see. The site at Jawahar Nagar, operated by Ramky Enviro Engineers on the outskirts of Hyderabad, for example, in 2015 had the required attributes—clay bedding, plastic liner, leachate catchment, methane capture, and an attached composting facility. The center also aimed to mine a preexisting dump and render it benign before the whole site was closed when it reached capacity, estimated to be 2035. But the Jawahar Nagar site, which on a good day could be presented as a model sanitary landfill, was bitterly criticized by nearby residents. "The filthy tale of Jawahar Nagar," the *Times of India* headlined a story in September 2015, and nine months later, there were accusations that leachate at the site was out of control.[20]

The difficulty of running an effective sanitary landfill underlines the need to reduce centralization and minimize reliance on burying waste, even scientifically. A principle of the Solid Waste Management Rules is that waste is segregated at the source. The 2016 version of the rules dictates that "every waste generator shall . . . segregate and store the waste generated by them in three separate streams namely bio-degradable, non bio-degradable and domestic hazardous wastes."[21] As household and commercial waste is collected, it should be sorted into various categories for recycling and composting, and this should be done as close to the place of origin as possible. Carrying waste long distances to central landfills burns diesel, costs money, pollutes the air, and angers citizens. The requirement to maintain separate streams of waste to enable recycling is repeated continually throughout the rules of 2000 and their new incarnation in 2016.

Transporting waste is expensive. When Mumbai was becoming a great city in the 1860s, it transported 110,000 metric tons of waste a year to its dump at Kurla and burned nearly 7,000 metric tons in small local fires. The cost was more than Rs 100,000 a year, which the authorities were keen to reduce, and for a time in the 1890s, they considered more local burning. That was rejected because of the annoyance it caused to surrounding neighborhoods, and by 1899, the Mumbai railway system was carrying waste each night from the built-up southern end of the island to the dump at Chembur.[22] The railways still carried waste in 2016, and nightly trains carried the waste of the city's railway stations to be dumped outside the city.[23]

Local authorities make similar calculations about transport costs today. It takes seventy journeys by fifteen-metric-ton trucks to carry one thousand metric tons of waste to a sanitary landfill. If the round trip is

50 kilometers (31 miles; landfills have to be some distance out of town), that's 3,500 kilometers (2,175 miles) a day, or fifteen thousand liters (3,963 gallons) of diesel. That means air pollution, wear and tear on vehicles and roadbeds, traffic congestion, and aggrieved local residents. Rail overcomes some of these problems, but railways seldom run to sanitary landfills.

Small-scale technologies offer cleaner, cheaper ways of dealing with a large proportion of domestic and commercial waste. Their disadvantage lies in their requirements for space, cooperation, relentless application, and systematic maintenance. The technologies themselves are simple. The people who do door-to-door collection need protective clothing and vehicles and equipment suitable to the areas where they work. In parts of Andhra Pradesh, Telangana, and Karnataka, towns use a rugged hand-pulled cart, designed and built locally and rolling on three polyurethane wheels, the same type used for roller blades. The carts have room for four sixty-liter (sixteen-gallon) bins for separating into biodegradable, paper, plastic, and miscellaneous waste.[24] The carts cope with uneven surfaces, maneuver in narrow lanes, and can turn tight corners. There is little to break, and repairs can be done locally and quickly. Cycle rickshaw frames have often been adapted for such work elsewhere, but the bicycle frame is more fragile, the vehicle is imperfectly balanced, and pneumatic tires puncture.

A biodigesting plant to turn wet waste into electricity-generating gas and compost uses well-known technology and requires relatively little space. The principles of biomethanation go back to their first application at the Matunga Leper Asylum in Mumbai in the late 1890s, developed by the engineer C. C. James (Chapters 1 and 7). The technology has been popular in parts of rural India for animal waste since the 1970s under the name of "gobar gas"—gas made from cow dung. A unit that digests three metric tons of wet waste a day can fit into the area of a couple of shops and produce 265 kilowatt hours of electricity a day, enough to power more than three hundred 100-watt bulbs for eight hours, a significant contribution to neighborhood street lighting or household uses.[25] Vegetable waste from markets and households, carefully segregated, is brought to the location and chewed up by machine into pulp and fed into a pit where it is stirred and agitated to accelerate its gas making. The gas fires a turbine that powers a generator that makes electricity. As with so many things concerning waste, there is a chain, and all the links need to be in working order. One of the problems in crowded cities is finding space for such plants and convincing neighbors that their lives are not going to be made miserable by refuse, odor, and disease. In the suburb of Yeshwanthpur in Bengaluru in 2015, such a plant operated opposite an Ayyappa temple with what was said to be relatively goodwill on both sides.[26]

Well-designed spaces are necessary to sort and organize recyclable waste. This does not involve high technology, but good design and amenities make such spaces more attractive, effective, and likely to be used. Small quantities of recyclables, retrieved by many collectors, need to be assembled into larger volumes to make it worthwhile to transport them to plastic factories, paper mills or other processing sites. As Bengaluru wrestled with multiple waste problems in 2015, it attempted to set up local centers—a large purpose-built shed with a concrete floor, showers, scales to weigh goods, and the opportunity for waste-collectors to be paid in cash, with rates of payment posted regularly and based on market prices. Such arrangements minimized the need to cart waste to distant landfills and improved the chances of regular daily cleanups because waste collectors got paid regularly and predictably and had a safe shelter with running water to deal with their collections.

The procedures for effective waste-management practices are well known, and the Solid Waste Management Rules require all local governments to "arrange for door to door collection of segregated solid waste from all households including slums and informal settlements, commercial, institutional and other non residential premises."[27] The rules intend to guarantee local sorting and processing of waste, and they insist that local governments establish places where segregated waste can be organized and passed onto dealers. The technology is simple; but the governmental and human sides of these equations are difficult, as we explore in Chapters 6 and 7. Bengaluru, for example, was said to have an influential lobby of transport contractors who had little interest in reducing the five hundred trucks required daily to cart garbage to dumps. The municipality paid Rs 400 crores a year (about $64 million) to transport the waste.[28]

In small towns, a study suggests, solid waste management may largely depend on the energies and interests of elected officials. Marginalized communities are far less likely to receive government-sponsored waste removal services.[29]

A sanitary landfill is one of the most expensive and technically sophisticated methods of dealing with waste. It assumes that many hectares of land are set aside and that hundreds of truck journeys will travel thousands of kilometers and burn thousands of liters of diesel each week. A sanitary landfill should be a place of last resort, especially in India, where more than half of household and commercial waste is biodegradable. Such waste can be cooked and composted, used to make electric power and turned into fertilizer. It does not need to go to a centralized landfill. Landfills, however, have attractions because they seem to provide a complete fix to a complex problem. "Someone" takes waste far away from households and businesses, carries it to an unseen place, and makes it the problem of other people. If a private company has been contracted to run the landfill, it will have negotiated an attractive agreement with governments that will probably reward it for accepting large, constant flows of waste through its weighbridges. The incentives to do things locally will be missing. Big cities probably need sanitary landfills, but the aim should be to make them last for as many years as possible by minimizing what goes into them.

Fire

Fire is a time-honored way of getting rid of waste, as the charred bones in prehistoric middens indicate. As towns and cities grew in Europe and North America in the nineteenth century, the industrial expansion that produced greater quantities of waste also generated industrial-style solutions. Nottingham in England introduced "the first systematic cremation of refuse at the municipal level" in 1874, and "large-scale implementation of incinerating devices" spread throughout Europe and the United States thereafter.[30] Mumbai toyed with local incinerators in the 1890s, but officials decided it was cheaper and less offensive to transport waste to landfills.[31] In the United States, the story of burning waste has played out in "three major waves." Since the 1990s, India has experienced similar trends and discoveries.[32]

In the United States, European-style incinerators arrived in the first wave in the 1880s, but by 1910, these had lost their attraction because American waste, like Indian waste today, was often too wet to burn effectively. Unlike India today, many U.S. towns and cities once had vast empty spaces where waste could be dumped. The second period of incineration in the United States, according to Edward J. Walsh and Rex Warland, authors of *Don't Burn It Here,* ran from the 1930s to the 1960s and had more effective incinerators and growing volumes of waste. By 1967, the environmental movement had provoked legislation that forced these second-generation incinerators to install scrubbers, pollution control devices, that controlled smoke and toxic gases. These add-on devices were "expensive enough to put most of the second wave of incinerators out of operation."[33] The third wave features expensive high-combustion furnaces that generate modest amounts of electricity, reduce the volume of waste by 90 percent, and leave an ash suitable for building purposes. They are designed, say their advocates, to ensure that poisonous gases are not released into the air. They provide a key method of waste management in Japan, Singapore, Germany, the Netherlands, and the Nordic countries. Europe has more than 400 such plants. Since the mid-1970s, more than 230 Mitsubishi-Martin incinerators have been installed in Japan, China, South Korea, and Singapore.[34]

In India, the first plant of this type opened at Okhla in the South Delhi Municipal Corporation at the end of 2011. Built and operated by a company of the Jindal group, one of India's largest conglomerates, the Timarpur-Okhla plant was a public-private partnership with the Delhi government.[35] Dogged by controversy, the plant provided a focus for questions about high-combustion incineration and its suitability for India. Construction began in 2010, and the plant was accepting garbage and generating electric power by early 2012. In 2016, it was taking 1,300 metric tons of waste a day to generate sixteen megawatts of electricity. One megawatt can power more than five hundred American homes for a day; Okhla's sixteen megawatts could provide power to perhaps eight thousand Delhi households.[36]

The National Capital Territory of Delhi is an administrative and political unit of India's federation, but its elected government has fewer powers than a full-fledged state, an aspect we discuss in Chapter 6. The National Capital Territory occupies a confined space of about 1,500 square kilometers (570 square miles), containing a fast-growing population of about eighteen million. There are no distant places in the territory to build new sanitary landfills, and every scrap of ground within the National Capital Territory's boundaries is jealously held. Even a hectare for a small recycling, composting, and biomethanation station is hard to find. Incineration of waste therefore looks attractive. But the Okhla plant and two comparable operations at Ghazipur in the east and Narela-Bawana in the north of Delhi were troubled, troublesome, and constantly criticized.[37] A landslide at the Ghazipur site in August 2017 killed two men.[38]

High-combustion incineration plants attract politicians and policy makers because they appear to provide a single solution to a wicked problem. An efficient plant reduces the volume of waste by up to 90 percent, which means a landfill, although still necessary, has a much longer life. High-combustion incinerators can produce heat and electricity, although in many countries these are subsidiary benefits, because the reduction in the volume of waste may be the most important aspect. High-combustion incineration, as described by advocates and manufacturers, offers desperate governments a seemingly magical solution to a compounding nightmare: growing volumes of waste and shrinking areas of land to accommodate it. A well-run plant will reduce the volume, leave a useful ash, and provide significant amounts of heat and electricity. This recipe is followed elsewhere in the world.

But high-combustion incineration has drawbacks and fierce critics. In *The Story of Stuff,* Annie Leonard, a longtime worker with the environmental group Greenpeace and the Global Alliance for Incineration Alternatives, offers a ten-point critique of incineration, which she believes is irrefutable.[39] Many developed countries, however, have built high-combustion incinerators, because the advantages seem to outweigh the deficiencies and dangers. But high-combustion incineration is expensive. A new plant near the prosperous city of Toronto, Canada, built to deal with only 400 metric tons of waste a day, cost US$215 million when completed in 2016.[40] Delhi and Mumbai each collect more than 8,000 metric tons of waste a day. The first plant along these lines in Australia was budgeted to cost US$285 million and would handle 1,100 metric tons of waste a day for the southern suburbs of the city of Perth.[41] The large plant at Tuas South in Singapore can handle 3,000 metric tons of waste a day and cost more than US$600 million when it was opened in 2000.[42]

A second limitation lies in the conditions such plants require. They need steady supplies of dry, high-calorie waste. Ideally, an incinerator burns twenty-four hours a day. If an incinerator shuts down, it needs external energy to restart it and heat it up for action. Costs of incineration rise in times of heavy rain because waste needs to be dried before burning. Any time an incinerator gets wet waste, fuel must be burned to dry the waste before it can be incinerated. Maintenance of incinerators has to be consistent, and modern incinerators must be shut down for maintenance every eight thousand hours, or about once a year. Multiple incinerators are necessary to keep a plant running constantly. In short, high-combustion incinerators need constant, close supervision.

High combustion is essential to minimize harm to environment and health. Highly toxic substances known collectively as dioxins are formed when materials containing atoms of carbon and chlorine are burned. Thus, PVC (polyvinyl chloride) plastic, benign in itself and widely used in industry (e.g., PVC pipes are used in plumbing), produces dioxins when burned under uncontrolled conditions. Tobacco smoke, smoke from forest fires, and smoke from peat bogs also release dioxins into the atmosphere.

Burning waste at high temperatures, above 850°C (1,500°F), reduces formation of dioxins. But there is a catch: after the materials are splintered into their constituent atoms and captured as their distinctive elements—for example, carbon and chlorine—unless the combustion gases are cooled rapidly, carbon and chlorine recombine to form dioxins. (Think of making jelly: if you don't pour the mix into molds when it's hot, it takes the shape of the bowl in which it was made.) Special equipment minimizes the reforming of dioxin molecules (but it is never entirely prevented) and mops up other chemical fragments resulting from combustion. In countries like Japan, Singapore, the

Netherlands, the Nordic countries, and Germany, the latest generation of incinerators appear to emit only tiny amounts of dioxins, especially when compared with emissions from forest fires or illicit burning.[43] Nevertheless, a number of environmental groups oppose incineration of any kind, because of atmospheric pollution and the belief that incineration discourages frugality and recycling.[44]

Although high-combustion incineration is frequently described as a waste-to-energy process that produces electricity, the amount of power generated is often secondary to the reduction in the volume of waste that goes to landfill. In Singapore, the large Tuas South plant produces sixty-five megawatts of electricity, 20 percent of which is used to run the plant itself; the remainder is sold to the Singapore electricity system.[45] That amount covers the needs of less than 3 percent of Singapore's domestic households and represents only a small contribution to its overall electricity needs.

Costs and rigorous technical requirements make complete-combustion incinerators unlikely to work effectively in India except under very special conditions. The expense of construction means that authorities will look for cheaper versions of the technology.[46] One of the criticisms of the Timarpur-Okhla plant in Delhi, which in 2016 was the only functioning example in India, was that it was a cheap and unsatisfactory Chinese design. India's underpowered local governments have difficulty raising enough money to buy the best equipment. If the expensive units were built, waste would have to come from far and wide to keep the furnaces burning and justify the expense. This puts hundreds of diesel-burning trucks on the road. A unit that deals with three thousand metric tons a day, such as the one at Tuas South in Singapore, adds up to three hundred daily journeys by ten-metric-ton trucks.[47]

Manufacturers are eager to sell cheaper forms of incinerators to hard-pressed and somewhat credulous local governments, which lack specialized staff and research capacity. The depressing experience of Thiruvananthapuram's mobile incinerator was not an isolated example. Local government is the least glamourous of administrative services, and employment in public sanitation is the ugliest duckling among ugly ducklings. Local governments have responsibilities that often exceed their capacities. Elected councillors and officials are desperate to solve their waste problems, satisfy disgruntled voters, and meet the requirements of the Solid Waste Management Rules of 2016.

If things go wrong with incineration plants, their size means the consequences are widespread. In cities like Delhi (with its tightly confining borders) and Mumbai (with its island limitations), there may be a place for a Swedish- or Singapore-style plant. Space is scarce, landfills overflow, and the daily volume of waste grows. But even in such circumstances, the costs, the low calorific value of the waste, the need for relentless maintenance, and the difficulties of directing hundreds of trucks to a single location are great. Bringing waste collectors and waste makers into effective cooperation to minimize waste and treat most of it close to home offers more beneficial possibilities for making India cleaner; but the quick-fix efficiency of mechanized mass destruction seems easier and more tempting than achieving such cooperation.

Water

Residents of Thiruvananthapuram, with whose travails this chapter began, have often used water, the third of the elemental resting places for waste, after earth and fire, to dispose of unwanted objects. Kerala has backwaters, rivers, the ocean, and a heavy monsoon, all of which were enough to carry away unwanted things in former times. But volume has outstripped capacity. After a waste-clogged canal near the center of the city was cleared over several days, "within a month the canal was partly blocked [again] because of the waste being dumped into it," a municipal councillor lamented.[48] Water bodies throughout the country are one of the first places citizens turn to when they have things to throw away and nowhere else to throw them. (See Map 3.1.) This is especially true of things that can be poured or flushed—anything liquid, and particularly urine and feces.

Water pollution is acutely harmful because clean water is a daily essential for every human being, and clean water is scarce. No Indian summer has passed for sixty years without reports of water scarcity. Dirty water spreads disease. But the sewage treatment plants of India's towns and cities treat less than 30 percent of the sewage the cities generate, and the treated water is usually released into polluted water bodies where it simply dilutes the mixture.[49] A leading minister in Narendra Modi's government declared in 2014 that "almost 70 percent of all [sewage treatment plants] in India are either not working or closed, because the cost of running these plants is high."[50] Most wastewater from rain, households, and industries flows untreated into lakes, rivers, and the sea.

The prospect of providing water-driven sewerage and treatment plants for India's four thousand steadily expanding urban areas is remote. The piped, underground, water-hungry sewerage built in Europe and North America a hundred years ago pose immense construction problems. Digging and pipe laying disrupt towns and cities. Pipes and drains must be laid across jealously guarded municipal boundaries and must empty into treatment plants. Many sanitation systems may now connect toilets to sewers, but the sewers empty directly into water bodies, not into treatment plants. (In this, Indian cities are not alone. Victoria, British Columbia, one of Canada's most genteel cities, has sent its sewage directly into the Strait of Juan de Fuca, to the annoyance of its U.S. neighbors on the other side of the strait, for more than a hundred years.)[51]

Sewage treatment plants require large tracts of land, big investment, community acquiescence, reliable power, and constant maintenance. In cities like Mumbai, aging sewers often mix their contents with drains that carry storm water, and the resulting concoction flows directly into tanks, rivers, or the sea. A Mumbai engineer described problems in 2016:

> We cannot put sewage pipes in the slum areas, with over 39 lakh population [3.9 million]. This is because they are located on the hills or near water bodies. It's also politically difficult; you cannot just raze the slums, and even if you try to put pipes it will be a zig-zag system, which makes it impossible to lay down fifteen-inch pipes for connections. This why about 40 percent of Mumbai is not connected to sewage line[s], but we cannot do it—it is a hell of a job![52]

The same engineer pointed out that "harvesting of water should be [a] higher priority [than sewage systems] in a state like Maharashtra, and here in the city we hardly recycle 4 percent of the water from the [treatment plants]."[53] Technology, imagination, and cultural insight can provide better ways to husband water and tame human waste.

The principles of capturing wastewater have not changed since the great sewer-building projects of Europe in the mid-nineteenth century.[54] In the old coastal cities, like Mumbai and Kolkata, where a few localities were sewered more than a hundred years ago, the ground beneath the streets is a snarl of pipes: sewer lines connected to toilets; stormwater drains collecting rainfall; a water system carrying drinking water; and more recently, cables for telecommunication.[55] Broken pipes, heavy monsoons, and industrial discharges sometimes cause the contents of sewage pipes to infiltrate water pipes, producing a noxious stew that may be served up as tap water.[56] In Varanasi, men who go into the sewers to clear blockages said that there was no accurate map of the city's underground pipes.[57] This failing made the work of sewer divers invaluable because they had the only verifiable knowledge of what lay underground.

For the past hundred years, the most common way for cities of Europe and North America to treat domestic sewage has been to channel it through a dedicated system of pipes to a sewage treatment plant where solid objects are screened out.[58] The "mixed liquor"—in the language of sanitary engineers—that arrives at the plant combines with oxygen-loving bacteria in tanks up to sixty meters (sixty-six yards) in diameter. The bacteria cause the tiny particles (think, fecal material) suspended in the sewage to coagulate and solidify. They fall to the bottom of a settling tank and eventually become fertilizer for agriculture. A small quantity of this oxygen-rich material—activated sludge—is injected into new sewage to keep the process going. The water at the top of the settling tanks may undergo processing to purify it further; but the initial treatment makes the water sufficiently harmless for agriculture or release into water bodies. In Singapore, NEWater, the brand name for one of the products of further processing, is sold as bottled drinking water.[59]

Singapore-style technology, however, is costly and complex, and sewage treatment plants operate effectively only if a number of conditions are satisfied. The World Bank summed up the problems: "[A plant is] expensive . . . , requires a constant energy supply, . . . trained operators . . . , [and] spare parts and chemicals. The track record . . . in the developing world is very poor, and few operate as designed or intended."[60] Surat in Gujarat illustrates the limitations, even for a relatively effective city. Surat recovered from the plague panic of 1994 to become, as we have seen, one of India's cleanest cities. It maintained its reputation and won an award in 2016 for having the country's "cleanest railway station."[61] In 2013 it had about 1,500 kilometers (932 miles) of sewers, which covered three-quarters of the city's area and 90 percent of its population. It had nine sewage treatment plants capable of handling daily more than 700 million liters (185 million gallons), the capacity of about three hundred Olympic swimming pools. The system was not total, however, and some sewage still flowed into the River Tapi. The plants took up space and cost money. The one at Bamroli near the airport in the southwest of the city covered more than ten hectares and cost Rs 290 million to build (Rs 29 crores, or about $5 million).[62]

Bengaluru in south India encountered greater difficulty than Surat, even though it was one of the country's most prosperous cities. In 2011, it had about 3,600 kilometers (2,237 miles) of underground sewerage serving a population of close to ten million people. It had fourteen treatment plants scattered around the city with a theoretical capacity to treat more than 80 percent of estimated daily sewage. But the plants were receiving about half their capacity because less than a third of the city's daily sewage was estimated to reach a plant. The city needed another 4,000 kilometers (2,485 miles) of pipeline to link up all its sewers to treatment plants.[63]

Sewage, wastewater, and treatment plants are inextricably connected to a town's water bodies, whether they are ponds, lakes, rivers, or the ocean. A report to the national Planning Commission in 2011 summed up:

> Today no city values its local water bodies as the function of its water supply—instead, these water bodies are seen as lucrative options for land—the hole in the ground is first filled with garbage and then taken over as real estate for housing and other developments. The catchment is encroached—by the poor, who are thrown out of the city and then by the rich who need it for everything from housing to airports. The essential role of water

> bodies as sources of local water supply and even potential spaces for sewage water treatment is never considered.[64]

New technologies that are thrifty with water, sensitive to cultural prejudice, and technically simple are needed to deal with human waste both in towns and in the countryside.

For rural areas, there are plenty of models for self-composting toilets, but their acceptance has been reluctant and patchy. Such toilets too often fall into the condition that Vinay Srivastava described when he wrote of his family's latrine in old Delhi in the 1960s: "extremely small, just enough to accommodate one person, dingy, almost like a dungeon, and poorly-lit and ventilated, without any facility of water inside."[65] It is misguided to think that a dingy outhouse is going to attract users. Such buildings were not popular when they were common in Australia and North America. Susan Chaplin, a scholar of public sanitation in India, grew up on a farm in the Australian countryside. She recalled that the outside toilet was a destination to avoid: "The danger was the hole, brown snakes and red-backs [poisonous spiders]. I tended to favour OD [open defecation] under the peppercorn trees with a shovel at hand [for burial]."[66] Research in three Tamil Nadu villages found that all castes, including Dalits, preferred open defecation and rejected the two toilet designs that officials and nongovernmental organizations had tried to introduce. These were viewed as "culturally inappropriate, unmanageable, rudimentary in design and . . . unusable." The chief defect was that the toilets required cleaning and maintenance; open defecation needed none. None of the people in the villages believed—or knew—that the random dispersal of feces transmitted disease.[67]

Can the internal design, even of rural toilets, be transformed so that they are easy to use and keep clean? Such an ideal toilet has not yet been invented. It will be achieved through clever design and suitable materials; it will be cheap, durable, attractive, and rapidly and easily cleaned; it will stand alone, not requiring sewers and treatment plants; and it will handle human waste in culturally acceptable ways and be easy to maintain. None of the current options fulfill all those conditions.

The favored design in India for rural toilets—the design being used for thousands of toilets built under the Swachh Bharat program—has two pits about 2 meters (6.5 feet) deep and 1.5 meters (5 feet) in diameter. A Y-shaped joint connects them to the toilet itself. Lined with bricks or masonry, the pits are spaced about 2 meters apart. Urine and feces flow into one pit until the pit is full. The pit is capped, the contents are left to break down into compost, and excrement is diverted into the second pit. After about two years (for a family of, say, ten people), when the second pit is nearly full, the matured first pit is emptied and its rich manure, now pathogen-free, spread on grateful fields.

Organizations such as Sulabh International, India's toilet champion for nearly fifty years, have built hundreds of thousands of two-pit toilets.[68] In some conditions, they work effectively, but they need land to build them on and skill and care to build them properly. The pits need to be dug deep and carefully lined. And who's to do the emptying? It is hard, cumbersome work, and it disrupts and dirties the neighborhood of the toilet. The chances are slim that a high-caste householder will do the job. Lower-caste laborers will be summoned, but today, they may not come.

Neater methods are needed to achieve the desired result of a clean, odor-free room for a toilet that is self-contained, not needing connection to a sewer, and producing a manure that is easily removed. The specifications are simple, but the task is delicate and complex.[69] "There are thousands of latrine designs," Rose George writes, but none of them quite works for rural or urban India.[70]

In dealing with tainted water and human waste, space is essential. In the countryside, structures intended as toilets become storehouses; in towns, small apartments skimp on plumbing to invest in the living areas. How do you provide satisfactory toilets in buildings thirty stories high and containing a hundred or more households? To be sure, Singapore and Hong Kong have built sewers, but these are city-states, and it takes four Singapores to equal the population of a Mumbai or Delhi.

The ideal toilet—urban and rural—would not need to be flushed with water (or would use only very little) or to be connected to sewerage. Feces would be contained within the toilet, not emit offensive odors, and would biodegrade into a container that could be sealed, easily removed once every week or two, and put out for collection as a separate category of waste. In urban areas, the collected bags could be processed at central locations, and the resulting manure put back into the land. In the countryside, this could be done by the household itself or at the village level. The manure would be benign and valuable.[71]

How achievable is such a picture? The Swachh Bharat campaign aims for 100 million toilets by 2019. But Sulabh International, which has installed 1.2 million toilets of various kinds since its founding in 1970, has yet to find a popular design that becomes an item in demand in virtually every household (like a mobile phone). Sarah Jewitt, an English geographer, surveyed toilet options worldwide in 2011 and found that biogas from animal and human waste was used in only 1.1 million Indian households (out of about 260 million), although the technology had been promoted since the 1970s. She summed up one of her key findings: "Improved sanitation systems have to 'capture the imagination of consumers as a life-improving benefit.'"[72] The fetish of the North American bathroom—a place of sparkling luxury and secure comfort—is a long way from capturing imaginations in India.[73]

Since the generation of electricity using biogas from human waste at the Matunga Leper Asylum in Mumbai in the 1890s—probably the first successful attempt—scientists, engineers, and ecologists have developed a number of options, but none yet fulfills all the requirements.[74] In Europe, the Terra Preta system promises to make fine compost, but the toilet requires daily attention, the separation of urine from feces, and feces need to be kept dry.[75] Such "ecosan" toilets were a flop in the three Tamil Nadu villages studied by Kathleen O'Reilly, Richa Dhanju, and Elizabeth Louis, partly because of the need to do *kai kaal*—thorough washing after defecation. "We can't do *kai kaal* inside ecosan [toilet areas]," a woman told the researchers, "so we don't use it for defecation."[76] The "ecosan" technique failed; the technology did not fit cultural practice.

Separation of urine from feces offers significant advantages. Urine has a high content of nitrogen and phosphorous, and one of Jewitt's sources contends that the 400 liters (106 gallons) of urine an adult excretes in a year "contains enough plant nutrients to grow 250 kg of grain."[77] Mixing urine and feces creates a much worse smell and limits the ways excreta can be turned into the most productive forms of fertilizer. But separating urine requires users to cooperate and systems that reliably remove both the urine and the feces, requirements that offer little hope for India's immense, complex, and urgent needs.[78]

The Clivus Multrum toilet, designed in Sweden in the late 1930s, is used around the world, particularly at tourist sites far from sewers and piped water. A concrete incline from the toilet slides excrement and urine into a composting chamber, with gravity separating the urine from feces. A fan circulates air through the chamber, and oxygen-loving bacteria decompose feces and create compost; urine becomes a nitrogen-rich, benign fertilizer. But the system needs space, fans, and maintenance.[79]

In South Africa in 2016, Ecosan, a company based in Pretoria, had installed more than nine thousand self-contained, molded-plastic toilet systems that appeared to meet some of the requirements of Indian conditions. In this design, feces fall into a chamber in which the contents are turned and aerated every time the toilet seat is raised. The movement exposes the excrement to outside air from a vent, and over the course of a few weeks the contents decompose into a benign manure that is guided into a collection bag. The bag is removed regularly, and a fresh bag installed, similar to changing the bag of a vacuum cleaner. The contents can be used by the household as fertilizer or collected and consolidated with bags from other households for agricultural use. The disadvantages are that a single unit is bulky (2.5 meters / 8 feet long, 65 centimeters / 2 feet wide), needs an external vent, costs about $750, and can accommodate the waste of only about eight people.[80] And in India, there will be resistance in many households to the idea of excrement remaining on the premises, even if there is no odor.

The first green corridor—a section of railway line on which toilets would no longer drop excrement onto the tracks—was announced in July 2016 on the line between Rameswaram, the pilgrimage site at the tip of India, and Manamadurai, the junction fifty kilometers (thirty-one miles) southeast of the great temple city of Madurai. An anaerobic biodigesting toilet, developed by Indian Railways and the Defence Research and Development Organization, was planned to be widely installed in railway coaches.[81] Indian Railways reported that 12,000 of its 55,000 passenger coaches had been fitted with biotoilets by January 2016. The target for 2015–2016 was to install 17,000 biotoilets, which would equip about 7,000 more coaches.[82] The 280 coaches operating on the Rameswaram line are now equipped only with biotoilets.

The chemistry of the biotoilet involves placing a cocktail of bacteria into the catchment tank under the toilets of each carriage. Sealed off from oxygen (anaerobic), the organisms reduce feces and urine to methane gas and harmless water. The water is released into drains or used for irrigation, and methane is expelled into the air. Although methane is a powerful greenhouse gas, the contribution of railway toilets to India's overall methane generation is thought to be minor. The bacteria in the catchment tanks need renewing only about once a year, and the major maintenance problem comes from passengers blocking the toilet with plastic bottles and every other imaginable object.[83]

Another promising contender in the slow race to create an acceptable stand-alone toilet system came from the Cranfield Water Science Institute at Cranfield University in the United Kingdom. Supported by the Bill and Melinda Gates Foundation's Reinvent the Toilet challenge begun in 2011, the Nano Membrane Toilet does not use water, separates urine and feces, burns the feces, creates electric power to run the toilet, and processes the urine through membranes to produce water for gardens or household chores. Unlike other contenders, the units are small and easy to move. The institute also envisages a business system in which small private contractors would make a living by regular servicing of the membrane and incineration features of the toilets. But, as with other entrants, there are disadvantages. The system needs servicing every three months, it can only cater to about ten people, the benign water has to be removed by the householder (in a reservoir rather like a clothes dryer without an external vent), and incineration suggests technical complications.[84]

Perhaps the most deceivingly simple sanitary solution is the Peepoo toilet, a concept developed by university researchers in Sweden in 2005 and having some success in Kenya. It appears to owe some of its inspiration to the notorious flying toilets—plastic bags into which people defecate and then throw away. In the Peepoo model, a biodegradable plastic bag, designed for easy use, contains a few grams of urea, which breaks down feces and urine. Once used, the bag is tied at the neck and buried. By the time the plastic breaks down, the contents have decomposed into a benign fertilizer. Bags cost about three cents, or two rupees. "Peepoo," the enterprise's website states, "offers a sanitation solution adapted to the needs of the user without endangering the environment."[85] It claimed some success in Pakistan and Bangladesh, but after brief experiments in India in 2010, it slipped from view.[86] Its deficiencies for Indian conditions are obvious. The cultural aversion to anything associated with excrement weighs heavily against the Peepoo model. How would one wash? Who would carry the bag to the fields? Where would it go to decompose if one lived in a one-room slum dwelling?

* * *

In June 2017, the website of the Swachh Bharat Abhiyan—the Clean India Mission—proclaimed the current count of household toilets built since October 2, 2014 to be 42,558,513—almost halfway to the goal of more than 100 million toilets and an India free of open defecation by 2019. The site also claimed 204,510 villages were now "open defecation free"—about a third of all villages in the country.[87] Experienced administrators will tell you that it is possible to achieve toilet-building targets if the pressures are strong and the funds are available, but it is another thing to ensure that the toilets are sound and that people want to use them.

Technology has a crucial role to play in improving public sanitation in India, and technology can range from simple improvements to elaborate breakthroughs. In the case of toilets and human waste, different locations and regional attitudes require different designs to be appropriate to each location and attitude, and the only style that seems generally acceptable is a flush-and-forget model. But as we have seen, making excrement disappear does not solve the larger problem of making it benign and useful. More efficient, cheaper methods of purifying water are essential. The standard current model of a sewage treatment plant, which requires large tracts of land, constant electricity, and relentless maintenance holds little promise for India's burgeoning towns and sprawling megacities.[88]

Technologies do not have to be on the mammoth scale of the high-combustion incinerators of northern Europe and other parts of Asia.

Small-scale improvisations, created to serve local needs, contribute to sustained improvements and changed practices. Carefully designed collection carts are one example. Smart uniforms and suitable equipment for sanitation workers impart dignity to the worker and a little more respect from the beneficiaries.

And technology alone is not enough. Cultural expectations and prejudices have to be accommodated or, sometimes, overcome. Creators of waste must become supporters of better methods, both of minimization and of disposal. Technical fixes by themselves become an excuse. They allow governments and those in power to avoid the glaring class divisions and failures of the state that make improved sanitation difficult to achieve.[89] Laws and regulations have to be enforced and well-considered investments made. All of this must be paid for, which leads to the role of governments, especially local governments.

6

LOCAL GOVERNMENTS AND LIMITATIONS

LOCAL GOVERNMENT, ESPECIALLY URBAN LOCAL GOVERNMENT, is inescapably about garbage and waste and the prevention of noxious activity near the dwellings of influential people. The *kotwal,* or magistrate, of a town, had such responsibilities in Mughal times, and in urbanizing England beginning in the seventeenth century, authorities struggled to deal with streets that were—as Southampton was described in 1601—"verye fylthely [filthily] kept."[1] By the nineteenth century, it suited British imperialists in India, whose own cities had begun to improve slowly as awareness of health science grew, to contrast the "cleanliness" of the "civil lines" where they lived with the dirt and disorder of "the 'native' quarter."[2] The local government reforms of the 1880s deftly transferred blame and responsibility for dirt and disorder from the rulers and onto the subjects with the pious explanation that this was a step toward self-government. But funds and authority were never there. After independence and addition of the seventy-third and seventy-fourth constitutional amendments in 1993, local governments acquired responsibilities but insufficient capacity to fulfill them.

"The British state," on the other hand, "was a *municipal* [emphasis added] project, and the state is now being unmade by the collapse of that project," according to a critic in 2016. The argument is that national governments, Conservative and Labour, reduced their expenditures by eroding funds to local governments that once provided "many of the features and functions of the state."[3] Dismantled local governments continue to bear the responsibility and face the frustration of citizens. That story sounds familiar, but the difference is that local government in India cannot be dismantled because it has never been "mantled": it has not had the legal, financial, and human capacity to perform tasks expected of it.

Indian local governments are unable to deal with the vast amount of waste their growing populations produce daily. The reasons have their roots in British rule. Changes after independence preserved structures in which local governments were expected to act simply as delivery mechanisms for programs devised by national and state governments.[4] When such programs did not materialize or did not work, local governments got the blame. The seventy-third and seventy-fourth amendments to the constitution made functioning local governments a required component of the Indian state. But the constitutional recognition did not overcome tangled and conflicting jurisdictions. "States," a tireless advocate of local government believed, "subverted or even outright flouted the provisions" of the constitutional amendments.[5]

Most local governments, dependent on state legislation, lack financial capacity. This in turn means a lack of prestige and reward for officials and elected councillors and a consequent lack of specialists in all aspects of local government, especially public sanitation. In these circumstances, a local government needs initiative and imagination if it sets out to improve the hygiene of its city, town, or locality.

The colonial state generated masses of data in the form of maps, censuses, ethnographic reports, and land surveys. These were designed to extract revenue and control potentially unruly subjects. Dealing with disorderly towns proved a practical and intellectual challenge. In British eyes, the street and bazaar festered in disorder, filth, and squalor, caused in part by "the domestic tasks and rituals of washing, changing, sleeping, urinating and cooking."[6] They aimed to distinguish themselves by imposing "an alternative metropolitan spatial order wherein a network of manicured, broad avenues [were] marked against the imagined disorder of the 'native' quarter."[7] But the problem of controlling an unruly landscape persisted.

The powers delegated to local governments during British rule were limited, and financial support was meagre. There was little substance to the proclaimed vision of local government as a milestone on a path to liberal modernity and perhaps even self-rule. The structures established from the 1880s on were, however, what formed the basis of urban and rural participation after independence in 1947.

These historical considerations help explain why local governments so often seem stymied and ineffectual. Their challenges range from jurisdictional wars between local authorities to shortages of suitably trained and motivated officials. Many are ill prepared to assess the technical quick fixes—and this applies especially to waste management—thrust at them by political superiors, aggrieved voters, and private industry. Such limitations undermine efforts to formulate coherent waste-management schemes, even as towns and urban centers struggle under the weight of their own waste.

History

Chennai, the capital of the southern state of Tamil Nadu, has changed many of the names the British gave to its buildings, roads, and bridges, even its own name (once, Madras), but one of its most imposing structures retains its original. Dazzlingly white in the sharp sunlight of a summer day, the Ripon Building houses Chennai's local government. Commissioned in 1909, it is named after George Robinson, Marquis of Ripon (1827–1909), viceroy and governor-general of India from 1880 to 1884. Ripon's name survives because his Resolutions on Local Self-Government, endorsed in 1882, are a landmark in the history of local government in India, and Ripon's ghost haunts offices, procedures, and even India's rubbish dumps today.

Chennai Municipal Corporation is one of India's largest local governments, with elected councillors representing each of its 155 geographical wards. Chennai is also India's oldest municipality. The East India Company's settlement at Madras got a royal charter from Charles II in 1687 that provided "a municipal constitution" for its European merchants. The intent then, as it was in Ripon's time two hundred years later, was to "facilitate the increase of taxation."[8]

Why should Ripon's initiatives more than 130 years ago be significant for campaigns to clean up India in the twenty-first century?

First, the reforms provided a long-lasting framework for local government, which has gone through many contortions but whose underlying assumptions continue. Second, the idealism that one can read into the Ripon reforms masked economic and political calculations about taxation and the provision of services that still affect the operation of local government. Before Ripon, "local government" had meant a British-appointed town council with few powers other than to advise the European official responsible for administering the town and its surroundings. The Resolutions on Local Self-Government, issued by the Government of India in 1882, enabled more than five hundred municipal bodies to elect a proportion of their members based on a very narrow franchise.[9]

Much of the rhetoric surrounding Ripon's local government resolutions referred to the "educational" aspects of enabling Indians—albeit less than 1 percent of them—to elect representatives who would be responsible for tasks of government. "Promoting gradually and safely the political education of the people" was how Ripon phrased it. This would, he hoped, "pave the way for further advances . . . as that education becomes fuller and more widespread."[10]

For the British, various benefits lay in transferring responsibility to Indian subjects for providing services that affected the everyday life of millions. Urban cleanliness was such an item. Under the guise of instructing people in self-government, a certain amount of blame and financial responsibility could be shifted to Indians. Some of these calculations were evident in a remark by one of Ripon's advisers: "We shall not subvert the British Empire by allowing the Bengali Baboo to discuss his own schools and drains. Rather shall we afford him a safety valve if we can turn his attention to these innocuous subjects."[11] The British vision of local government, somewhat camouflaged in the Ripon reforms, was that local governments existed to take pressure off higher levels of authority and should work in response to the needs of such authority. This attitude has remained widespread.

In the 1890s, conservative British governments and their appointees in India withdrew some of the prerogatives that the Ripon reforms had bestowed on elected local councils and returned powers to British officials. British rulers argued that the Ripon reforms had failed and local government was best handled by superior officials.[12] At the time of independence in 1947, most Indian towns and cities had only sporadic experience of local government. A few larger cities, like Kolkata, Ahmedabad, and Allahabad, had had national celebrities as mayors, but these were largely ceremonial offices, useful for putting pressure on the British as part of the national struggle but less useful for building sewers and cleaning streets.[13] "The progress of local government . . . for the past quarter century," concluded *Indian Year Book 1930*, "has been disappointing . . . the powers entrusted to local bodies were insignificant and the financial support was small."[14]

Disdain and distaste for local government grew partly from detritus being at its core. Dead animals, human excrement, and rotting vegetables have to be dealt with every day if a town is to be tolerable. In the sixteenth century at the time of Emperor Akbar, the *kotwal* was instructed to ensure "the open thoroughfare of the streets . . . and secure freedom from defilement . . . [and] allot separate quarters to butchers, hunters of animals, washers of the dead and sweepers."[15] About four hundred years later, Philip Oldenburg concluded that "sanitation . . . is the most salient problem with which local government has to deal."[16] Such work seldom had glamour or reward, and British rule had not been notably effective in keeping towns clean, as Florence Nightingale had told the sanitary inquiry so caustically in 1863.

Independence

The framers of the constitution of 1950 omitted local government and panchayats (village councils) from early drafts. Eventually, pressure to pay attention to M. K. Gandhi's vision of revitalized village communities led to a directive principle—one of fifty-one add-ons, including references to motherhood and world peace—being added to the constitution. It referred to the need for state governments to "organise village panchayats and endow them with such powers and authority as may be necessary to enable them to function as units of self-government."[17] The emphasis, too, was on *rural* local government. The Gandhian vision of a purified village life lingered into the 1980s, and development of towns and cities was often seen as something to be discouraged.

Gandhi continually mused about the improvement of rural life that would create an ideal India. In the first decade after independence, community development programs, run by officials who rode in jeeps and lived in towns, "failed to evoke people's participation," which led to renewed calls for genuine local government of the kind Gandhi had advocated and romantics believed had existed in a distant past.[18]

The Balwantrai Mehta report of 1959 recommended creation of a three-level system of panchayats, or panchayati raj. But the constitution of 1950 had left to individual states of the federation the legislation of the terms under which urban and rural local governments would operate. Contrary to the recommendations of the Mehta report, these new units of government were not given powers to raise funds or to decide what the needs of their localities might be.[19] Their role, as spelled out in most states, was to provide a local institution to carry out the plans of officials and state governments.[20] What was true of panchayati raj in the countryside was largely similar in towns and cities. "Most municipal administrations are not strong enough to carry out these functions," was the conclusion in *Third Five-Year Plan* in 1961.[21] As a consequence, "the initiative for urban policy formulation," Rodney Jones, an American political scientist, wrote in 1974, "is therefore preempted by politicians and bureaucrats in state governments."[22] State legislators had little interest in creating a tier of elected politicians who might rival them for patronage and influence.

In the space of a generation, between 1961 and 1981, India's urban population doubled—from 79 million people (18 percent of the total population) to 160 million (23 percent). The capacity of towns and cities to manage schools, public health, and sanitation was never great, and the increase in density exposed deficiencies that were galling to urban dwellers.[23]

Four government inquiries in the ten years between 1978 and 1988 eventually led to a proposal for a constitutional amendment to strengthen the powers of local governments, but in 1989 it failed to get parliamentary approval. Liberalization of the economy in the 1990s compounded problems of housing and infrastructure in urban India.[24] To transform metros like Mumbai and Delhi into world-class cities became a primary goal as private enterprise increasingly looked to international collaborations.[25] In this rapidly changing landscape, civic bodies appeared to be lethargic institutions, unable to cater for the needs of aspiring middle classes. A key problem was that local governments were still beholden to the states for financial and structural support. Local governments were expected to do things, but they lacked authority and financial resources. In some states, elected local governments often did not exist, held in suspension by state governments not wishing to constitute potentially troublesome forums. The state of Tamil Nadu, for example, avoided holding local government elections for twenty years.[26]

Structure

The seventy-third and seventy-fourth amendments, which came into effect in 1993, made it mandatory for each state to constitute rural and urban local governments, to establish mechanisms to fund them, and to carry out elections every five years.[27] If states failed to do so, their authorities were in breach of the constitution, and citizens could take them to court. The seventy-third amendment spelled out the rules for the countryside; the seventy-fourth amendment did the same for urban and semiurban areas. It now was unconstitutional for state governments to keep local governments in abeyance.

The seventy-fourth amendment prescribed three levels—municipal corporations for populations of more than one million, municipal councils for areas of less than one million, and *nagar* panchayats for "an area in transition from a rural area to an urban area."[28] It also provided for "metropolitan planning committees" that would coordinate development across a number of jurisdictions. Every state was to constitute a finance commission to ensure that federal and state funding flowed equitably and predictably to local governments. The details of these initiatives, however, were left to the individual states, and responsibility for a number of key decisions was vested in the state's governor, a senior public figure appointed by the national government but expected to act primarily as a ceremonial official accepting the advice of the state government.[29]

These jurisdictional complications affect waste management crucially, because sewerage schemes and sanitary landfills—not to mention contentious and expensive matters such as high-combustion incinerators—have to serve large populations and wide areas. One might guess that larger units of local government would be able to raise more revenue and coordinate planning. Local government in Delhi, however, was revamped in 2012 to divide the single Delhi Municipal Corporation into three municipal corporations—South Delhi, North Delhi, and East Delhi. The argument was that a single corporation could not deal effectively with Delhi's vast population. In contrast, local governments in Hyderabad were consolidated into a single Greater Hyderabad Municipal Corporation in 2007. In Bengaluru, the celebrated information technology center, an enlarged municipal corporation was created in 2007, but by 2015, this was found to be inadequate to deal with a mushrooming city, and an inquiry committee recommended creation of five entities to replace the single corporation.[30]

The powers of local governments depend on the law of the state in which they operate. The constitutional amendments that required states to set up local governments do not specify the rules, and some states do their best to ensure that "local bodies remain mere agents of the [state] government." Other states, notably Kerala, devolved substantial funds and powers to its one thousand units of local government in the 1990s.[31]

Jurisdictions: Small Collisions

Pammal is one of thirty-seven units of local government that make up the greater Chennai area.[32] The Pammal experience underlines the pressures and contradictions that citizens encounter when they look for ways to make their environment cleaner and to manage waste sustainably.

When the seventy-fourth constitutional amendment came into force in 1993, Pammal was classified as a *nagar* panchayat, a locality no longer rural but not yet fully urban. It attained municipality status, and the additional powers that go with it, a few years later. As greater Chennai grew, so did Pammal—from 36,000 people in the census of 1991 to 76,000 people living in 18,800 households in 2011.[33] Although the locality has polluting industries like tanning and leatherwork, Pammal also has neighborhoods of tree-lined streets and comfortable householders.

Pammal's contests with waste are widely known among people who work in public sanitation in India. In 1994, a group of women, responding to constant problems with garbage, banded together to improve waste disposal in a single ward of the municipality.[34] At the center of the group was Dr. Mangalam Balasubramanian, an experienced development professional who had returned to Chennai after a career partly spent as an adviser to one of the foreign embassies in New Delhi.[35] The group did not collect waste themselves but "began by hiring a few workers, buying a tricycle, and collecting waste from 264 households" in a single ward.[36] They appealed to residents for cooperation, staged street theater about garbage and pollution, and eventually requested each household to pay ten rupees a month toward the wages of the workers who collected the waste.

From their efforts in a single ward, they discovered one of the deficiencies of local government. Before 1996, Pammal did not have an elected local government. The low-level officials who administered rudimentary services were pleased to see a clean corner of the locality. They cooperated with the residents' association and sent a vehicle once a week to clear the skips (Dumpsters) where house-to-house collectors deposited the rubbish gathered in their daily rounds. The truck carted away the waste to an unspecified destination. The residents' group was satisfied to be keeping their ward clean and did not concern themselves with where the collected garbage went.

In 1996, the first elections to the *nagar* panchayat introduced unforeseen political dimensions. As one of Pammal's twenty-one wards, the area now had its own elected representative. On the face of it, one might have expected strengthened cooperation between citizens and governments to improve sanitation. But this did not happen. The elected councillors were members of state-level political parties, and the ward representative with whom the residents' association had to deal was "not well educated," meaning that he was a creature of his party and not prepared to take up the association's sanitation cause.[37] Because the ward was kept relatively clean, the new council withdrew the truck that came each week to cart away the ward's waste. The reasoning was that dirty wards needed the vehicle more urgently. Annoyed at the pileup of garbage around the collection skips, householders blamed the residents' association. The association blamed the ward's councillor for his silence. "He never thought," one of the members said to Bharat Dahiya, "that cleaning has to be done on a continuous basis."[38]

No locality is an island, especially when it comes to waste. The residents' association in Pammal depended on the local government to remove the waste it collected in its ward. Forced to innovate or give up, the association began segregating waste for recycling and turning wet waste into compost. This required space—a place to sort recyclable materials and to build composting beds. A private hospital offered a location, and from these beginnings, the association grew into a full-fledged nongovernmental organization.[39] The organization joined with an umbrella all-India NGO, Exnora Green, in 2005, and Exnora Green was contracted by the municipality to collect and manage the waste of all Pammal's twenty-one wards.[40] The municipality paid the NGO a fee for each household, and out of these fees regular wages were paid to the workers who did the daily collection.

Pammal told a promising story. The NGO had grown in twenty years from a small association of exasperated residents seeking to clean up their immediate neighborhood into an organization contracted to provide services to an entire municipality. It had projects in other parts of India and enjoyed international recognition.[41] In spite of its notable successes, however, Pammal's experience also illustrates the administrative collisions that impede attempts to improve public sanitation and waste management. One of the earliest was the confrontation between the well-meaning residents' association and the newly elected Pammal municipal council. Why send a truck to carry away waste from an area that was cleaning itself? It was clear that ward councillors had to be turned into active supporters of waste-management schemes.

Pammal also found itself in dispute with a neighboring municipality. Tamil Nadu has more than 700 urban local governments, 152 of them municipalities like Pammal.[42] A neighboring municipality with rough-and-ready waste-management practices began spilling its unsorted rubbish into open land next to Pammal's composting and recycling yards. The Pammal operation got the seepage, the spillover, and the blame. Pammal's managing director explains:

> When you go to the compost yard, you will see a lot of rubbish there. That is not our municipality's rubbish. Both municipalities belong to the same political party, so the neighboring municipality has been dumping a hundred tonnes every day. They don't have the space at all and they are spoiling our work.
>
> We always have a problem. We want to do good work, but there are a lot of problems.
>
> I had to go to the courts. I got a stay order from the courts to prevent them [the neighboring council], but whatever the damage—they have done it. It is huge. But now they are not doing anything. Again now I am going to the courts to remove all those things [rubbish] and give me a neat place. So it takes time. Any legal battle always takes time. But at the same time I'm working with the government, with the political party, so I cannot hurt their feelings. I have to do it in a very subtle manner . . . so the local party people know I only went to the court to get it stopped . . . and they are very happy. But they want me to take all the initiatives.[43]

The Pammal experience highlights key problems of local governments and waste. Elected councillors, who face various political compulsions, need to be supporters, convinced of the importance of the task. Residents and waste workers need to be motivated to adopt new methods. Local authorities have to find sites where recyclable waste can be sorted, wet waste can be composted, and least desirably, where unusable waste can be dumped in sanitary landfills. A further lesson from Pammal is the need for persistence and sustainability. Finally, the conflict with the neighboring municipality underlines the need for superior authorities who are able to resolve disputes, promote cooperation, and create large facilities—such as sanitary landfills and sewage treatment plants—to serve the needs of different local government units.

Jurisdictions: Big Collisions

Jurisdictional problems are not exclusive to small municipalities like Pammal. In the National Capital Territory (NCT) of Delhi, the official name for India's capital, local government is a labyrinth of authorities. They collide with each other in a confined area of 1,500 square kilometers (570 square miles), in one of the world's most rapidly growing cities. The NCT's population is estimated at 16.8 million,[44] giving a density of about 11,000 people per square kilometer (28,600 per square mile). The city-state of Singapore has a density of about 8,000 (20,800 per square mile). A metropolitan area like Melbourne, Australia, has a population of about 4.4 million and density of only 400 (1,040 per square mile). More important for purposes of waste management, however, is that Melbourne is part of the state of Victoria, which has a vast hinterland beyond the urban boundaries. Even Mumbai, although an island, is part of the state of Maharashtra, which has jurisdiction over the hinterland. Delhi is bounded by two states of the Indian union (Haryana and Uttar Pradesh), neither of which has an incentive to help solve the problems of the national capital. Delhi bursts at its seams.

Local government in Delhi has a complicated history. After independence, an attempt to establish elected local government was abandoned in 1956, and the capital was administered directly by the national government. The creation of the NCT in 1991 by the sixty-ninth amendment to the constitution was a landmark in the growing awareness of politicians and officials that urbanization was irresistible and local government was desirable. The sixty-ninth amendment provided the NCT with a chief minister and an assembly with many—but not all—of the powers of a state of the Indian union. Reasoning that the country's capital needed to be under the ultimate control of the central government, the Government of India retained various powers over the NCT. The NCT has as its formal head a lieutenant governor but not a full-fledged governor as do states of the union. The national government also retains control of Delhi's police. As well as its elected NCT government, Delhi has municipal governments. In 2016, decision-making in the NCT involved eight jurisdictions, close to four hundred elected representatives, two ministries of the government of India, and dozens of appointed representatives. (See Map 6.1.) The list of governmental entities includes the following:

- the Delhi Development Authority (DDA), under the national government's Ministry of Urban Development[45]
- a lieutenant governor, appointed by the Government of India, as the more-than-ceremonial representative of the president of India and chairman of the DDA
- a legislature of seventy members, elected from territorial constituencies and empowered to form a government under a chief minister
- three municipal corporations, which account for more than 95 percent of the NCT's area and together have 308 representatives elected from territorial wards
- the New Delhi Municipal Council, covering the small area of New Delhi built by the British in the 1920s and 1930s, where the president's palace and many government offices are located
- the Cantonment Board, presiding over the military establishment in the heart of the NCT and under the authority of the directorate general of Defence Estates in the Ministry of Defence

With the NCT's crushing population density, complicated by the unsympathetic states of Haryana and Uttar Pradesh on its borders, this proliferation of authorities leads to constant unresolved collisions and has major implications for waste management.

Space is vital, and no one has enough. The use of land in the NCT is controlled by the DDA, which is under the authority of the Ministry of Housing and Urban Affairs in the central government. Its minister often comes from a faraway state: "Delhi waste is not his concern."[46] The municipal corporations are responsible for waste management and deal with Delhi's citizens each day. In 2014, the South Delhi Municipal Corporation took the DDA to the Delhi High Court to demand that it release 650 hectares of land on which to create a new sanitary landfill and waste-management facilities. "I cannot take a gun and put it [to] their

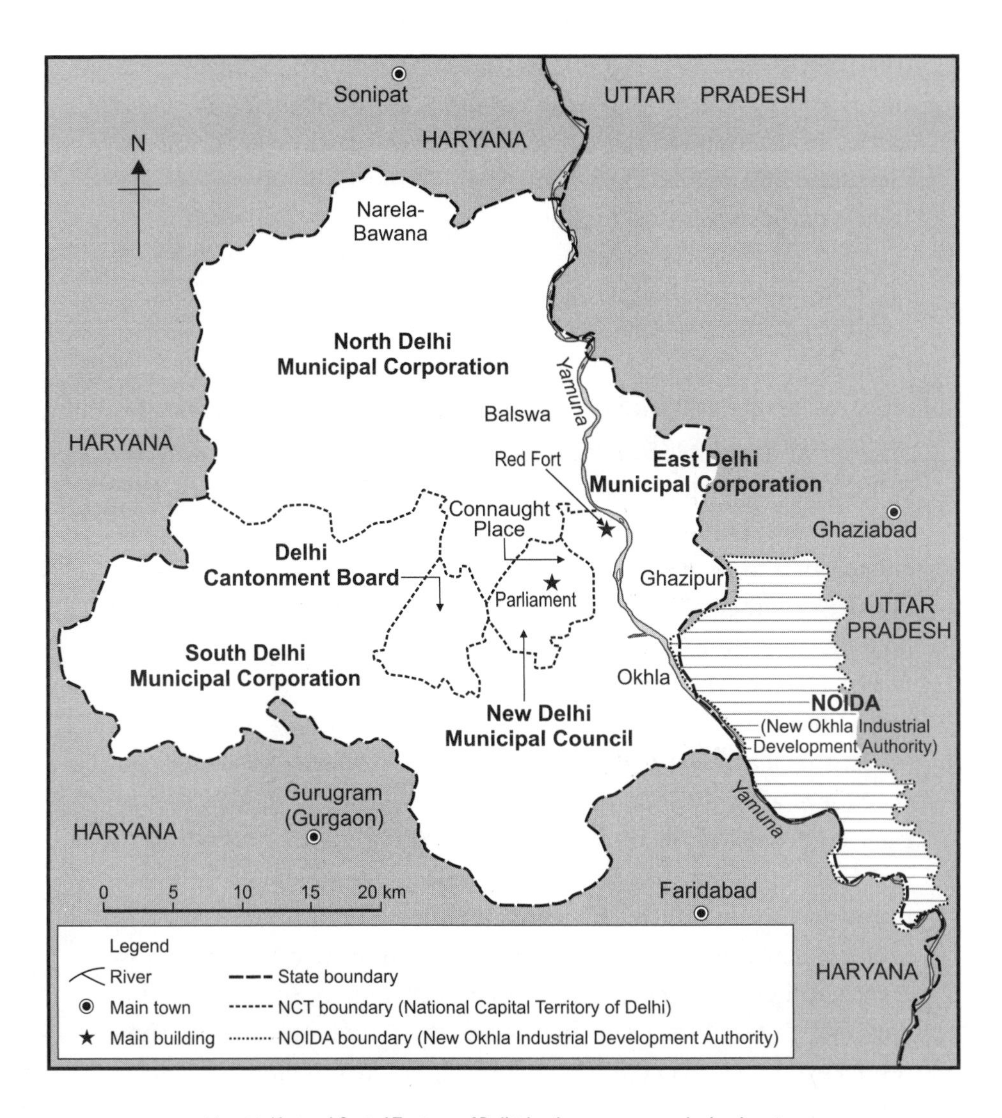

Map 6.1 National Capital Territory of Delhi: local governments and select locations

[the DDA's] head," said an exasperated senior official of the corporation.[47] Two government agencies confronted each other in the courts, just as tiny Pammal had moved the courts against its neighboring municipality. Meanwhile, Delhi's citizens continued to make waste, and Delhi's dumps continued to grow.

Finance

"But who is to pay for it?" is a universal cry when expensive sanitation projects with multiple beneficiaries are mooted. From Ripon's time, the British were happy to transfer responsibilities for local amenities to local bodies, but their funds and powers were never equal to the tasks. And it is one thing to have the legal authority to collect local fees and taxes, but it is another to extract payment from reluctant merchants and householders. "While direct taxation produced protest widely all over India," Douglas Haynes, a longtime historian of Gujarat and its urban life, writes of the nineteenth century, "perhaps no city was so consistent in resisting it as Surat. . . . A license tax on local businesses in 1878 provoked several days of rioting."[48] It took the plague panic of 1994 to bring rigorous tax collection and compliance to Surat.

Collection of revenues—house and business taxes and other dues—proves fiendishly difficult for municipalities. Even in the twenty-first century, many do not have reliable records on which to base assessments, and even when they do, evasion is common. In Hyderabad in 2015, employees of the municipal corporation, under pressure to show results from their tax collection efforts, attempted to induce a hotel to pay "property tax to the tune of Rs 1 crore [about $200,000] and after their efforts went in vain, they staged a sit-in in the premises. This move resulted in collection of a part of the payment i.e., Rs 50 lakhs [$100,000]."[49] The Hyderabad Municipal Corporation had to deny in court that it had "given instructions to the tax collection officials to dump garbage bins in front of the premises or buildings of property tax defaulters."[50] Placing skips in front of defaulters' premises to bully them into paying tax arrears also reminded them of the connection between their taxes and public sanitation. The corporation denied the charges, but shaming defaulters had worked elsewhere. In Ahmedabad and

Surat, where tax collections were at one time less than they should have been, the state government had given its blessing to beating drums in front of defaulting premises and publicizing the names of owners.[51]

In some municipalities, "as much as 30–50 per cent of the Municipal Corporation budgets are being spent on solid waste management,"[52] estimated Kiran Sandhu, a scholar in Amritsar, in 2015. Such estimates may be on the high side, but most local governments collect only a fraction of their tax demands and spend more on waste management than any other budget item except salaries and administration. The weakness of revenue collection, and resulting constraints on sanitation projects, was illustrated in a review in 2009. It found that local governments lacked accurate information about the number of residential and commercial premises within their boundaries. Because their chief source of revenue, independent of grants from state and national governments, came from property taxes, this was like owning assets but not knowing that you owned them. Delhi, for example, was estimated to contain 2.5 million properties, but only 960,000 were "on the municipal tax register."[53] The review estimated that, across the country, local governments in 2007 managed to collect only 37 percent of the property tax they demanded. Cities varied. Bengaluru and Chennai collected about 85 percent. Delhi, on the other hand, managed only about 20 percent. The 2009 report recommended a national survey of India's property tax systems, but it was never carried out.[54] Lack of reliable information remains a major handicap for most local governments in their struggle to raise revenue to pay for the services their voters expect but are reluctant to pay for.

Various studies highlight "the persistent weak financial condition of municipal governments," which are "unable to generate adequate funds" and sometimes unable "to even pay salaries to their employees."[55] To tackle this "acute urban crisis" and the "extremely unsatisfactory state" of "municipal finance," Prime Minister Manmohan Singh's government set up the ponderously named Jawaharlal Nehru National Urban Renewal Mission (JNNURM) at the end of 2005. The program recognized that "urbanisation . . . has come to stay." But the prime minister also found it necessary to genuflect to the Gandhian ideal that "India by and large still lives in our villages."[56] Within four years, the JNNURM committed Rs 50,000 crores (about $7 billion at 2017 exchange rates) for projects aimed at "reshaping our cities."[57]

From 2014, the Bharatiya Janata Party (BJP) has emphasized urbanization unequivocally and without rhetorical bows to Mahatma Gandhi (although Gandhi was retained as a symbol in the Swachh Bharat campaign). "India is moving away from villages," the Minister of Urban Development wrote. "Urbanisation drives economic growth," but "long years of vacillation . . . have taken a very heavy toll of life in urban areas."[58] Water supply and sewerage were high priorities, and Rs 14,643 crores (close to $2.2 billion) was allocated to "making cities clean." The minister claimed that "over 500 cities and towns have already become open defecation–free." He asserted accomplishments in areas that urban analysts had often identified as crucial: "citizen participation" and "bottom up" planning, "technical capabilities" of local governments, and cities empowered to raise funds by issuing bonds.[59]

Cities had been able to offer bonds to finance projects from the late 1990s, but only a few local governments had done so, usually to finance big projects for sewerage, water supply, or roads. Ahmedabad, the pioneer in 1998, used the method most frequently.[60] The Government of India exempted such investments from income tax, and by 2005 ten cities had sold bonds to finance projects. But initial enthusiasm waned. Investors were skeptical about the financial systems and efficiency of most local governments, and assembling the paperwork for a public offering needed skilled people and continuity of administration. After 2010, no local governments offered bonds, although the Government of India tried to reinvigorate interest in 2016. "Sadly, Indian states do not empower their cities," an investment banker explained.[61]

Capacity: Politicians and Professionals

Local governments lack the powers and finances to fulfill the responsibilities expected of them. But even if funds and authority become available, elected representatives and employees lack training, expertise, and motivation. In some places this may result from freezes on the hiring of staff.[62] But there is a paucity of trained and committed individuals attracted to careers in local government, and too few of India's one hundred thousand elected urban councillors are informed about, or interested in, the mechanics of running their town.

Local government is not a popular career choice, probably anywhere in the world and especially in India. Waste management, which is an inescapable aspect of local government, generates a distinctively Indian stigma, and the salaries and incentives are not notably attractive, even in metropolitan cities. Cynics may say that the potential for bribery and corruption provides plenty of compensation, but not everyone is inclined to graft and, in any case, not everyone has sufficient influence to peddle profitably.

The neglect of local sanitation and government was a theme recognized in Florence Nightingale's time. In 1862, she exploded at the lack of attention to, and clear responsibility for, keeping Indian towns clean: "No good will be done unless it be made some competent person's business."[63] In the 1890s, British officials with genuine interests in public health "declared the urgent need for a 'sanitary service' for India." They believed that without a cadre of specialists working with local governments, local government itself would be discredited for not performing tasks allotted to it.[64] "Municipal service," Hugh Tinker, one of the first scholars to focus on local government, wrote of the British period, "attracted few Indians of ability."[65] The Third Five-Year Plan in 1961 lamented that "most municipal administrations are not strong enough to carry out these functions" of looking after a town, because "resources and personnel" were lacking.[66]

Local governments are still underpowered in revenue, authority, and expertise. Whereas the government of India has a cadre of high-status administrators in the form of the Indian Administrative Service (IAS) and state governments recruit their own state services, local governments get the administrators that state governments assign them. Work in local government is often regarded as a punishment, a sinecure, or a rung on a ladder leading elsewhere. For an IAS officer, being a municipal commissioner is something you do for two or three years on the way to something else. At lower levels, "ad hoc methods of augmenting . . . staffing requirements are followed," contends a 2014 report recommending creation of dedicated cadres for work in urban government. "Lack of training had rendered most of these staff grossly inadequate." States with dedicated municipal cadres performed better.[67]

Career possibilities in local government are different in countries like the United Kingdom, Canada, or Australia, where elected municipal governments advertise key positions.[68] Applicants are usually on contracts, and during their careers, they move a number of times, take on greater responsibilities, and receive higher salaries. In Australia, for example, the City of Yarra, one of the thirty-two councils that make up the area of greater Melbourne, has a population of ninety thousand. The chief executive officer in 2017, who happened to have begun her career with the Reserve Bank of India before moving into local government in New Zealand and then to Australia, was on a five-year contract and earned a salary exceeding A$350,000 (about Rs 2 crores, or US$260,000), comparable with the chief executive officers of Melbourne's thirty-one other municipalities.[69]

In India, local government suffers from administrative prejudices inherited from British rule and the reluctance of state politicians to lose patronage and create rivals. These deficiencies have been compounded in some cities by ill-considered acceptance of privatization as a panacea. Lisa Björkman in her penetrating book *Pipe Politics* describes how consultants, employed at the instigation of the World Bank, concluded in 1997 that the department in charge of Mumbai's water supply was overstaffed. According to the engineer who was Björkman's informant, the conclusion was reached on the basis of comparison with Singapore. The World Bank's review, he said, "told us that Singapore was operating with two workers per connection, and we've got forty. . . . But . . . in Bombay we count one connection per . . . *housing society;* in Singapore they have separate connections to each apartment in the building."[70] The comparison seems absurd and the absurdity obvious to anyone acquainted with the two different systems; but staff cutbacks resulted nevertheless, and Björkman was told in 2009 that staffing levels had not changed since the 1970s, though Mumbai's population had more than doubled.[71]

The skepticism about the usefulness of government employees, which accompanied neoliberal economic policies, reinforced an enduring disdain for local government. A report from Odisha, one of India's least developed and urbanized states, found that its towns and cities needed about 7,000 municipal staff to begin to perform the duties expected of them; the state employed 1,500.[72] Another report from Odisha concluded that officers working in local government are "not interested to take the job seriously" and are "not at all interested in Municipal work."[73] If it was true that the IAS had lost its glamour and that state administrative services did not have much glamour in the first place, working at the local level represented the lowest rung on a rickety ladder.

Social conditions—literacy and education, for example—result in some states producing a larger proportion of people with the skills needed to make them effective elected officials. A study in 2005, for example, found that close to 90 percent of councillors in Kerala bought newspapers, but only 10 percent did in Tamil Nadu, and almost none in Madhya Pradesh.[74] Investing in a newspaper suggests some exposure to a wider world. More than 90 percent of Kerala councillors had more than ten years of education, but the proportion was as low as 11 percent in Madhya Pradesh and 28 percent in Tamil Nadu.[75] Places in all local governments are reserved for women (about half of places in some states and a third in the rest), Scheduled Castes, and Scheduled Tribes. However, the study in 2005 found that women were frequently puppets of male relatives.[76] "Success stories" of women playing active roles, "are few and far between," a 2013 report concluded.[77]

Throughout the country, various efforts are made to improve capacity. In Bengaluru, the Bangalore Political Action Committee (B.PAC), an NGO founded in 2012 "to convert urban apathy into positive urban engagement" and provoked by the city's problems with waste, began a "civic leadership incubator program" to equip likely candidates for local elected offices.[78] The aim was to train a thousand people, over five years, in cohorts of about fifty. "We run classes every week over Friday and Saturday," Revathy Ashok, B.PAC's chief executive officer, said.

> They're all working people, but they come in the evening. . . . Everybody can come and understand and participate in the program provided [they meet] our selection criteria. Education is not a bar. The bar that we have is [that] they must be politically inclined. They should have done some active work in their community, [and] they should be recommended by at least a hundred people in their community to enter the program. What we want to see is their power to influence. . . . We impart further training on civic issues and many such

> government issues. It's not thoughts and ideas: . . . [it] is implementation.[79]

Twenty of the program's graduates contested elections in the Bengaluru municipal corporation in August 2016, and one of them, Mandara Sampath Kumar, won in Ward Ninety-Three. Born in 1967, Sampath Kumar had been an activist in movements to promote the Kannada language and ran as a BJP candidate. "They can be from any party," Revathy Ashok said. "It puts pressure on the government that a group of trained people are now contesting elections. . . . It raises the bar." Sampath Kumar had a polished website declaring that his major election promise and postelection achievement was "waste segregation." His tactics included "going door to door, awareness camps and initiating massive cleanliness drives."[80]

Changes at a local level require "an engaged political leader," according to N. S. Ramakanth, a member of the B.PAC board.[81] The government of Maharashtra came to similar conclusions. In identifying four small towns that had become cleaner, a senior official noted that "the common feature . . . was that elected leaders made a decision to depoliticise cleanliness services. After that they made efforts to build trust in their ability to deliver."[82] In Alappuzha in Kerala, a once-smelly city improved its sanitation and the lot of its waste workers when local Communist Party and Congress Party politicians put energy into a program to compost and recycle. "We, the people's representatives, led the movement from the front," one of them said proudly. "When you mean business, that gives a certain degree of confidence to the people."[83] In 2016, Alappuzha was named one of India's "three . . . cleanest cities" by the Centre for Science and Environment.[84]

People make waste, and people have to mitigate it. Local governments, and the people who run them and work for them, constitute an institution that can make the taming of waste possible, as the hopeful story from Alappuzha suggests. But at all levels, if the work of sanitation is to be done effectively, people require training, incentives, recognition, and authority. At the grinding, ground level of informal ragpickers, there is potential to organize to achieve better income and conditions in return for systematic collection and disposal; but this requires willing local authorities and dedicated organizers. In most jurisdictions, waste collectors directly employed by local governments have some security of income, but equipment and training are rare.

Reliable income is a necessity for waste-collecting families and an incentive for thorough work. Changes, depicted as beneficial, can undermine conditions. A study in a town in West Bengal found that efforts to improve segregation of waste and effective recycling were undermined by a local NGO. (Not all NGOs are on the side of the angels.) The NGO offered to do the work more cheaply by replacing the municipal staff and their union. Wages for the NGO's workers would be lower, and the NGO

> proposed that the workers themselves would be responsible for collecting the user fees . . . [putting] the mostly poor and low-caste workers into a difficult system where they were responsible for forcing non-poor and often higher-caste people to pay. The union rejected this proposal, demanding higher wages and the employment of separate people for the collection of fees. With these demands, the union went on strike.[85]

Successful programs make council-employed workers into something more than mere sweepers of muck. In Alappuzha, Kerala, where the municipality supported local recycling and composting and achieved notable success, one of its employees, placed in charge of an aerobic composting unit, spoke of a new dignity: "Earlier I used to mop up and load the dirt in trucks. Everyone looked at me with scorn. Now I find dignity in my job. I have to help people deposit their domestic waste in bins and fill these with dry leaves for processing."[86] Regular payment of wages, appropriate uniforms and equipment, and meaningful responsibilities are benefits that municipalities can offer their workers in return for reliable service.

Capacity: Where Can We Get Some?

What does a local government do if councillors, citizens, or officials want to improve sanitation? A random but revealing example from

Karnataka throws light on the requirements and discoveries of one small city in its attempts to deal with mounting volumes of waste.

The city of Raichur lies about four hundred kilometers (250 miles) north of Bengaluru in the state of Karnataka and two hundred kilometers (125 miles) southwest of Hyderabad, in the state of Telangana. Until 1956 and the reorganization of India's states on a language basis, it was part of the old princely state of Hyderabad, which had had a Muslim ruler. Today, Raichur's population of 230,000 is 30 percent Muslim. Raichur's population places it among India's four hundred largest cities. Raichur's struggles with waste illustrate some of the administrative, technical, and human problems that cities encounter when they attempt to improve public sanitation.

The structure of Raichur's local government is not as complicated as Delhi's, but it has its own intricate charm. The city has an elected municipal council whose members represent thirty-five geographical wards. The councillors elect a president from among themselves, but the municipal commissioner—the chief executive officer—is an appointee of the state government and a member of the state's administrative service. The *city* of Raichur, however, is located in the *district* of Raichur, which has an area of 8,300 square kilometers (3,200 square miles) and a population of about 2 million. Raichur city is the headquarters of the district. The commissioner of Raichur district is also appointed by the state government, but he or she is a member of the IAS, the much more prestigious national service. The powers of the district commissioner can override those of the municipal commissioner. Raichur suffered from turnover of its key executives: it had fifteen district commissioners in the ten years between 2005 and 2015, and municipal commissioners might have changed as often.[87] A dry district, 400 kilometers from the bright lights of Bengaluru, was not a prize posting.

The Raichur municipality had a blemished past. Charges of fraud and nonpayment of workers went back at least to 2004, and an Asian Development Bank loan for sewerage improvements could not be spent in four years prior to 2012 because of administrative indecision and lack of commitment.[88] However, in 2015, the Swachh Bharat campaign was being trumpeted around the country. The IAS commissioner of Raichur district, a young officer on the way up, was aware that achieving Swachh

Bharat goals and showing results would be a career boost, and he looked for ways to clean up the city of Raichur. The municipal commissioner, however, was a member of the Karnataka administrative service, approaching retirement, and not much attracted, it was said, to the troublesome demands of public sanitation.

Raichur is a striking city with an old city wall and a commanding fort sitting on top of a hill. But Raichur was not a clean city. It had a typical sprawling, unmanaged dump on what was once the fringe of the town. In the town itself, squadrons of pigs did much of the street cleaning, and residents warned of the pig menace if one got in the way of hungry pigs who sniffed fragrant, newly dumped edibles. From the town's famous city wall, people on an evening walk looked down into a moat that doubled as a cesspool for some of the town's sewers and a snack bar and bathhouse for the pigs. The district commissioner determined to put Raichur in step with the Swachh Bharat program, even if the municipal commissioner was unenthusiastic.

Technical considerations arose. Where did an ambitious officer who wanted to carry out national policy begin? Officers of the IAS or state administrative services are rarely specialists in a particular area. They move from one department of government to another, often at short intervals and the whim of politicians or influential citizens. This is especially true of local government, and public sanitation and waste management are among the problems least likely to attract ambitious officials until forced to deal with them, either by pressure from above or significant community anger.

Seeking advice, the district commissioner consulted a retired member of the Andhra Pradesh administrative service who had a wide reputation for having cleaned up the towns in which he had worked.[89] Now a freelance activist and consultant, Khader Saheb (see also Chapter 7) had a well-known and detailed program for waste management. It emphasized doing things locally—daily collection; predictable payment and proper equipping of workers; organized composting of wet waste to keep it out of the mouths of pigs; diligent segregation of recyclable materials; and cooperation with traders in plastic, paper, and metals to carry away recyclables and get a reasonable price for them. The aim was to make towns cleaner by reducing the rubbish produced, earn income from segregation of waste, and improve the conditions and earnings of waste collectors. It stressed motivation, monitoring, equipment, and training.

Khader Saheb had a plan, but Raichur lacked an organization to carry it out.[90] The city's employees would need to be augmented, motivated, and given clear tasks and rewards. Khader Saheb put the district commissioner in touch with a nearby NGO that had been created to deal with the fly ash from a coal-fired power station. The district commissioner engaged the NGO to plan and oversee the cleanup of the city of Raichur and its uncontrolled garbage dump.

As a result of its work with fly ash, the NGO had a reputation for recycling.[91] However, as one of its officials said, they had had no knowledge of other facets of waste management when they were asked to take on the Raichur cleanup. In consultation with Raichur officials and Khader Saheb, they implemented a program to collect and segregate waste and to rehabilitate Raichur's chaotic old dump and turn it into a recycling and composting center.

Daily door-to-door collection and on-the-spot separation of waste began, and by March 2015 it seemed to appeal to householders. When a councillor led a door-to-door stroll to ask householders in his ward how they liked the new system, the women who came out to talk were pleased with the collections. But they took the opportunity to question the councillor about when the storm-water drains running down their narrow streets would be cleaned.[92] The district commissioner believed there had been an improvement in the sanitation of the town in the three months the program had been operating. He had, he said, developed a presentation called "The Malnourished Pig," based on his observation that the town's pigs, deprived of much of their daily menu, were losing weight.[93]

In the short term at least, things in Raichur seemed to go well. The redoubtable Almitra Patel, who pursued the legal action that led to the Solid Waste Management Rules of 2000 (Chapter 5), visited Raichur ten months after the new system began and described waste management in the town as "quite good"—better than in Bengaluru. The manager of the former dump, which was reengineered as a waste segregation and composting center, reported progress, which included a whittling down of the refuse from the old dump site and steady processing of the daily collection from Raichur.[94]

* * *

State governments have the legislative power to arm local bodies with more fund-raising power and authority, but few—Kerala may be one exception—have done so. Local governments suffer from collisions of jurisdictions, antiquated financial systems, and insufficient incentives for those who work at all levels and especially in public sanitation. One of the results is a scarcity of trained, equipped, and motivated people. That a collection of best-practice studies of urban waste management was not published by the National Institute of Urban Affairs until 2015 helps explain why Raichur turned to an NGO whose unlikely experience was in reusing fly ash. "Much needs to be done," a 2016 study concluded, "in regard to the capacity building."[95] Around the country, local initiatives arising from virtuous coincidences of citizens, councillors, and officials provide a patchwork of promising methods and techniques, as we explore in the next chapter.

7

OCCUPATIONS AND POSSIBILITIES

ANYONE WHO HAS READ KATHERINE BOO'S memorable book *Behind the Beautiful Forevers* about families of waste-pickers in the Annawadi slum colony of Mumbai will need little convincing about the human complexity that accompanies waste. In this chapter, we illuminate that complexity by focusing on people and their institutions. To give order to this discussion, we have created four categories of occupations that deal with waste—professionals, handlers, recyclers, and facilitators. The categories are artificial, and in real life, people slide from one to another. But the categories have some value in revealing the interests and pressures that motivate those who work with waste.[1]

Waste professionals are the people that local governments turn to for managing waste. These include scientists, engineers, private-enterprise executives, and the public-service administrators and finance managers who go with twenty-first-century bureaucracy. They vary in their enthusiasm, knowledge, and commitment, but the best of them bring skills, networks, and institutional understanding necessary to improving and maintaining public sanitation in growing towns and great cities. Even for those who never touch a bin or clean a toilet, work associated with garbage brings little prestige and only modest rewards at best. As we have seen, India has always been short of expertise in local government and public health.

At the other end of the waste chain—or the bottom of the pyramid—are the handlers of waste. These are the people who scratch a living largely by dealing with the expelled materials of their fellow citizens. How many people make livings in this way? No one knows for sure, and the category depends, elastically, on definition. The census does not have an occupational category for ragpickers or waste-pickers. In New Delhi, a common estimate was that between 200,000 and 350,000 people worked as waste-pickers in an urban area of 16 million people in 2011.[2] Rough calculations suggest that India's 53 cities with populations of more than 1 million support close to 2 million waste-pickers, and its 465 cities with populations between 100,000 and a million sustain a further 1.5 million.[3] At that rate, urban India in 2011 had at least 3.5 million people handling waste every day, and these calculations do not include the manual scavengers who clean the dry latrines described in Chapter 3.

The way people who collect waste derive their income varies. Some are completely on their own—they find what they can in the streets, around rubbish dumps, and around the skips, or Dumpsters, at street corners of towns and cities. They confront feral animals, (pigs, stray dogs, monkeys, and rats, to name a few), police, and better-resourced competitors for items of value. Better-off collectors may be full-time employees of local governments and enjoy some benefits, including regular wages (although often paid irregularly) and even ghetto-style housing. Other collectors may be employees of contractors who work for local governments or for recyclers.

As well as a hierarchy of employment conditions, there is a hierarchy of status. At the very bottom are the manual scavengers of human waste. They are mostly women; their male equivalents descend into India's sewers to unblock them and keep them flowing. "We," they say, "are the lowest of the low."[4] What is certain is that the foulest jobs are done by Dalits and very poor Muslims, and it would be rare indeed—although in India nothing is impossible—to find a higher-caste person working at any hands-on task in waste-picking.[5] The exceptions might be in the shopping malls built in the past twenty years where maintenance tasks may be carried out by uniformed staff. Scholar-activists have argued that the salaried work sometimes overcomes caste.[6] In terms of mobility, a few waste collectors may become *kabaadiwalas* themselves—able to assemble sufficient items of value and sell them at a profit to larger *kabaadiwalas* or to processors of plastic, paper, glass, or other materials.

Recyclers (*kabaadiwalas*), the third of our categories, buy items of value from householders, merchants, and waste-pickers and carry them to places where they are reborn. India's long-standing culture of frugality rests on at least three pillars. Certain systems of Hindu belief and practice celebrate asceticism and renunciation, and since the nineteenth-century, Hindu revivalists have emphasized the spirituality of India over the materialism of the West. During the nationalist movement, Mahatma Gandhi made spiritual characteristics key aspects of his program for national redemption. The rural life that characterized most of India until the 1990s meant that most people had little to throw away. And the controlled economy for the first forty years after independence produced few consumer goods. The door-to-door recycler can still be found in towns and cities, and many *kabaadiwalas* have gone far beyond hauling bags on a bicycle to become substantial middlemen of a kind Adam Minter, author of *Junkyard Planet,* would recognize at once.[7]

The last category we call facilitators—nongovernmental organizations or self-help groups, which thirty years ago were often called action groups.[8] India is rich with such organizations, usually run by educated, middle-class activists who aim to improve their environment by bringing skills and organization to disadvantaged workers. Such organizations are often at the center of stories of improvement in public sanitation. They suggest promising possibilities, if only. . . . If only the work of the best of them could be scaled up; if only they were capable of surviving the loss of a dynamic founder; if only governments interfered with them less; if only more powerful interests had not muscled in on activities they had made effective and profitable; if only some of them were less enthusiastic about purely market-based solutions.[9]

An examination of these categories of activity and people suggests rich possibilities for a cleaner India if the skills of the professionals, the networks of the recyclers, the energy of the NGOs, and the willing labor of the collectors could be synchronized. Coupled with advocacy networks and propaganda aimed at waste makers, such a combination has the potential to find ways to improve lives by vastly reducing what goes to waste.

Professionals

Drainage Problems of the East is a book that might have been an invention of P. G. Wodehouse, the sort of volume Lord Emsworth of Blandings Castle might have consulted in his researches into agriculture and pig rearing. In fact, however, *Drainage Problems* represents a landmark in Indian public sanitation on a par with the *Report . . . into the Sanitary State of the Army in India* (1863), the *Scavenging Conditions Enquiry Committee Report* (1960), the Solid Waste Management Rules (2000 and 2016), and the prime ministerial statement of 2014 that set out the program for Swachh Bharat, or Clean India.[10]

Engineers

C. C. James, the author of *Drainage Problems,* as well as four other books (*Oriental Drainage, Notes on Disposal of Sewage at the Matunga Leper Asylum, Notes on Sewage Disposal,* and *Further Notes on Sewage Disposal*), is the spiritual great-grandfather of the admirable men and women who bring science and good management to India's urgent problems of waste.[11] Born in 1861, James was educated as an engineer at a time when the struggle between "miasma-ists" and "infection-ists"—between those who believed that bad air transmitted disease and those who understood that germs caused disease—was being won by the germ walas. James arrived in India in 1887 to work for Indian Midland Railway, based in the princely state of Gwalior.[12] How he moved from railways to public sanitation is not clear, but his generation of civil engineers was the first that had no doubt about germ theory and the dangers from contamination of food and drink by polluted water.

Drainage Problems consolidated the knowledge of a new class of professionals—people responsible for applying scientific research to policies intended to improve health in tropical countries. These professionals came from varied backgrounds, including medicine, commerce, government bureaucracy, and engineering. But they were invariably trained professionals in one field or another. They emerged as an identifiable group as a result of urbanization in Europe and North America and discoveries of the relationship between dirt and disease. A medical doctor's research in New York City led to the formation of the American Public Health Association in 1874, and it was a drainage engineer, the legendary Colonel George Waring, "a pioneer in the field of sanitary engineering," who began to clean up New York with his uniformed White Wings in the 1890s.[13]

Technicians and administrators who work on waste usually distinguish between solid and liquid waste—garbage versus sewage. James, however, appreciated the connections between the two. Human excrement was just another biodegradable form, and it contained energy that could be used productively at the same time the repugnant material was made benign. *Notes on Disposal of Sewage at the Matunga Leper Asylum* describes biogas from human and animal excrement being used, for perhaps the first time, to generate electricity at Matunga in Mumbai.

These days the Matunga leper asylum has an outpatient clinic and more than a hundred inpatients. James is still remembered. Dr. Pandya, a long-time volunteer at Matunga, describes him as a visionary. But what drove his quest to turn waste into energy was the threat anxious neighbors posed to the leprosy hospital. "They were afraid that legal action would be mounted against the asylum," Dr. Pandya said,

> because they were permitting leper waste matter to flow into the neighboring fields and contaminate them. At the time, the *naalas* were open and they were afraid of infection. . . . C. C. James . . . had the idea of using the effluent and excreta for energy, and for fertilizing soil, and growing grass which they directly sold to the municipality for fodder and, some say, for flowers for the Taj Hotel. In the end the asylum even made profits.[14]

The technology that Matunga and James pioneered laid the groundwork for the biogas operations that provide one weapon in public sanitation efforts today.

Professional people who take up the causes of public sanitation and health often find they have to become advocates and event organizers. Making places clean needs investment and organization, but perhaps most of all it requires public awareness, which may need to be created.

It was true in James's time. He was a networker, keen to show off what modern engineering could achieve. He endeared himself to Mumbai's people of influence by building an artificial river for a carnival in aid of a women's hospital and persuaded the Bombay Municipal Corporation to spend a million rupees (Rs 10 lakhs) to build sewerage for three Bombay localities, including today's wealthy Malabar Hill.[15]

Students at one of India's best technical universities needed a research topic for their annual Engineer's Day in 2011. They nominated "plastic management in Ahmedabad," their home city. As their speakers, they invited two nonengineers, both of whom were graduates in commerce. One had been a deputy director of solid waste management for the Ahmedabad Municipal Corporation for more than fifteen years. There was significance in the choice of topic—plastic management—and of a nonengineer with as unglamorous a title as deputy director of solid waste management. Would-be engineers realized that plastics posed a growing challenge, and they looked for a speaker known for experience, authority, and conviction.[16]

Two years later, Jeffrey spent a day with the same deputy director. He was an appealing waste zealot whose day began early. He provided visitors with a formal briefing and polished PowerPoint presentation, followed by visits to local waste collection sites, a water treatment plant, and three waste-reclaiming operations. Of the latter, two were not being well run and not making money, but at the third the deputy director and Jeffrey were greeted by a young man in a sweaty T-shirt who looked like an ordinary worker. He had a slightly American accent and said to call him Sandy. He was an engineer. Sandy and the deputy director talked the same animated language about waste. "This," Sandy said, "is probably one of the only sectors where your raw material is free. You can run the industry only when you look at it as a proper industry and you look at waste as a raw material rather than looking at it as a complete waste. This is an ever-evolving process where every day there [are] changes." His company was based in Mumbai and had focused on real estate and labor recruitment for the Persian Gulf before making this foray into wealth from waste. Sandy had chanced on waste management and found satisfaction in using engineering skills to establish a profitable industry and contribute to more sustainable practices in his country. "For anybody who thinks about a generation ahead . . . ," he said, "landfill must come to a complete stop." The future lay in composting wet waste and turning combustible waste into refuse-derived fuel that could be sold to generate electricity. But it would take five years, the deputy director said later, for this site to make a profit.[17]

The dedicated municipal official and the ambitious entrepreneur are recognizable characters in the theater of Indian waste. Critics will say that for every official who understands the importance of the work, there are dozens of slackers who work only when it is necessary and extract bribes whenever they can. And for every idealistic entrepreneur, there are others who exploit their workers, cheat on their contracts, and evade the Solid Waste Management Rules with slippery impunity. Zealots and their methods can, however, change attitudes and practices.

Fifteen hundred kilometers (930 miles) south of Ahmedabad, the city of Bengaluru struggles to cope with a population of 11.5 million that had more than doubled in the fifteen years before 2016. One aspect of the local government's attempt to deal with the growing volume of waste was to establish seven substantial waste treatment centers around the perimeter of the city. The aim was to minimize transport costs, use wet waste to make compost, and to segregate recyclables and divert them for productive use, including refuse-derived fuel.

One of the plants was at Thippenahalli, about fifteen kilometers (nine miles) west of the city's center where eighteen acres, including an ancient dump, were walled off, permanent sheds erected, and heavy equipment installed to enable large-scale composting and preparation of refuse-derived fuel. The young engineer in charge of the site was called Prince. He was from Tirunelveli in Tamil Nadu but had trained in Coimbatore and now worked for the Coimbatore engineering firm that operated the new site.[18] He wore the uniform of young, hands-on technicians on new and ambitious waste sites—a dusty T-shirt. It was about eight thirty the morning Jeffrey arrived in the company of the nattily dressed zonal joint commissioner, an official of the municipal government.[19] The manager was an employee of the company contracted by the municipal corporation to operate the site, which had been open less than two months. Its eventual cost would be close to Rs 60 crores (about

$10 million). Prince spoke proudly about the hefty investment the local government had made to build the site and lined up his team of three dozen workers for a group photo.

The covered sheds prevented dust and smells from escaping to annoy neighbors and kept the rain off two-meter-high, twenty-meter-long (6.5-foot-high, 65-foot-long) windrows where biodegradable waste dried, decomposed, and became compost. The windrows were turned regularly to let contact with the air hasten the transformation of fruit skins and vegetable peelings into rich compost. The concrete floors captured and drained leachate, the fetid liquid that percolates from decaying material. Giant cylinders with fine-mesh filters shook the composted material to remove nonbiodegradable items and reduce each grain of compost to pinhead size, no single grain larger than four millimeters (one-sixteenth of an inch) in diameter. Unwelcome items, including coconut husks, mango stones, and renegade plastics, were ejected, and if they were combustible, they were shredded, compressed, baled, turned into refused-derived fuel, and sold to cement factories eighty kilometers (fifty miles) away.

"It's a little complicated," Prince said as he explained the connections necessary to make the plant work effectively. Sorting and segregating were essential. Inbound trucks were inspected and turned away if they contained large quantities of mixed waste—hard waste, such as plastics or batteries or metals, that would not break down. The likelihood, however, was that a truck with a rejected load, unless supervised, would simply dump its contents in the first vacant lot outside the treatment center. Segregation of waste was best done during the initial collection, ideally by householders cooperating with waste workers who collected door to door. But even when waste worker and householder did their parts, stories abounded of truck contractors, the next link in the chain, throwing carefully segregated waste all together and arriving at processing centers with a steaming stew of mixed-up garbage.[20]

Bloating cities like Bengaluru added another dimension. As they burst beyond their administrative boundaries, villages on their periphery became semiurban with poorly planned but eagerly sought after housing complexes built around them. Such villages became the neighbors of waste treatment plants. Desperate municipal officials, faced with growing

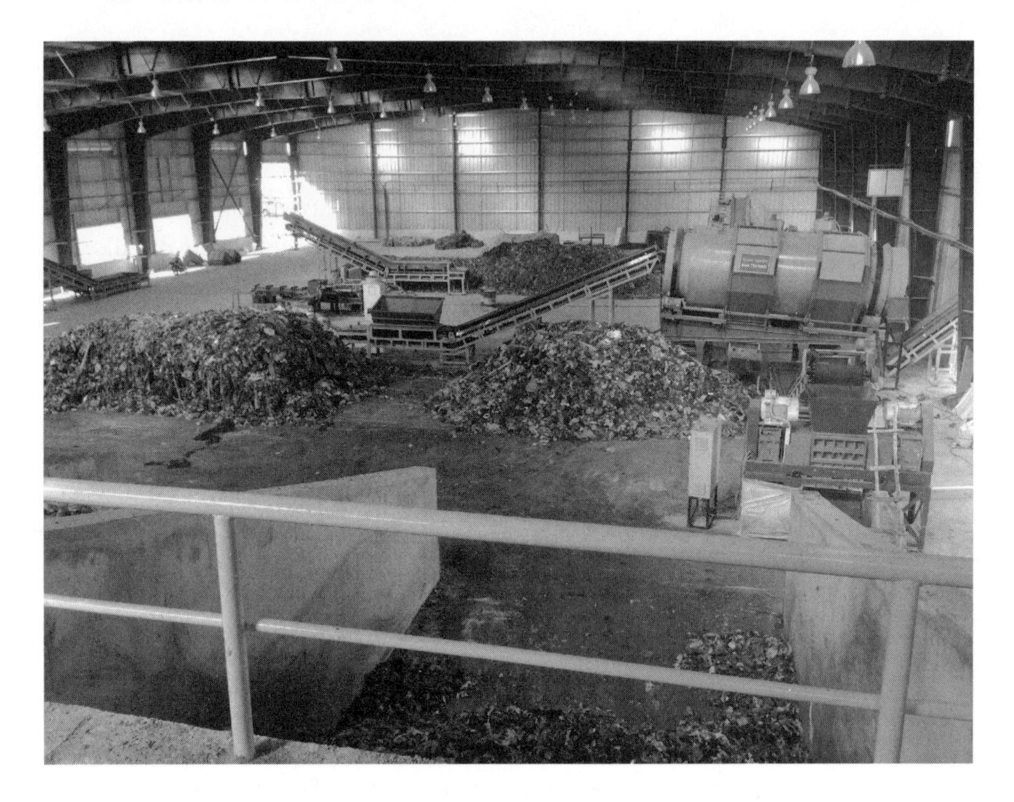

Fig. 7.1 **Roofed processing center for separating dry and wet waste and making compost and refuse-derived fuel at Thippenahalli, Bengaluru.** Photo © Robin Jeffrey, 2015.

daily waste collections and with fierce opposition from local people living near overflowing dumpsites, diverted truckloads of unsorted garbage to the new processing centers. When that happened, the new centers were swamped with unsorted mixed waste that had to be stored and then segregated for processing. These renegade accumulations produced smells, flies, mosquitoes, rodents, contaminated groundwater, and skies full of fugitive plastic bags. The failure to ensure that segregated waste stayed segregated contributed to a catastrophic attempt to set up a waste treatment plant outside Thiruvananthapuram in Kerala at a village called Vilappilsala. The plant became a sore that bled for fifteen years.[21] In Vilappilsala, villagers lamented that they cannot arrange marriages for their children. "No one is willing to move to this area, the flies, the smell,

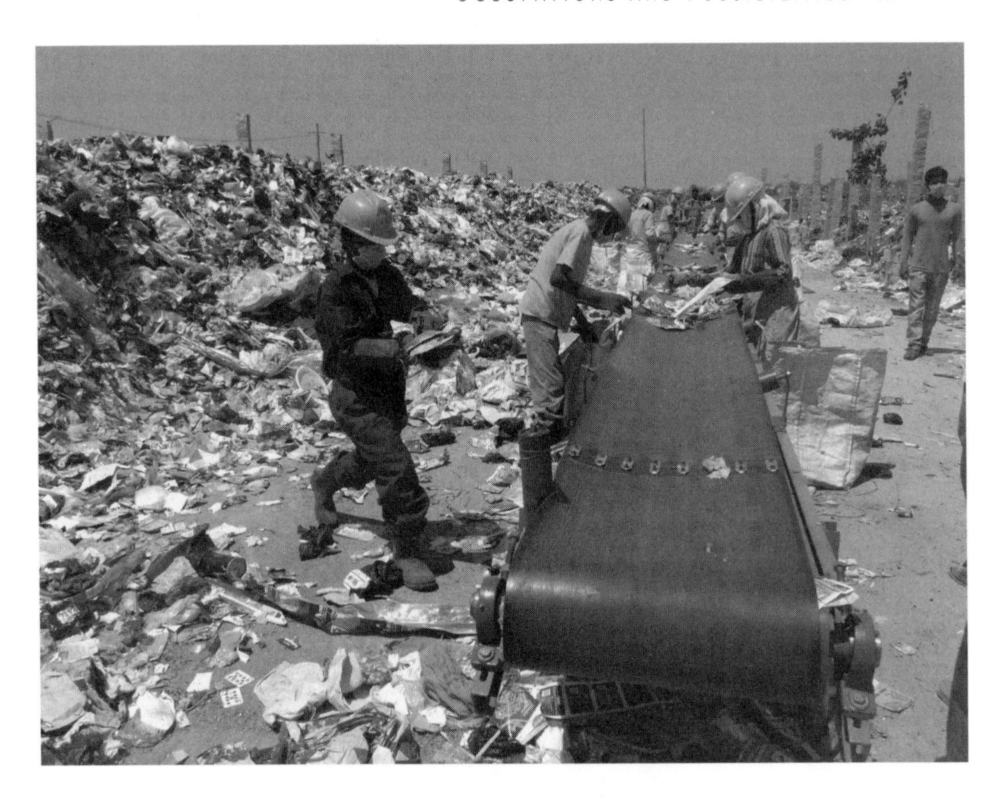

Fig. 7.2 **Extracting compost, refuse-derived fuel, plastic, metal, and paper from a neglected dumping ground in Raichur, Karnataka.** Photo © Robin Jeffrey, 2015.

the bad water," a villager told Doron when they went to view the defunct recycling plant. "The damage is done," he added, "and it will take time for things to go back to normal, even if the plant is now closed."[22]

At a smoothly working site, these side effects could be controlled, but this was impossible when a center was faced with huge quantities of mixed waste. Garbage generation does not take holidays. Waste piles up and becomes more noxious every day. In Bengaluru, waste treatment centers faced this problem of accumulating loads of unsuitable mixed waste. Nearby villagers, troubled by the detritus escaping from dozens of garbage trucks and worried by the arrival of crafty property developers looking to acquire cheap land, protested. "The contractors [running a new waste processing center] . . . should have taken the villagers into confidence," lamented a Bengaluru municipal official questioned about protests, "and shown them that the processing plant is safe and bad smell will not spread."[23] His forlorn remark—"should have taken the villagers into confidence"—underlined the relationships, cooperation, and person-to-person communication needed to make waste-management plans work.

Prince at Thippenahalli was an engineer, but during his time in Coimbatore, he had had to dabble in agricultural extension. Composting puts biodegradable materials back into the ecosystem and prevents wet waste from merely rotting in space-gobbling landfills. But there is no purpose in turning wet waste into compost if no one wants it, and a waste processing center does not have the space to store hundreds of bags of spurned compost. To farmers, the compost often seems both old-fashioned and, if it comes from a suspect waste processing center, newfangled. Farmers have bought chemical fertilizers at subsidized prices for years and are accustomed to its predictable results. "In Coimbatore," Prince said, "we conducted a program for the local farmers. We gave them the samples [of our compost]—forty kgs or a hundred kgs—free samples. They used it for a particular area of their farm, and the particular area got a very good growth compared to the other areas of their farm." He explained further: "We had to teach them. We had a particular five acres for demonstration [of types of crops grown around Coimbatore]. We only used our manure. . . . They come to know through practical things. Farmers . . . are open-minded now. More than 50 percent . . . turned to our manure."[24] Success required not merely well-funded and designed facilities but also the ability of professionals to take "the villagers into confidence."

The need for advocacy is inescapable. The compost produced in centers like the ones in Bengaluru has to compete with the chemical fertilizers subsidized since the 1960s as part of the green revolution. In some areas, peasants might once have been keen to tap the degradable waste of nearby towns. But those habits have slipped away and been replaced by harmful overuse of chemical fertilizer. Advocates of compost from waste processing centers argue that the price of chemical fertilizers should be raised and farmers required to buy natural compost along with the much-loved (and subsidized) chemical fertilizer.[25]

Administrators

Few engineers and executives looked forward to a career in garbage and sewers when they began their work. A number, however, found satisfaction wrestling with an urgent challenge. "In India," the municipal commissioner of Ahmedabad said in 2013, "none of our policy-makers . . . , not a single political system here, realize the gravity of the [waste] problem. . . . [It's] even worse than nuclear warfare [because] nuclear warfare is not likely at all. This is inevitable. After three years, Ahmedabad will have no place to dump."[26] In Surat in 2013, the executive engineer for drainage and solid waste management had been in the service of the local government for twenty-seven years. He had joined before the plague panic of 1994 and been part of the transformation of Surat from one of the dirtiest to one of the cleanest cities in India. His understanding of technologies for managing waste was coupled with detailed knowledge of his city and its waste workers at all levels.[27]

The potent combination for promoting public sanitation requires authority, resources, and motivation. Authority is necessary because change needs enforceable guidelines. Resources are necessary because waste does not magically disappear. Even humble householders wanting to compost wet waste at home need containers in which to do it. Most important of all is the motivation of those who see the possibilities for change and are able to communicate their awareness to the people they deal with. It is not difficult to find sleepy bureaucrats sitting in offices with "Waste Management" written on the door, but many had a prophet's passion even before the prime minister called for a Swachh Bharat in October 2014. Young employees of profit-making businesses were not the only ones to understand their role in improving the waste chain.

A former state-level official illustrated some of the possibilities. State government employees do not enjoy the status of the Indian Administrative Service, the elite national cadre. In towns and smaller cities, state government employees carry most of the administrative responsibility. They are also natives of that state.[28] The local language is their mother tongue, and they have grown up with the geography, customs, and relationships of their fellow citizens.

Khader Saheb, who advised on the cleanup in Raichur (Chapter 6), retired in 2013 as a joint director in the administrative service of the state government of Andhra Pradesh, which was divided into the states of Telangana and Andhra Pradesh in the following year. He had been a municipal commissioner for fourteen years, appointed by the state government as executive officer of small cities and towns around the state. He had, he said, always been interested in cleanliness and vowed, "I'd keep my town as [if it were] my house."[29] In 2002, he became municipal commissioner of Suryapet, now in Telangana, with a population of about a hundred thousand. Two years later, the city won a national award for cleanliness and adherence to the Solid Waste Management Rules.

In Suryapet, it was not money that made the difference. It was, according to Khader Saheb, "attitudinal change," In the past, the municipality's waste workers were not paid regularly, and when they were paid, the cash went to liquor or repayments to the moneylenders who had been tiding them over with loans. The new regime set up the workers with bank accounts. It started regular yoga classes. The municipal commissioner was on the street each morning at six to hold meetings and talk to residents while overseeing the daily door-to-door waste collection. "In history, no commissioner has moved into the streets in early morning," Khader Saheb said as he explained what he regarded as the recipe for cleaner towns and cities. "I used to wake them [the residents] up." The commissioner set a target: remedy residents' complaints the same day and report to them the following day. At eight o'clock, the commissioner or an assistant was in a school to give a five-minute talk on disposal of waste and why it was important. On Fridays, he induced imams in mosques to speak about waste disposal; on Sundays, he got clergy to speak in churches.[30]

On the streets, the commissioner and his subordinates encouraged householders to cooperate with waste collectors. When householders handed over unsegregated garbage, the workers segregated it in front of the householder and politely asked them to segregate it themselves in future. Within a few days, Khader Saheb claimed, 80 percent of householders in a street or colony would cooperate. Within three months, the system functioned effectively. Local artisans designed the three-wheel pushcart described in Chapter 5. Its tough wheels and sturdy, welded frame meant it was "a tool that will give no problem even in a year."[31]

Fourteen years later, and long after Khader Saheb had left, the Suryapet system survived. The town was ranked eighth in a survey of waste management conducted in 2016 by *Down to Earth,* India's leading environmental magazine. The town got high marks for waste collection and an appearance of cleanliness; however, the survey found that segregation and recycling had fallen off and were almost nonexistent.[32] "It's painful to realise," Khader Sahib told a reporter, "that they are now wasting their waste which was once composted religiously." It is a common story: effective practices are driven by individuals, not systems, and when the person leaves, practices falter.[33]

Because planning and enthusiasm can fade quickly, a sustainable system requires motivation—profit, discipline, need, pride, or some combination of the four. A notable event in the city of Warangal in 2012 illustrated the complexities, as well as the use, of attention-grabbing events to promote new attitudes and behavior. In Warangal, the Indian Premier League, a national cricket competition that generates immense interest, inspired the use of similar intercity rivalry to promote waste management in the towns of Telangana. At that time, Khader Saheb was a senior official in the Andhra Pradesh government. As a prophet of waste management on the lookout for consciousness-raising activities, he and others extracted government support for what came to be called the Clean Cities Championship. Hosted by the city of Warangal (population six hundred thousand), the weeklong event drew more than 380 teams from fifty-seven local governments in Telangana and was preceded by three weeks of announcements and preparation. Teams of four members collected and processed the daily waste of five hundred Warangal households for a week. The most effective teams won cash prizes of up to Rs 30,000 (about $600). Warangal gained national prominence as an example of relentless collection and processing.

Almitra Patel, a leading activist in the campaigns that led to the Solid Waste Management Rules of 2000, wrote a glowing report on Warangal's achievements, and at first glance, the Warangal story appeared entirely positive. However, as Prince, the engineer in Bengaluru, had said about making a plant work effectively, "It's a little complicated." There were losers in Warangal: informal ragpickers were left out. The eager competing teams collected all the solid waste and amassed large volumes of recyclable, saleable material—three hundred metric tons of it in seven days, according to Patel's report.[34] "I don't know what to do," one of the excluded waste-pickers told the journalist Keya Acharya. "No paper, no plastics and no money."[35] The organizers said the waste-pickers would be included in Warangal's future waste program as it developed. That was all very well, but freelance waste collectors live from day to day. Civic initiatives tend to overlook people who are barely considered citizens.

Ragpickers had unexpected sympathizers: employees and contractors who did quite well by the old system. Acharya wryly describes the scene "at Warangal's dry resources centre" during the Clean Cities Championship:

> The sanitary inspector on duty looked disgruntled at the plastics being baled. When asked for his view of the proceedings, his expression changed to disgust. "Too risky," he said, his distaste at his "new" job overriding his need for caution in front of an audience.
>
> An aide whispered snidely that the man had never had to work so hard before. "They come for work at 9:30 a.m. or so, sign their registers and leave for the day by 11:00 a.m.," complained the young aide. Elsewhere, a senior health officer was disgruntled at having to change old methods. Her comment that things would go back to "normal" once everyone left after a week reached her bosses' ears.[36]

Procedures often decayed quickly when people were transferred, resigned, or lost interest. In 2016, the pages of the Warangal Municipal Corporation's website devoted to cleanup had not been amended since 2012, the year of the championship.[37]

Municipal officials of big cities stressed the difference between smaller places and metropolises. Unrelenting door-to-door collections, local segregating of recyclables, neighborhood compost making, and constant awareness campaigns could not be sustained in great cities, they said.[38] In Hyderabad, officials also pointed to the contests between rival unions of city employees, who were spread across five trade unions and had interests they keenly protected. If one union signed an agreement, others would set out to sabotage it. In July 2015, a strike involving most of the unions stopped waste collection for more than a week.[39]

Companies

Indian companies also found the waste business "a little complicated." But three reasons drew a few of them to waste management. The first was obvious: profit. If companies elsewhere in the world made money from waste, then surely Indian companies would too, especially because in India there were few corporate competitors and a growing awareness that garbage needed managing. Second, the Companies Act of 2013 requires any company making a net profit of more than Rs 50 million a year to devote 2 percent of that profit to corporate social responsibility (CSR) via projects that benefit the community. Waste-related work may satisfy CSR criteria. Third, directors of a few companies had training that persuaded them of the importance of environmental sustainability and the benefits that expertise and investment can bring to waste management.

Long ago, ITC was the Imperial Tobacco Company. As global attitudes changed, "Imperial" became "Indian" in 1970 and then "Tobacco" faded away like the Cheshire cat in *Alice in Wonderland* and the "Fried" in KFC. The company became simply ITC in 1974. One of India's biggest companies, ITC still dominates India's tobacco industry but has diversified into hotels, fast-moving consumer goods, agriculture, information technology, and paper manufacture. ITC wanted to build a favorable reputation for its various brands and to leave the "T" in its name far behind. And it owned four paper mills with an enormous appetite for wastepaper. By 2014, ITC was spending more than Rs 100 crores (about $15 million) in its Wealth Out of Waste project to meet standards for CSR. A significant portion was invested in a project to reduce landfill, improve waste-pickers' incomes, and feed ITC's paper mills.

ITC's Wealth Out of Waste project illustrates not only the motivations of corporations and sympathetic executives but also the varied qualities they could bring to the waste chain. Jogarao Bhamidipati, the senior ITC executive in charge of the project in 2015, laid out the economic attractions for ITC. India's six hundred paper mills, he said, were producing twelve million metric tons of paper a year, half of it from recycled paper. In the past, *kabaadiwalas* had collected wastepaper from households and small businesses, but as the economy grew, so did the use of paper—by about 9 percent a year.[40] It was estimated that eight million metric tons of wastepaper was going to landfill at a time when India was importing four million metric tons of wastepaper from the United States and Europe as pulp for production of new paper.[41] The scope for more comprehensive recycling was immense.

Possibilities and potential benefits became clear. ITC surmised that if India's waste-pickers and small-scale *kabaadiwalas* were better organized and supported, they would capture more discarded paper, increase their incomes, and feed hungry paper mills. In 2007, ITC began a program in Coimbatore in Tamil Nadu where the company has a paper mill. The company first tried offering householders a small payment of about sixty rupees a month (about one dollar) to keep their paper for a monthly collection, but the reward was not enough to induce people to clutter small households with a month's worth of scrap paper. Waste-pickers, on the other hand, could collect more frequently and cover scores of households. More paper would be collected, and waste collectors would make more money.

ITC brought skills and advanced technology to waste collection. It had businesses in fast-moving consumer goods—candy, chocolates, school supplies, cosmetics. It knew how to introduce products to customers, conduct research, and run marketing campaigns. Working with the Coimbatore Municipal Corporation and NGOs, ITC followed a well-understood procedure for the launch of new products in India. "We engaged social-work [students] and college students who wanted some project work" and launched "door to door campaigning." ITC and its partners trained the temporary workers, linked them to local waste-pickers, and assigned each of them blocks of about 150 households and shops. The temporary employee and the regular waste collector went door to door, spoke to occupants, handed out free recycling bags, and explained that careful separation of different items and regular transfer to a waste collector would benefit the collector and help the country. "That," Bhamidipati said, "touches an emotional chord."

The scheme, renamed Waste to Well-Being, fitted neatly with the concept of decentralized processing of waste. The municipal corporations of Coimbatore and Bengaluru gave small parcels of land for local hubs where waste-pickers could sort and consolidate material and sell it in bulk to the recycling dealers who were the next link in the waste chain. On about a third of a hectare of land (about two-thirds the size of an American football field or four-fifths of an acre), an ideal hub provided showers and toilets, shelter from rain and sun, and regular payment to waste collectors. By 2015, the ITC program operated in a dozen municipal wards (out of 198 wards) in Bengaluru and 30 wards (out of 100) in Coimbatore. More than three thousand collectors were involved, and most of them now had bank accounts into which earnings were paid. ITC was getting inquiries from other organizations about how the program worked. "Every company has to spend 2 percent of profit on CSR," Bhamidipati explained. The model fitted well with ITC businesses and with the Swachh Bharat campaign—and 60 percent of the collection tended to be paper, which went directly to ITC's Coimbatore paper mill. The ITC efforts are significant not for what they say about the much-debated CSR legislation.[42] Rather, the ITC initiative highlights the organization, incentives, and sustained implementation needed to improve recycling rates and the lives of people who live from waste collecting.

The waste chain extends from the poorest worker searching for enough saleable waste to pay for a day's food to senior bureaucrats and private corporations. Elsewhere in the world, waste collection has become big business, with smaller contractors increasingly bought out. In India, however, the biggest corporate families, such as Ambani, Birla, Tata, and their rivals, are yet to enter the waste-management business, and foreign corporations show little enthusiasm. The French-based multinational Veolia has public-private partnerships in water management in Maharashtra and Karnataka but not in solid waste. The two American waste company giants, Waste Management and Republic Services, confine their operations to North America.[43]

Few other Indian corporations aspire to become rubbish rajas. A list of companies "involved in sewage and refuse disposal, sanitation and similar activities" in November 2017 totaled 791, most of which were small private companies. Only 82 were public companies, and even among these, only 65 were active. The list was inflated by inclusion of companies like the intriguingly named Regency Diaper Industries of Hyderabad, which was described as "under liquidation."[44] Corporate investment in waste management was modest. Three-quarters of the listed companies had paid-up capital of less than Rs 500,000 (about $8,000), and only eight had paid-up capital of more than Rs 25 crores (about $4 million). Of those eight, three were controlled by representatives of the Ramky Group, based in Hyderabad. Ramky is the corporate group most deeply involved in garbage and waste in India.[45] It asserts on its website that "Ramky Enviro Engineers Limited is Asia's leading provider of comprehensive environment management services."[46] The Ramky Group had other business interests. Why had it made a commitment to waste management?

Ramky executives lived at the top end of the waste chain. When the group's founder, Alla Ayodhya Rami Reddy, contested the Lok Sabha (lower house of Parliament) elections in 2014, he declared his family assets at Rs 648.7 crores (about $100 million).[47] With engineering degrees from two Indian universities, Rami Reddy began his career working for firms building water-treatment plants. He set up the first Ramky company in 1994.[48] M. S. Goutham Reddy, the chief of Ramky Enviro Engineers, has a master's degree in environmental engineering from the University of Nevada.

At the extremities of the waste chain, experiences were very different: dumpsite at one end, jetset at the other. Ramky has business interests in Singapore, and Ramky executives will fly from Singapore for a day's work, taking the night flight from Hyderabad and returning on the night flight from Singapore.[49] "We are still at a very nascent stage," Goutham Reddy said, explaining that, unlike Europe or North America, no one expected to make large profits from waste management in India. Rami Reddy

> always has been an environmentally oriented person. He worked, himself, in various companies, building effluent treatment plants, building water treatment plants. That was his orientation towards environmental infrastructure. He also built

> some landfills in the initial days. So that gave him initiation towards waste management and he started the concept of developing waste management in India.[50]

Goutham Reddy had worked with the Andhra Pradesh government's Environment Protection Training and Research Institute before taking jobs in private industry.

Both extremes of the waste chain view waste strategically. The wastepicker looks for ways to ensure future meals; executives and engineers think about technologies, government policies, and balance sheets. Explaining why foreign waste-management companies shied away from India, Goutham Reddy pointed to the complexities: "Lot[s] of things to manage. One is social-political. Two, you have the labor force involved. Then there is the technology. The tipping [dumping] fee. All of these have to be balanced. It is going to be some more time before these [foreign] companies can establish their footprint." He believed that the Solid Waste Management Rules of 2000 were unrealistic. "The law says source segregation is mandatory. Which country in the world has achieved it well? The best of the countries are perhaps able to get to 30 percent or 40 percent." Similarly, the rules called for door-to-door collection, elimination of poorly managed neighborhood skips, and transport of waste in covered vehicles. "Sixteen years after the law is framed, we don't have one good example" of a town or city meeting all the stipulations of the rules.[51]

Why, then, did some companies persevere when "in general the experience for most companies in municipal waste in India has not been great"? First, international experience indicated that waste could be profitable. When conditions changed, those already in the business would reap benefits. It was also possible to turn modest profits: "The margins are competitive but not very great. But [they are] still there."[52] Finally, some executives, as well as being driven by the demands of capitalism, judged that their companies and enterprises had solutions to some of the problems of public sanitation. For an organization whose leaders believe in the worthiness of the cause as well as the potential for profit, the top of a well-run landfill could be seen as high moral ground.

This was particularly true in the case of modern and deadly subcategories of waste—medical and hazardous, which pose a threat to people who have to deal with them. Until 1989, when the first specific legislation was passed, there was little recognition that some thrown-away things were more dangerous than others. To begin with, disposable medical equipment was unusual in India until the 1980s. Hypodermic needles were reused until they were too blunt to penetrate. If a patient visited a careful clinic, equipment was sterilized by boiling, sometimes in a saucepan over a kerosene burner. Bandages and similar hospital debris were thrown away or burned.

The rapid expansion of profit-driven private hospitals since the 1990s, a significant aspect of economic liberalization, rapidly accelerated the use of medical technology and disposable products in India.[53] Quantities of exotic-looking medical waste with valuable components like steel and plastic increased. In 1998, the Bio-Medical Waste (Management and Handling) Rules generated a need for specialized plants to handle such materials. Ramky's first venture, in 2000, into waste management was a medical waste center.

By 2016, India had 198 approved centers for disposal of medical waste to serve 169,000 hospitals and clinics, according to the central government.[54] These included some of the most sophisticated waste-management operations in the country, requiring investment, infrastructure, administration, and maintenance, qualities expected from doctors, executives, and engineers. Goutham Reddy believes that medical waste was dealt with more successfully than other categories: "At least we [India] are trying to meet [safely dispose of] 65 percent of medical waste."[55] That might have been optimistic. A national survey in 2009 found that 54 percent of main hospitals were not meeting the required standards. More than 80 percent of primary health centers failed to do so.[56]

The temptation to maximize returns from medical waste is substantial, for both hospital executives and old-style waste-pickers.[57] A case in Chennai highlighted the possibilities. The National Green Tribunal, set up in 2010 to expedite decisions on environmental cases, found twenty-one hospitals guilty of "gross violations" of the medical-waste rules.[58] The conduct in one hospital exemplified the complex questions of ownership, cost, and value. The hospital, which should have been *paying* an accredited agency thirty-nine rupees a kilogram to dispose of waste, was *selling* its waste to a freelance dealer for forty-nine rupees a kilogram. What would have been a thirty-nine-rupee cost became a gain of forty-nine rupees.[59] For waste-pickers at the bottom of the chain, medical waste was valuable and the dangers from cuts and disease, although known, were a scant deterrent.

Hazardous waste—materials that can harm people or the environment—is the other specialized category that grew with the economy starting in the 1990s and required special care from professionals. An inescapable by-product of mass production and economic growth, hazardous waste is costly to deal with safely, and producers are required to pay for its correct disposal. By 2015, the country was estimated to produce 7.5 million metric tons of hazardous waste a year from forty-four thousand industries. (The United States produced about five times as much.)[60] Goutham Reddy of Ramky estimated that "out of about 7 million metric tons of hazardous waste, we are probably managing [neutralizing] about a million metric tons as a country."[61]

A treatment center for hazardous waste reveals the complexity of dealing with toxic material. In 2015, the states of West Bengal and Sikkim in eastern India had only a single hazardous-waste-disposal center. Located near the city of Haldia on the western bank of the Hooghly River about 125 kilometers (78 miles) southwest of Kolkata, the plant was built by Ramky and began operating in 2006. Ramky's website states that the company was the largest processor of hazardous waste in India, with twelve centers handling 60 percent of "of the total industrial waste generated."[62]

Escorted around the Haldia precinct by Snehangshu Chakraborty, Ramky's coordinator for its eastern zone, Jeffrey was shown the record keeping, science, and technology required to meet legislative standards for neutralizing hazardous waste.[63] Brief visits do not demonstrate how sustained an operation may be, but they help explain what best practice might look like. The first step in safe processing of hazardous waste is to induce producers to take action that would cost them money. "In many places," Chakraborty said, "waste used to be dumped openly, and as a result it contaminated surface water bodies and in some places groundwater." He continued, "When it started, there was not much response from the industry in disposing of this waste, because the culture was not there. The culture was either [for] storing it or [for] dump[ing] it somewhere else." The government-owned Indian Oil Corporation brought the first waste to the Haldia plant on June 5, 2006. Chakraborty noted the date as a landmark. Other government-owned industries followed, along with a Japanese multinational and the Exide battery company. Awareness had to be built up by Ramky and the West Bengal Pollution Control Board. "Once [companies] found that, by paying a minimal amount, they are getting their premises clean," numbers increased, and by 2015 the Haldia site had 820 registered users from West Bengal and Sikkim and processed thirty-five thousand metric tons of waste a year.[64] But West Bengal had close to fourteen thousand registered industries and produced at least 5 percent of India's estimated seven million annual metric tons.[65] At that rate, the Haldia plant captured about 10 percent of West Bengal's hazardous waste.

Neutralizing the detritus of industrial mass production is complex and dangerous. As trucks come through the gates, samples of their cargoes are removed and analyzed. Within four hours (according to the rules), the cargo is assigned to appropriate processes to make it harmless. Scientists work in shifts in the plant's laboratory. Sludge from iron and steel industries could go directly to the sanitary landfill. Other substances could be treated to render them benign—a process called stabilization and chemical fixation—before being deposited in the landfill. High-combustion incineration using a U.S.-built Alstom incinerator is the third option for organic waste, leachates, and medical waste. This is not a waste-to-energy incinerator but one designed for handling hazardous waste. Ramky uses a similar incinerator at its hazardous waste plant in Mumbai.[66] The incinerator at Haldia got only about four thousand metric tons of material a year, not enough to keep it going around the clock, so it was fired up only when the quantities justified it.

"I am an environmentalist," Chakraborty said, explaining that as a student he had been admitted to a master's degree program in business administration, but his father, a schoolteacher, had said he should do something he could feel proud of, so, he said,

> I studied environmental management. I started my career in an NGO in Dehra Dun. There I was engaged in air pollution

> training in Dehra Dun city. Also water quality monitoring. Then I shifted from Dehra Dun to Bengal and worked in a water management company engaged in wastewater treatment plant construction . . . in Kolkata. And my third job was Ramky. I found it interesting, and for last nine and a half years I am with Ramky.
>
> From what I have seen in the last nine and a half years, the awareness level was zero when we started. But now people are much more—especially the young generation—they are much more aware about the importance of waste management. But there is a culture issue.[67]

Not every executive in the waste-management business matches Chakraborty's ability to talk feelingly about challenges and urgency. Nor do private corporations offer cure-all solutions to the problems of waste. But their successes and failures illustrate the need for investment, scientific application, and efficient administration—accompanied by motivated people, attitudinal change, and local flexibility—to tame the waste of an urban, industrializing society. Engineers, administrators, and executives are essential, but enduring improvements must include and reward the millions of people who cull livelihoods each day from the existing, unsatisfactory ways of managing waste. These are the handlers, the people at the bottom of the waste pyramid—socially and economically, the weakest link in the waste chain. Improvements in their lives will signal fundamental change in attitudes and practices related to waste.

Handlers

On the frontline of rubbish recovery are the people who collect waste. Scavengers, waste-pickers, ragpickers—by whatever name they are called, they carry a burden of poverty and prejudice. They are commonly regarded as dirty people, dislocated migrants, indifferent to basic hygiene. Their scavenging of open dumps is taken as an affront to social order and urban sanitation. And the fact that they work in places that were once regarded as no one's land, or the commons, but now are often claimed by the state or private owners makes them ready targets for police harassment. Little is mentioned about the effects of their work in reducing the amount of rubbish destined for landfills.

The most vulnerable scavengers work in grim conditions on mountainous landfills, such as Deonar in Mumbai, Okhla in Delhi, Dhapa in Kolkata, Kodungaiyur in Chennai, and less prominent dumps like Belgachia at Howrah in West Bengal. Estimates put scavengers' life expectancy at thirty-nine years.[68] In their search for defecation space and salvageable materials, adults and children have learned to tread lightly.[69] At Deonar "there are cracks and crevasses" that can trip, and even swallow, waste-pickers, Doron was told when he visited the smoldering mountain, "and kids inhale the toxic fumes" spewed by the mountain. In 2017, a landslide at another site, East Delhi's giant Ghazipur dump, killed two people.[70]

The usual competition on open dumpsites comes from rats, dogs, pigs, monkeys, and birds—all thriving on mixed rubbish. For ragpickers, sporadic fires generate an acrid haze that makes breathing difficult and presents the greatest health risk. Waste workers register high levels of tuberculosis.[71]

To extract value from the Deonar landfill, families and individuals are routinely confronted with an inventory of risks: economic exploitation, social stigma, ill health, harassment, and violence. Even when the landfill was on fire in early 2016, leaving many Mumbai residents gasping for breath, ragpickers were still scouring the dump, as a reporter observed:

> Kamble's first thought wasn't to escape the fire. In fact, both she and her husband ran towards it—desperate to salvage gunny sacks of glass, plastic and paper, which they had left at the dump the night before because no garbage truck was available to ferry them out. "All the stuff we had collected in the last few days got burned," said Kamble. . . . "We spent the morning sifting through it in the smoke."[72]

To try to understand the lives of people at the bottom of the waste pyramid, we have to ponder the pyramid itself and the paradox that

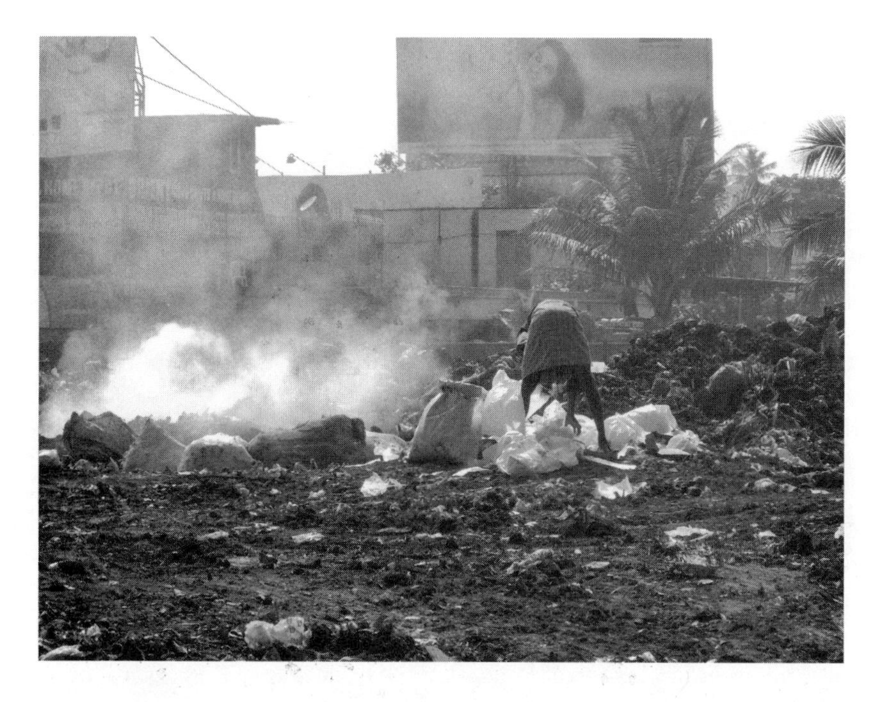

Fig. 7.3 **Overseen by an advertising billboard, a waste-picker collects recyclables at an open dump in Thiruvananthapuram.** Photo © Assa Doron, 2014.

underpins it. The paradox is that waste is mobile but people who collect it seldom are. Waste-pickers assemble items that can be hauled up a pyramid of value. But the men, women, and children at the bottom of the pyramid rarely have the chance to move to less hazardous and more rewarding work. The pyramid weighs down those at the bottom, who begin the whole process by handling waste in its most raw state. Hair gains value spectacularly as it moves from a gutter in the street to a factory in the city and to a wig in China or the United States, a journey that humble hair handlers cannot imagine. This mobility of things depends on the immobility of people and is compatible with a parallel pyramid-like structure—the caste system. At the top of the caste pyramid, upper-caste purity is maintained and reinforced by having those at the bottom, low castes and untouchables, available to perform unclean tasks. No doubt there are very poor people among higher castes, but few of them will be found among India's millions of waste-handlers.[73]

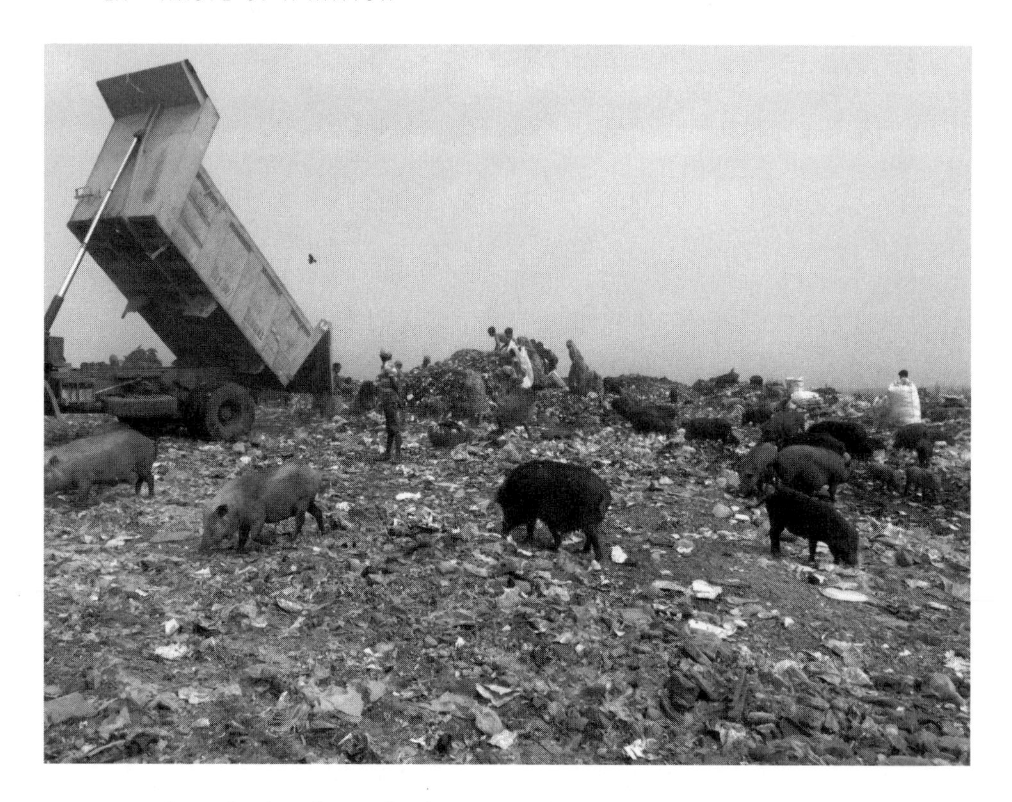

Fig. 7.4 **Rough recycling: people and pigs search the Belgachia dump in Howrah.** Photo © Robin Jeffrey, 2015.

Although they experience searing prejudice and discrimination because of their profession, waste handlers cannot afford to discriminate about the places they work or the materials they pick through.[74] They mine municipal bins (*dhalao*), open skips, and roadside rubbish. Some venture into restricted and more lucrative sources of waste in office buildings or shopping malls. At the bottom of the pyramid, courage and gumption are useful skills. Risks are high, and rewards are uncertain and unlikely to be large. The perils of waste-picking were summed up in report prepared by a Pune-based NGO with long experience: "Cuts and wounds, animal bites, chemical burns and inhalation of toxic gases, falls and traffic accidents, musculo-skeletal problems, sexual violence and mental trauma are all part of a waste picker's daily burden."[75] A scavenger's body often bears scars, and even small cuts can turn into long-lasting deformities or life-threatening infections.[76]

One of the biggest occupational threats for scavengers is the police—more threatening even than stray dogs. For the police, waste handlers are easy targets when arrests and scapegoats are necessary. They are seen as itinerants and almost-criminals. Even the more formal garbage men (*kuudewalas*) who do daily work for housing societies (also known as colonies, many of which lie behind gates and walls), local governments, or contractors are suspect and need to establish rapport with residents.[77] However, waste handlers have a significant advantage: they get the first and authorized access to good garbage, as well as occasional perks such as a monetary bonus from householders and shop owners at the time of festivals.

Santosh, now in his thirties, came to Delhi from Bihar. As a child he scavenged for waste from open dumps. Now he holds a more official role as a collector of rubbish from a relatively affluent neighborhood in Shivpuri, north Delhi. He explained,

> There are rules; you can't just go and pick garbage anywhere you want. In most places there is already someone who controlled the area [*ilaaqa*]. Or if you collect here, the police will chase you. So we work for Sushila, and she pays us 300 rupees per month for collecting the rubbish in this area from about forty-five households. The rubbish I collect I then sell to the *kabaadiwala* [dry scrap dealer], and on a good day I can get up to 250 rupees, so in a month earn about 9,000 to 10,000 rupees. In Diwali I usually get additional money from the people [householders].[78]

Santosh's job involved elaborate arrangements. Sushila, a local Dalit (a Balmiki), had had informal authority for collecting in the area for the past forty-five years. After Doron spoke to Santosh, she sold her territory to her daughter, Rani, and son-in-law for Rs 70,000. Rani mostly supervises the work and might collect rubbish occasionally, but she pays Santosh out of her income (which she did not specify but we can speculate as being roughly Rs 10,000 to 12,000 a month). Santosh was in effect her subcontractor but with no legal standing. He removed rubbish from about 230-odd houses, which were under the jurisdiction of three separate bosses, including Sushila (or Rani), and from which he earned Rs 1,500 a month for collecting rubbish. He then sold the valuable items from the daily collection, from which he averaged about Rs 250 a day.

Santosh worked with bare hands and carried the bags of mixed rubbish (*kuuda kachra*) to his pushcart (*redi* or *thela*). It was parked on the main road, where he sorted the rubbish for sale (*chhataai*). He dumped worthless rubbish at the local rubbish station (*kuuda khaana*), where small skips collected whatever residents and waste-pickers like Santosh dumped in them, or more often, around them. The skips were carted away by municipal employees to transfer stations, and the contents eventually would find their way to a landfill. Santosh and his family lived several kilometers away. His room had no running water or toilet; the rent was Rs 2,000 per month. Water cost another Rs 500. His family of four used the community toilet. "I've always worked in rubbish," he told Doron. "Since I was young I have worked in Delhi, and I'll grow old here. But doing this work gives me peace of mind; even though the earnings are meager, I prefer that to being a thief. Because if someone does something wrong (*galat kaam*), they will be scared twenty-four hours a day, someone can catch us or beat us up or even hit and kill us (*maar dega*)."[79] Santosh emphasized that he was trustworthy, never lied or committed crimes, and preferred the peaceful life of a hardworking waste collector. This was a common refrain among domestic workers, such as maids and garbage collectors, whose association with middle-class households meant they needed to reassure householders of their good character.

Waste handlers' status as social outcasts stems from a combination of circumstances. The majority are Dalits, poor Muslims, or migrants whose caste is uncertain and is therefore assumed to be inferior. They are assumed to have been born into a Dalit *jati*. Such assumptions are reinforced by the uncertain and irregular nature of their work, the sullied material they collect, and the dangers and encounters they face in collecting it. Waste is contaminating and contagious. A study of recycling in India found that even poor upper-caste recyclers were considered to be polluted by their work in transforming waste.[80] Mixed wet waste (*geela kachra*) is more ritually polluting and usually collected only by those who must—employees of local governments or contracted workers for governments or housing societies. Touching wet waste violated one's personhood and imperiled one's ritual and social status.[81]

Waste-pickers all over the world share some characteristics. "Waste work," writes Joshua Reno of a garbage dump in Michigan in the United States, "exposes people to bodily pollution, which they must learn to manage lest they bring traces of their occupation home with them." But Reno's colleagues on the landfill drove home in cars to comfortable houses, and their neighbors were not particularly concerned about how they earned their living.[82] No one suggested their jobs, their birth, or their "purity" were connected.

The most troubling and distasteful of the waste handling tasks that must be carried out to keep a city clean is maintenance of the sewers. This work is different from collecting excrement from dry latrines or cleaning septic tanks. It involves going underground to prevent or remove blockages that send backed-up raw sewage into the streets. This dangerous work requires elaborate equipment to do it safely. When the British writer Rose George was taken into the London sewers, she listed her wardrobe and the dangers:

> [I wore] overalls, with hood. Crotch-high waders. . . . A hard hat with a miner's light. . . . Rubber gloves. . . . Emergency breathing apparatus, . . . along with a backup battery. . . . A safety harness. . . . The hazards include bacteria and viruses such as hepatitis A, B, and C; rabies and typhoid; and leptospirosis . . . from rat urine. . . .
>
> There are also the gases. Methane, obviously. Hydrogen sulphide, known as sewer gas, which . . . kills by asphyxiation.[83]

George is cautioned to follow instructions carefully. "No one gets killed in my sewers," the boss of the gang tells her. "It causes a hell of a lot of paperwork."[84]

It was different in Varanasi when Doron met four men working to clear a blockage at the Bhelupur Crossing. They were contract workers, employed by a subcontractor of the state's Jal Nigam (water corporation). All were Dalits. Work, they said, was constant, but the pay was poor and often irregular, even though they were supposed to be paid daily. Before descending into the city's sewers, they needed alcohol to muster courage and block out revulsion.[85]

Their hard-learned knowledge of the system was invaluable, because Varanasi has no reliable map of its sewerage, which has been built piecemeal over a hundred years. A first stage had just been completed when the redoubtable C. C. James visited in 1906 and commented on the sewer lines having been "laid at a great depth in lanes which do not average more than six feet in width."[86] The greater the depth, the harder it is to get a sewer diver out if he encounters trouble from built-up gas, toxic material, or sudden flooding as a result of heavy rain or clearance of a blockage.[87] For local authorities, it is expedient to put sewerage work out to contractors who may in turn hire subcontractors who hire men like those Doron met. Responsibility is shifted to the bottom of the pyramid and away from officials of the local government.[88]

Doron's encounter with the four men was at midday with the temperature approaching 40°C (104°F). Sewage was gushing into the busy road crossing, and a large Jal Nigam tanker was parked on the roadside, having tried to clear the blockage with jets of high-pressure water. It didn't work. Using yellow police railings, the men fenced off the center of the intersection and removed a manhole cover. Vinod stripped to his loincloth. He was young and handsome and well aware that his lean, muscular body was on display amid the noon dust and traffic chaos. Before entering the narrow shaft, he wrapped a pink plastic bag on his head to ensure his neat mop of hair was protected. (See Figure 1.2.) His lifeline was a rope that his peers tied to a railing to help guide his descent. In less than a minute, he disappeared down the hole. His friends said he knew his way around the reeking underground labyrinth. He emerged twenty minutes later, smeared with sewage, and began reporting to the team about his expedition.

Similar groups of Dalits work for different contractors across Varanasi. None had the elaborate deep-sea-diver gear that Rose George wore in London or that Doron was later to be shown in Mumbai. They went into the sewer with no more than what Vinod wore: a plastic bag to keep the worst muck out of his hair. Employment conditions were hard. One of the group explained that although he had completed the tenth standard (year ten or grade ten) at school, he could not find any other work. His brother, who converted to Christianity, was more fortunate and had a job with the church; but then, he added, others who converted in their *basti* (hutment) were still jobless.

The situation in Mumbai in 2013 was similar. Dalits did sewage and sanitation work, and most worked as contract laborers. Some were direct employees of the Municipal Corporation of Greater Mumbai (Brihanmumbai Municipal Corporation), which provided accommodation for them and their families. But such employment was something of a trap, because promotion was impossible, even for the educated, and if a man quit his job, he lost the housing. The work was sometimes passed on from one generation to another.[89] Piyush Garud from the Tata Institute of Social Sciences interviewed sewage workers:

> The life expectancy of these workers is between 50 and 55 years. The profession is extremely hazardous and scavengers often suffer from respiratory diseases, gastrointestinal disorders and trachoma, a disease often resulting in blindness. Deaths due to tuberculosis (TB) are also common. On an average, 25 sanitation workers of the BMC [Brihanmumbai Municipal Corporation] die every year due to these illnesses. Liquor consumption among the workers is also high, owing to the inhuman conditions in which they are expected to work. . . . For most workers consuming alcohol makes them temporarily immune to their work conditions.[90]

Garud's article was accompanied by Sudharak Olwe's stark and distressing photographs of sewage divers and their work.[91]

By 2016, there was in Mumbai an awareness of how sewage workers *should* be equipped and supported. In the eastern suburbs, Doron was taken on a tour to view sewage equipment, including truck-based mud suckers and powerful jetting machines, and protective gear for workers. Despite the array of machinery used for the work, ordinary sanitary workers remained crucial to ensuring the operation of the network. The premises had an office with a sign—"Diving unit"—on the door. It was staffed by Dhasu Chandrakant, a diver, who showed the items he used in his work, including a full set of scuba-diving gear, recently purchased by the municipality. Only if mechanical methods failed, he explained, did he venture into the sewerage network. Before entering the shaft, he assessed the level of oxygen by lowering a lit candle. The civic body employed three divers, who worked in eight-hour shifts. All belonged to the fishermen Koli community. Their salary, he said, was about Rs 12,000 a month after deductions.[92]

Across India, however, casualties continue to rise. According to calculations of the Safai Karmachari Andolan, the organization fighting for the rights of manual scavengers, ninety people died in sewage lines in the first eight months of 2017 alone. A headline read, "It's Safer Being a Soldier Fighting in Kashmir Than a Sewer Worker. What Does That Say About India?"[93]

Stigma accompanies work with waste. Robin Nagle's striking book *Picking Up,* about the "san men"—sanitary workers—of New York City, devotes more than a dozen pages to discussion of the stigmatization they experience. Those experiences range from simply being rudely ignored to abuse: "Get away from here, you smelly garbage men." Nagle learns from one of the men that "after decades on the job, he still hasn't told the neighbors what he does for a living. His wife is happier that way. So is he."[94]

This may sound a little like the experience of waste handlers in India. But Nagle's informant also told her that the work has "let him build a life rich with social, educational and professional opportunities for his children."[95] Contrast that with Vinod, the Varanasi sewer diver, whose high school education did him no good, and consider the Mumbai sewer workers interviewed by Piyush Garud who hid their year twelve and post-high-school qualifications from the authorities for fear of being declared overqualified.[96] Attitudes related to caste inform everyday practice. The "menial tasks" dealing with waste are, asserts the sociologist P. S. Vivek, "so impure, profane, degraded and disgraceful in the eyes of the twice-born as to condemn them [waste handlers] as 'achhut' [untouchable]."[97] To be *achhuut* means that, unlike Nagle's New York san-man, chances of building "a life rich . . . with opportunities" are remote.

Waste handlers are essential in every society, and the millions who earn livings in this way represent a key component of India's best hope for building a healthy, sustainable future. And improvement in the conditions of waste handlers, and in the thoroughness of the work they do, will undermine ideas of caste. Better work requires predictable payment, recognized credentials, and appropriate equipment, including advanced machinery. All of these begin to give people dignity. The award-winning U.S. film *Fences* revolves around the character of a man who becomes the first African American to be allowed to drive a garbage truck in Pittsburgh. Bengaluru had a comparable (and real) moment in 2016 when it got its first woman waste-picker garbage-truck driver.[98]

Recyclers

Kabaadiwalas do not pick through piles of garbage. They are very different from waste handlers—higher in status, the next tier in the waste pyramid. Householders who have things to get rid of, and waste-pickers who have items of value, need a *kabaadiwala* to convert their holdings into cash.

Even a lone *kabaadiwala* needs knowledge, connections, and space—knowledge of the prices that the things he (or rarely she) buys will bring, connections with traders who will buy such commodities, and space to sort them and store them until he has sufficient volume to present to a scrap-trading business specializing in items like glass, paper, or metals. A *kabaadiwala*'s shop might be a tiny hole in the wall close to where he operates. Or it could be something larger in the *kabaadi* bazaar next to similar shops or in bazaars specializing in specific commodities such as metal, glass, paper, or plastic.

Relationships between *kabaadiwalas* and waste handlers vary. Some waste-pickers work as freelancers, and others have ties to a particular *kabaadiwala*.[99] Because *kabaadiwalas* pay cash, they can be a source of high-interest loans, which bind a waste-picker to work for them as they scratch a daily living. Economically, a *kabaadiwala* is better off and more secure than the waste-pickers they source their goods from.

Access to space is one of the key assets of *kabaadiwalas*. They require somewhere to store, sort, and prepare their acquisitions until they have assembled large enough volumes. Efficiency in moving materials up the chain is critical for a profitable turnover, as is knowledge of current prices for particular commodities.

The work presents its own challenges, especially given the increasingly complex range of waste materials that are characteristic of consumer society. To maximize returns, waste needs to be sorted into refined categories—glass by color, plastic by color or composition, metal by type, paper by quality, and so on. Such careful preparation makes for better prices at the next level. Larger *kabaadiwalas* employ very low-paid workers who strip insulation from copper wire, separate plastic bottle caps from plastic bottles, and perform similar tasks (see Figure 4.8 and all Chapter 7 figures). Hands-on labor adds value to the recyclables.

Storage spaces vary from large godowns to makeshift sheds. In 2015, on the main Mahatma Gandhi Road in Thiruvananthapuram one could find dealers whose shops were labeled *akri* or *akri kada,* meaning a "shop dealing in waste." More specialized shops dealt solely with one or two types of waste, such as cardboard or rubber from old tires. A dealer explained that "some [buyers] pick them [the tires] apart to extract the steel wires that make the insides of the tires. Then the rubber itself is recycled for all sort of things, from electric-box insulation to buckets, and even the inner tubes are used as improvised footwear for construction workers to protect themselves against the acidity in the lime and cement mix."[100] His was a small business, he added, but the bigger waste dealers sent thousands of tires to recycling plants in Tamil Nadu. To be renewed and gain value, waste has to move.

Movement

The routes that scrap travels are not always known even to scrap dealers, let alone scavengers. Devaraj, a small-scale scrap dealer on the outskirts of Thiruvananthapuram, knew only that his scrap was trucked to the neighboring state of Tamil Nadu, somewhere near the city of Coimbatore, where many recycling facilities operate. Indeed, news reports often decried Kerala's systematic dispatch of its waste to Tamil Nadu.[101] According to Devaraj, the main reason was that Tamil Nadu had more space for recycling factories.[102]

Devaraj himself was from Tamil Nadu and a Nadar—once regarded as a lower caste but today successful in business and other walks of life. He came to Kerala early in the first years of the twenty-first century from the district of Tuticorin, hoping to peddle garments from house to house on credit. But chasing creditors proved too difficult, and he followed his brother's advice and began a waste-trade business. His brother was already dealing in foreign waste in Tuticorin, a hub for waste and recycling in Tamil Nadu. Its port is notorious for smuggling waste into India, much of it hazardous waste from Western countries, often, he said, from Australia.[103]

During his door-to-door selling days, he noticed how much stuff people hoarded in their homes and the potential for the waste trade. From the outset, he realized that space and location were critical for running a waste business. His shop had a large roadside sign in Malayalam announcing "Raj Waste Paper Store" (Raaj Vesttu Peepar Stor). In fact, any type of waste was welcome if Devaraj could see value in it. Because newspapers are among the first things such shops collect, many dealers call themselves wastepaper traders, even if they also deal in metal, plastic, electronic waste, and other profitable items.

Devaraj rented his shop's two rooms at a cost of Rs 3,000 a month. His roadside shopfront meant that householders and business people could readily stop and sell their goods. Waste-pickers sold their daily collection to him regularly. Trucks found it easy to pick up the bundles of sorted goods destined for Tamil Nadu. Unlike similar scrap dealers in big cities, Devaraj had little competition and ready access to waste.

Devaraj did not have any long-term relationships with waste-pickers, although such relationships are common in some cities where waste work is enmeshed in social relations and local politics.[104] According to him, the fact that he paid well and did not cheat meant that waste-pickers, many of whom were semiliterate, trusted him. He therefore had a regular stream of material.

Several people came into the shop during the time Doron spent with Devaraj. They carried a variety of waste, including a car battery, stacks of newspapers, and a large sack full of plastic bags, brought by a boy. The items were assessed and weighed on the digital scales at the front for all to see, and payment was settled. When asked about what would happen to the car battery, Devaraj replied that it would be reconditioned. "Except your mind," he said, "everything can be reconditioned!"[105]

Devaraj's rented rooms were covered with asbestos sheets that stretched about a meter (thirty-nine inches) outward to protect the sacks and shield clients from biting sun and monsoon rain. Once the waste was processed, it was put into the concrete-floored storerooms. Bundles of newspapers were stacked high near one of the walls, and electronic goods and scrap metals were piled in another corner. Along a third wall lay gunnysacks full of beer bottles. The next room was filled with gunnysacks of different sizes holding varieties of plastic and glass. These were piled up in rows to await pickup that evening.

Sorting and separating were the essence of the trade. Devaraj did little of the sorting himself, something one could judge from his dress, trousers and an ironed shirt. As he explained, the waste-pickers themselves generally did the sorting when they brought their goods. "If I need to do the sorting, then I will pay less."

Devaraj's claim was confirmed soon after, when an old woman appeared from the roadside, carrying a large polypropylene sack on her head. Her silver hair was in a loose bun, and she wore a colored lower garment (*kayali*), a blouse, and a stained white shawl over her shoulder (*thorttu*), all of which suggested she belonged to a lower caste. When asked where she collected the goods, she smiled, revealing missing teeth, and replied that this was just a day's catch from the area. This was a lucky day, she said, because the bus driver agreed to let her on the bus with her sack and dropped her off not far from Devaraj's shop, so she did not need to walk far in the pounding heat.

She emptied the contents of her bag on the dirt floor that extended off the concrete slab, sat on the ground, and began sifting through the various types of junk. Some of it was tangled in plastic-coated copper wire, itself snarled within much longer strands of metal string. She shook the worst of the items and patiently disentangled them. All this was done bare-handed. The items were separated into three small piles: a bundle of wires, a small pile of scrap metal including a deodorant can and several tin boxes, and the largest pile, which contained plastics of all types, from bottles to Vaseline tubs, and various broken coverings and containers. Devaraj took the items and placed them on the digital scale, jotting down some letters, with the weight and price per kilogram. The woman said she was illiterate but trusted Devaraj's calculation. He handed her Rs 140.

A man in his midfifties arrived. He was pushing an extraordinary bicycle, stacked with sacks of junk and on top of which were tied two large plastic chairs. He was in a good mood; his eyes were bloodshot, and he seemed happily drunk. He wore a tucked-up *kayali* and a shirt. He carefully untied the ropes that held his treasure. One bag was full of school textbooks and old notebooks. Another had twenty plastic paint containers. A third held empty milk sachets. He had been doing this work for more than three decades, he said, and was accustomed to it. What he had collected was a record of the places he had visited over previous days, testimony to the knowledge that enabled him to gather such an array of goods. There was also miscellaneous scrap—a dozen cement sacks, aluminum whisky-bottle caps, a container filled with rusty bolts and nails, parts of a car's steering mechanism, two folded sheets of corrugated iron, and a heavy metal railing. Once all this was sorted and measured, he was given a receipt on a scrap of paper that detailed the value according to type and weight. He was paid the acceptable sum of Rs 619.50.

Devaraj had standard prices for various items, which were usually paid by the kilogram: paper (Rs 15), plastic (Rs 15), scrap metal (Rs 17), milk sachets (Rs 8), and jute, plastic sacks, and cement bags (Rs 1–3 per bag, depending on quality). Good cement bags fetched Rs 3 each. Beer bottles were Rs 1.5 per bottle. The price, Devaraj said, had recently dropped from Rs 4. Prices vary on the basis of the quality of the waste, the waste-picker's care in segregating it, and the demand for the product from higher up the waste pyramid.

In contrast to Devaraj's shop, which was characteristic of a small-scale *kabaadi* business, was a waste dealer that Doron stumbled across. It was one of the largest waste dealers in southern Kerala near the town of Varkala. Behind what appeared to be a small shopfront lay a world of used goods that eventually found their way up the waste pyramid to the recycling factories of Tamil Nadu. After entering the shop's narrow opening, a visitor could see a huge covered backyard, filled with junk of all kinds and divided roughly into processing zones. A constant hammering came from a man sitting on the ground and stripping the interior parts from a computer. He was surrounded by six or seven drums filled with different computer parts, including copper wire, plastic casings, nails, screws, and pieces of aluminum and other alloys. He marked his territory with two separators made of large metal washing-machine casings. Opposite him, two men waded through a sea of paper—magazines, newspapers, notebooks, books, and office documents. A mound of paper was slowly sliding toward them. Stacks of X-ray film were piled up in another area, ready to be sent to a factory to recover the silver content. Hanging on a metal pipe above all this were the workers' clean clothes, which they changed into after work.

Other zones in the shed held household appliances in various stages of dismantling, with about twenty men undoing, measuring, stacking, and packing. The uncovered area of the backyard was littered with scrap. Big items filled the yard: metal railings, appliances, a towering stack of plastic chairs, bicycle parts, and degraded water tanks. There were hundreds of large, tightly packed gunnysacks sewn up with nylon rope and awaiting dispatch. But to where?

Mr. Raman, the owner and manager, had been in the business for fifteen years and employed fifteen or twenty men on a regular basis. "Things have changed" he said. "We never used to take computers and TVs before, but now we can break them apart and sell those parts to a different place, like Madurai, for the alloys or plastics, and the metals to towns in the north of Kerala, especially Palakkad. We also buy motherboards for about thirty rupees per piece. The markup is five rupees per unit."[106] Mr. Raman's establishment seemed to trade in every conceivable piece of junk. He was a licensed waste trader, attested to by the tax books he showed Doron in his tiny office overlooking the road. He emphasized the importance of his location. His location in Varkala was a prime spot, he said. Although there were smaller junk traders all around the area and closer to the villages, his establishment paid the most for scrap. "Sometimes," he said, "I will pay twice as much for things like copper and paper, depending on the demand." The scale of his operation meant that he had a much higher turnover than smaller traders like Devaraj.

Mr. Raman's shop buzzed with activity, and his role was to deal with a caravan of people bringing waste for sale. Unlike Devaraj's smaller business, goods arrived by motorized transport, especially auto rickshaws. Mr. Raman explained that some of the sellers "are smaller scrap dealers," but many others were individual waste-pickers. They accumulated specific types of waste and, once they had enough, came to Raman to sell it.

Scrap flowed from various directions. A Bihari laborer loaded with sacks full of bottle caps came into the shop. He worked for one of the hotels near Varkala beach and collected the bottles left by affluent local and foreign drinkers. He fetched large rice sacks brimming with aluminum caps from bottles of domestic and imported hard liquor. Another was full of less profitable beer-bottle caps. Aluminum fetched seventy-five rupees a kilogram, but beer caps were worth only fifty-five rupees.[107] Mr. Raman explained that these caps would go to the town of Tirunelveli in Tamil Nadu for recycling.

Doron tried to trace the bottle caps, but following the sorted waste to its destination in Tamil Nadu proved more challenging than anticipated. It was not so much the secrecy shrouding the industry but rather that waste traders often transport their waste on a truck that collects metal and paper from other traders and carries them to different destinations. With a name and vague address, Doron traveled eight hours to Tirunelveli in Tamil Nadu in search of a recycling plant. To his surprise what he found were more than a dozen such plants, all located in one place—a walled industrial park officially referred to as an industrial estate.

Rebirth

The sign above the meter-high walls around the industrial estate read "6 SIDCO Industrial Estate, Pettai." SIDCO is the acronym for Small Industry Development Corporation, a creation of the government of Tamil Nadu that promotes small industries. SIDCO provides "infrastructure facilities," "work sheds and developed plots," "guidance to entrepreneurs," and assistance in accessing raw materials and finding marketing opportunities.[108] Indeed, the key word was "entrepreneur": the centerpiece of the neoliberalism that has gripped India since the 1990s. "Enterprising citizens" needed only—it seemed—to take the initiative and embrace the opportunities afforded by state support to launch a successful small business. Rebirthing waste seemed to be precisely such a business.

These formal arrangements were intended as a public antidote to the common perception of small-scale recycling industries that typically operate unregulated in dark, overcrowded slums; hide waste work from the eyes of the state; and illegally procure utilities by, for example, tapping power lines and water pipes. In contrast, the industrial estate in Tirunelveli looked nothing like a slum. Its spacious layout had well-paved roads, streetlights, and neat blocks of buildings lining the streets. These were legal structures set up to promote productivity and were supported by the state. Yet the streets were oddly empty: there was none of the usual bustle of vendors and passersby.

Signs indicated some of the activities that took place in the estate. One declared the presence of the Office of the District Environmental Engineer and the Tamil Nadu Pollution Control Board. Another specified the approved quantities for hazardous chemicals handled in the estate, such as nitric acid and sulfuric acid, as well as the quantities of hazardous and nonhazardous industrial waste products (liquid, solid, slurry, sludge) that could be discharged and how they were to be safely contained.

It was already two o'clock when Doron began exploring the estate. The emptiness was puzzling, and he began to doubt the location of the supposed recycling plants. A closer look, however, revealed that the estate was substantially involved in recycling. Piles of gunnysacks full of metal scrap lay outside high concrete walls, behind which were smoking chimneys and the drumming noise of furnaces.

There was no signage, it was difficult to judge where entrances might be, and Doron was able to enter a plant only after negotiating with a security guard. The interior contrasted sharply with the stillness outside. Dozens of workers, mostly women, sorted and hammered scrap metal on a dirt floor. The manager of the plant did not like the idea of a visitor and asked Doron and his friend to leave. Similar encounters followed throughout the day.

In the street, a uniformed worker emerged every so often. Men and women were covered in black dust, as if they had come out of a coal mine. After persistent inquiries about Sri Maharaja Industries, the name he had been given by one of the scrap dealers in Thiruvananthapuram, Doron found the place. The guard at the gate confirmed it was a recycling plant, but there were no signs. Knowing the scrap dealer in Thiruvananthapuram enabled Doron to gain entry, meet the manager, and see the small plant.

The noise from the furnaces made it impossible to talk, and the manager, Ganesh, led Doron to his office in the center of the plant. Glass walls muffled some of the noise. Ganesh described the recycling process and offered a tour, but cautioned Doron against straying from the path they would follow. Fumes immediately caught in the throat, and it was hard to breathe. The first section of the shed had several machines, one of which rolled sheets of silver metal. Another cut the sheets into round pieces suitable for the base of a large plate, or *thali*. A few women squatted beside the machines, sifting through scrap metal and discarded pots and pans.

In the foundry, the largest area of the shed, the sound of the furnace was bone shaking. Barefoot, shirtless, and gleaming with sweat, two men swirled a molten silver-colored concoction in huge vats heated over the furnaces. Every so often they drew out the molten metal in giant ladles and poured it into molds to make ingots. The furnaces were fired up every morning at four. The foundry men had no protective gear.[109]

Ganesh explained, "The scrap metal comes from aluminum and stainless steel materials. This is what we recycle here. And much of it is from Kerala because they don't have space for such plants." Doron's research assistant later suggested that it was equally likely that such plants did not exist in Kerala because the state had stronger regulations and labor unions than Tamil Nadu. In another section of the shed, aluminum bottle caps that once crowned liquor bottles were dumped into the bubbling metallic stew and slowly dissolved into silver liquid.

Back in his office, Ganesh explained the process: "First we have women who sort out the scrap, then we melt it and mold it into ingots, which are pressed to make the long metal sheets that are cut to round plate-like shapes." The final product lay in stacks: Frisbee-sized sheets of shiny silver metal. Packed in fifty-kilogram bundles, they were wrapped in jute bags ready for dispatch. "These go to another factory nearby which makes different utensils, mostly cups and plates," Ganesh said.

Ganesh was in his midthirties and originally from Chennai. He had arrived in Pettai at Tirunelveli about a year earlier, sent by the parent company to manage the plant for two years. The small plant employed twenty people, four of whom were women. They worked a six-day week from 8 a.m. to 4 p.m. for an average wage of Rs 200 per day, which included a lunch break. They received an extra Rs 20 an hour for working overtime. Overtime was common, because of the high demand for metals. The plant purchased the scrap for around Rs 120 a kilogram. Once processed, it could sell for Rs 180. Even after paying for electricity, fuel for the furnaces, salaries, and food for workers, Ganesh estimated his turnover of around a ton of aluminum a day made a daily profit of Rs 30,000 (roughly $600).

Sri Maharaja Industry is only one of many small to midsize recycling plants in Tirunelveli's Pettai. Similar small-scale processors of metal and plastic operate all over India. Jeffrey saw tiny plants remaking plastic in the Tiljala area of east Kolkata in 2015.[110] The ingots from Tirunelveli's Pettai probably contained scrap picked up by scavengers on the roads of Varkala, channeled up the pyramid to waste traders, eventually reaching the foundries in Tamil Nadu. Near the top of the reuse pyramid are large-scale aluminum and steel industries, usually hungry for scrap.

Waste collectors come in many sizes. At the high end of the scale are the ship-breaking companies of Alang that bid for waste—unwanted oceangoing ships—in a world market. At the low end are the lone, bicycle-riding, door-to-door *kabaadiwalas* whom every Indian born before 1995 is likely to remember. Somewhere in between is Sanjay, whom Doron met in the Varanasi metal market. Sanjay was an enterprising waste trader who relied partly on scavengers to source his scrap. But Sanjay also spent several hours a day sifting through the pages of *Auction News Journal* in search of materials being sold off by governments. Common items included transformers, air-conditioning units, vehicles of all kinds, office furniture, and an array of metals. On one occasion, he was preoccupied with dismantling a whole building—a police station built during the British period. At the site of the demolition, men from Bihar were pulling the building to pieces. "I resell everything," Sanjay explained, "from the cabinets and pipes inside to the bricks of the building, which are very good quality."[111]

Seasons

In some parts of India, local conditions produce larger quantities of valuable thrown-away things. Kerala on the southwestern coast became an international tourist destination in the 1990s, and the value of rubbish in tourist areas provides incentives for keeping such areas clean, tidy, and attractive for visitors. Kerala also has a high rate of literacy and active trade unions.[112] In such slightly more prosperous places, waste handlers can become part of a more rewarding recycling chain.

In Kerala, Doron chanced on a large clearing filled with garbage in the village where he was living near Kovalam beach. Amid the coconut and banana groves were piles of rubbish bags several meters high. At the center sat a team of women, emptying bags of undifferentiated rubbish and sorting it into categories—plastics, paper, glass, and so on. But this was not village rubbish. Villagers typically burned their nonbiodegradable rubbish every evening. (It was said the smoke drove away mosquitoes.) Rather, this was tourist refuse, and there was plenty of it.

The rubbish came from Kovalam beach, which had become a magnet for tourists from all over the world. In recent years, Russian tourists were among the most numerous. They arrived by chartered flights to escape the winter cold. Increasingly too, middle-class Indians frequented Kovalam. Tourists are itinerants, rely heavily on consumer goods, and leave large quantities of rubbish.

Teams of women were responsible for keeping Kovalam clean by collecting the valuable tourist waste. The teams had different tasks. Some were sent to collect rubbish strewn along the promenades and beaches. This was a punishing job, especially so because it was carried out in the heat of the day. They carried the bags to a collection point to be picked up by a small truck and taken to a sorting center, the village clearing Doron had seen, a few kilometers away. The sorting area was a self-contained rubbish depot, its boundaries were clear, and odor and leakage were tightly regulated. What arrived here was rubbish that was going somewhere—waste on the move. The place relied on three key elements: containment (to avoid being a nuisance to neighbors), movement (to get it quickly to the next link in the chain or tier in the pyramid), and profitability (to realize a return as soon as possible). The site was orderly. Neighboring villagers, Doron was told, would not tolerate it otherwise. The women on the site said the waste was heading for "return making"—recycling. It was destined for Tamil Nadu, they said, although no one knew exactly where.[113]

This was seasonal work, a contract-based job, seven days a week; their pay was Rs 4,500 per month. "Rubbish never takes a break," said one woman, repeating a theme of waste workers all over the world. "We work every day, from eight to four, and if we don't come to work, the boss will not pay, and if you miss more than a day or two, you are likely to find yourself without a job when you get back." But there were also some concessions for workers, and during the day, the women got a tea break of half an hour and an hour for lunch. This was Kerala, and workers had rights, even when working for a government subcontractor. It was hot and humid, and the work involved carrying heavy bags and bare-handed sorting of their contents, which ranged from baby diapers and bottles to sodden newspapers, plastic food containers, and coconut shells. Among the dozen or so women who worked on the site regularly, all but two were lower-caste Hindus; those two were Christians, probably Latin Catholics or Protestants.

Usha, a woman in her early thirties, ran the operation for the contractor, who was awarded the contract by the tourist authority. She had been working there for more than eight years. According to Usha, the contractor convinced the villagers to lease him the land on the condition that it would be strictly regulated and that locals would be employed. However, no village women worked at the site. Some of the local men worked the night shift, but that was a different type of work. "Women should not work at night," exclaimed Usha. "That is when the men work." Such a division of labor aligned with the type of waste that the men were best qualified to deal with: mixed, wet waste, good for compost and biomethanation. The night shift also loaded the bags of sorted dry waste prepared by the women during the day onto the trucks that would take them to Tamil Nadu. But the main work during the night shift was the collection of the food scraps from the tourist restaurants and hotels along the Kovalam coastline.

Raju was one of the few men from the village who worked the night shift. It began about eight o'clock when Raju and his six or seven colleagues met at the junction leading to the tourist promenade. A truck with about forty crates waited for them. Each man picked up an empty crate, placed it on his head, and walked along the promenade before disappearing into one of the alleys leading to the backdoors of the restaurants. Minutes later he would reappear with a crate filled with food waste. Each crate could be as heavy as ten or fifteen kilograms (twenty-two or thirty-three pounds). Raju eased his way past the throngs of tourists and into the lanes. When he arrived at the backdoor of a restaurant, a kitchen hand, often a migrant from north India, quickly emptied buckets of slimy organic waste into the crate. The crate was now full of liquid and food waste, some of which began to drip through the cracks onto Raju's head and clothing. He was unfazed and professional and warned Doron not to slip in the winding alleys leading to the main thoroughfare near the truck. He unloaded the crate, picked up an empty, and continued the nightly run. The system seemed well tested, and the restaurant's food waste was always ready for collection. Each of the men did at least a dozen trips back and forth to the truck. When a section of hotels and restaurants was cleared, the truck moved to the next stretch.

The team drove up a hill and stopped at a large hotel. Here, however, the kitchen hand seemed unaware of the arrangement. The waste had been put into a large plastic bag, which tore when the contents began to be transferred to the crate. This was unacceptable to Raju and his colleagues. The team refused to pick up the waste, reprimanded the kitchen hand and hotel staff, and left them to deal with the mess. There were rules and a system, and they had to be maintained.

Four hours later, the truck was fully loaded. The team headed back to the "office," as they called it, located in a bungalow near Kovalam Junction. When they arrived, a smaller truck with Tamil Nadu license plates was already waiting to take delivery. The men quickly moved the crates from one truck to the other. The destination of the food waste was the piggeries on the other side of the border in Tamil Nadu.[114] This was a sensitive issue. Pigs that are fed on untreated waste, slops, can carry disease, and strict regulations in Kerala prohibited feeding slops to animals.[115] As the night came to a close, the men washed their feet and hands at a small tap outside the office and headed home.

The people who process the waste of Kerala's thriving tourist industry are poor, and most were born into groups with low social status. But Raju's example suggests that it is possible, as Robin Nagle's New York City san-man said he does, to extract some benefit and even dignity from the work if certain conditions are met. Confidence and an understanding of the purpose of the work are two conditions. The pickup team felt able to tell the restaurant staff to clean up their own mess when the improperly prepared bag fell apart. The driver of the team's truck said he worked "365 days, each day, every day. Waste does not wait for anyone!" When asked if he ever missed a day, he gestured to his nose, as if to show the bad smell that would result if he or his team missed a day's work. His salary of Rs 1,000 a night was markedly higher than that of the other men, but to encourage thrifty driving, he had to pay for the fuel himself. Each member of the pickup team earned Rs 275 for a four- or five-hour shift, almost twice as much as the women.

A reader might ask, Why discuss Raju's role as if he were a recycler, a *kabaadiwala*? He's a waste handler. It's a fair question and illustrates the limitations of attempts to put people into categories. But there is a reason. Raju and his team are an essential component of a systematic program of recycling that offers predictable incentives to everyone in the chain. Raju's team is informal in the sense that its members have no security and no enforceable contract, but they provide an efficient, skilled service. They know the geography of the Kovalam tourist areas, the characteristics of each restaurant, and the dangers and pitfalls of the job. They are committed to their work. Before Raju got married and was absent for a few weeks, every night for a week he trained his brother to fill in for him. No doubt this was to ensure he kept his job, but it was also, he said, because he had a responsibility to see that the work was done properly and on time.

India has the capacity to use existing foundations to build sustainable ways of dealing with waste. The *kabaadiwala* tradition—the custom of trading some forms of waste—is one of India's strengths in the struggle to tame the detritus of prosperous urban life. Having millions of people depend on processing waste for their livelihood can be an advantage, because human labor makes reuse and remaking of thrown-away things more effective. Visionary policy, however, will aim to make this moment fleeting and draw those who depend on waste into comprehensive systems that reward them adequately and ensure that their children can aspire *not* to become waste handlers.

Facilitators

Indian public life has another characteristic that offers promise. It lies in its thousands of NGOs, the various groups we refer to—imprecisely but conveniently—as facilitators. Many of those have turned their attention to dealing with waste. Their activities provide scattered examples of what can be done when the skills of collectors, recyclers, and professionals are synchronized. Governments can sometimes do this, but private citizens often do it better.

India's remarkable array of NGOs has some of the most promising models for containing mushrooming waste. Their activities show promise because they are usually local, and they try to connect individuals—waste handlers and waste makers—as citizens in common causes to improve the lives and environment of everyone. NGOs are invariably founded and led by educated, middle-class women and men, but the goal of the best of them is to empower people at the bottom of the waste pyramid.

In New Delhi railway station, Ajay was on his mobile, directing his team of waste-pickers to incoming trains and relevant platforms. He was one of three supervisors overseeing about fifty men at the station. As a train entered and passengers alighted with their baggage, about fifteen uniformed men with gunnysacks boarded Ajay's assigned coaches. Five minutes later they returned with bags full of litter. Ajay was already on a different call on his cell phone, a new one with a camera that helped him report irregularities and accidents. He directed men from a second team to another platform, where the Kolkata train was about to arrive. The first team disappeared to a shed to unload their haul for sorting and recycling.

Even amid the multitude of passengers that rushed through New Delhi station, Ajay's luminescent green polo shirt was easy to spot on the platform. He and his team wore shirts with the name of the

NGO—Chintan (Contemplation)—printed on the back. ID tags around their necks identified them as licensed workers of the station.

This official status was secured with the help of the Delhi-based Chintan, which began championing waste-pickers in the late 1990s. One of Chintan's stated goals is to align institutions, technologies, and policy to empower communities working with waste. As well as collaborating with people on the ground, Chintan researches and publishes reports on waste-related issues to try to influence policy and enhance awareness in the national capital.[116]

At New Delhi railway station, Chintan was working with Ajay and a member of the Safai Sena, "a registered group of wastepickers, doorstep waste collectors, itinerant and other small buyers . . . and junk dealers."[117] They engaged in a number of projects, including partnering with Indian Railways to clean the platforms and coaches at New Delhi's main railway station, as well as the stations of Old Delhi (Delhi Junction), Hazrat Nizamuddin, and Anand Vihar.

Ajay and his teams of waste-pickers at the railway stations were connected to wider networks of support that linked them to NGOs, government agencies, social movements, and international charity bodies. In trying to bring knowledge, confidence, and organization to some of the most deprived groups, these groups perform a role that the government finds almost impossible to fill. Governments look for straightforward solutions that emphasize technology, welcome public-private partnerships, and favor a limited number of formal partners who can sign contracts.

The "anti-politics machine" of development is a term coined by the anthropologist James Ferguson to describe a similar process in Lesotho in southern Africa. The depoliticizing thrust of development schemes, he argues, favors neutral expert knowledge and technical interventions while leaving structures of inequality unchanged.[118] In Indonesia, Tanya Li found that problem and solution were paired from the start in many development schemes. All too often, she argues, the diagnosis, prescriptions, and techniques fitted together, and complex social relations and political processes were "render[ed] technical." In other words, the manner in which the problem is defined is "intimately linked to the availability of a solution."[119] NGOs dealing with waste, on the other hand, often grow out of the complexity that exists on the ground where waste begins. At their most positive, they challenge purely technical solutions and prevent those who depend on waste from becoming more vulnerable to social and environmental risks and exploitation. At the same time, they help create more effective ways of managing waste in specific localities.

Back at New Delhi station, Ajay led the way to the waste and recycling shed and pointed to the large fenced area where the station kept its highly prized scrap. Inside, piles of discarded steel rails, wheels, axles, and stacks of old concrete sleepers (railroad ties) were securely stored to prevent theft. Railway scrap is big business, a far cry from the small-scale recycling facility that Ajay and his team managed. Their facility was a shed. Painted green, it stood out in the gray industrial setting. A large sign declared "Chintan Material Recovery Facility" in Devanagari script and had the international triangular recycling logo beside it. The shed was divided into rooms, each serving a different material—segregation of paper, metals, plastics, or glass. A plastic-shredding machine feasted off the mountain of PET bottles at the back of the shed. A whiteboard had a scorecard in Hindi recording the quantities of waste collected the previous day. For February 2, 2015, the collection was

- bottles, 170 kilograms
- paper (newspapers, magazines), 45 kilograms
- other paper (*raddi*), 65 kilograms
- cardboard, 40 kilograms
- Tetra Paks, 10 kilograms
- plastic, 14 kilograms
- aluminum bags and foil, 37 kilograms
- total rubbish from the platform, 575 kilograms

Several men and women delved through waste on a blue tarpaulin. The neat setting provided a playground for large rats that scurried in and out of the mounds of waste. The sorters ignored the rats, the rats ignored the sorters, and the segregation continued. The segregated waste, explained Ajay, would be taken to a larger facility outside the station for further sorting and from there for recycling.

Chintan billboards provide information in English. One describes the nature of Indian trash, emphasizing that most of it is biodegradable. Chintan boasts a small composting plant nearby and sells the compost to farmers. Another billboard notes the amount of waste collected every day in the capital: 8,500 metric tons. "Of this, 2,000 metric tons, or nearly 22% is recycled by waste-pickers and kabaris [*kabaadis*], the rest is sent to three polluting landfills or sent to waste-to-energy plants, which are costly and release toxic gases." The NGO was unimpressed with the technologies of waste management favored by municipal authorities. Another sign highlights the environmental benefits of recycling and states that "recycling means waste-pickers get jobs, their children go to school and the municipality saves money spent on disposal." The signs convey to visitors the value of the work carried out in the green shed.

Chintan's recycling shed is part of a wider project for achieving a degree of legibility—recognition that waste workers are uniquely qualified to collect, measure, codify, record, and trade in waste. The shed is also a symbol. It demonstrates a relationship between local knowledge and practice (what waste-pickers offer) and procedures endorsed by governments (what systematic policy demands). Founded in 1999, Chintan's mission is to connect waste-pickers, the state, and foreign donors and increase awareness of the value that waste workers bring to cities wallowing in waste.[120]

In New Delhi railway station, Ajay and his Chintan-trained team of workers were licensed and had privileged access to the station's rubbish. But they were not alone in vying for valuable railway trash. Young children rummaged in the dustbins, collected overlooked rubbish from the platforms, and sneaked into the carriages in search of leftovers. Other, adult waste collectors worked in an adjacent plot. Ajay emphasized that these men worked for contractors and were independent of Chintan. The contrast was revealing. These men had no uniforms or protective gear, and their plot looked like an open dump, similar to many found across India—fenced off by concrete slabs and exposed to the elements. Dogs lay among piles of rubbish, and a couple of men sifted through it bare-handed. "These guys," noted Ajay, "are not licensed like us; they did not go through a police check." Their contractor had a separate agreement to collect waste from the railways. These men, Ajay asserted, are worse off than his team, who had protection, recognition, and employment conditions secured through their membership in the Safai Sena in partnership with Chintan.

Employment security and recognition are rare for waste handlers. Many belong to marginalized groups, part of the vast pool of informal workers trying to eke out a living in the cities. Most live in huts cobbled together from rejected materials. They are commonly viewed as vagrants and criminals who use shady markets and dealers to sell goods they collect by questionable means. In Delhi, some are also foreigners—Bangladeshis—and this raises the question about the extent to which they can be legible and interact with the Indian state.[121] Many are indebted to waste traders from whom they take loans and seek protection. The founding director of Chintan, Bharati Chaturvedi explained,

> Most waste-pickers are illegal immigrants—Muslims, Bangladeshis—and they need protection, which is given to them by the *kabaadiwalas* whom they work for. The police are paid off by the *kabaadiwalas,* and it works well for them because the police are reluctant to chase every waste-picker they see in their area. . . . The police are excellent at mapping every vulnerable person in the colony for extracting money and favor. But the police are also under huge pressure to solve problems in their areas, especially theft. So they will go to the godown [the *kabaadi*'s shed] and ask the owner for suspects, which he is expected to deliver every so often for finger printing, etc. This is the way of criminalizing these waste-pickers.[122]

Waste-pickers also become "criminals" by foraging in municipal waste bins, which in legal terms are the sole preserve of the local government and its workers.[123] Unless payoffs are made, informal waste-pickers can be arrested. They are thus easy prey for periodic shakedowns. Chaturvedi explained, "We [Chintan] soon realized that we must break this kind of police domination." They helped waste collectors gain official recognition through the provision of ID cards. However, this could succeed only if the police on the ground were willing to cooperate. Chintan began a program of training police to understand the type of work involved in waste collection and to "stop pursuing, and humiliating waste-pickers, verbally or physically." Chaturvedi continued,

> We worked with the Paul Hamlin Foundation for five years, as well as lawyers like Prashant Bhushan and others, and devised training programs that we ran for years. . . . Eventually we managed to get the police to employ an orderly who would be responsible to oversee any violations, and as long as waste-pickers had some form of ID card that would identify them they would be fine. Waste-pickers often say that they are fine with this work, but they want to ensure that it is safe, legitimate, and secure; that it's a dignified job; and that they can give an education to their children.[124]

"Dignity is important," Chaturvedi said. "Waste-pickers often say that all manner of people abuse them; it's a kind of institutional abuse from householders and their domestic workers, who imbibe the values and biases of the middle-upper-class people." But the problem with official abuse by the police is that they can strip waste handlers of their only asset: rubbish. "Once the authorities seize their goods," Chaturvedi said, "they are helpless. . . . Many waste-pickers tell us that this is the worst, because waste work helps set them apart from mere beggars."

The nature of waste-picking is subject to market fluctuation and seasonal changes. Impoverished and stigmatized waste handlers damage their bodies through irregular hours, hazardous conditions, poor nutrition, and little medical aid. The almost inexhaustible supply of cheap labor has made it difficult for them to form rights-based organizations, such as trade unions.[125] It has often been NGOs that have sought to shield them from some of the risks. Various models of collaboration between grassroots organizations, waste workers, and the state have been tried. Some are more NGO driven, as with Chintan's activities, whereas others place greater emphasis on unionizing and mobilizing waste-pickers. The Pune-based Kagad Kach Patra Kashtakari Panchayat (KKPKP; Paper, Glass, and Metal Workers Organization), a trade union of waste-pickers and scrap buyers, is such an example.

The KKPKP's website is movingly written and provides a reminder of the costs of waste work across generations:

> We pick up what someone has discarded as having no value and give it value through our labour. Long ago in 1990, we were treated like the trash we collect. People would shoo us away like they would dogs. They would cover their noses when they passed us. It hurt. We were not sitting in garbage because we enjoyed it! We were there because we wanted the recyclables. We mostly worked alone, sometimes with friends who did not care too much about it either. Our mothers and grandmothers had done it before us. It was this work that brought us money to feed ourselves and our families, so we did it.
>
> One summer's day in 1993 all of us gathered in a hall to talk. We talked like we never had before, giving vent to our anger and frustration at the way we were treated like trash! That was the turning point for us. That day we decided to stand tall. That day we decided to walk with dignity on the road we had never travelled, as human beings. Kagad Kach Patra Kashtakari Panchayat KKPKP is our trade union. It brings together waste pickers, itinerant waste buyers, waste collectors and other informal recyclers. We recover, collect, categorise and sell scrap materials, such as corrugated board, paper, plastics, metals and glass for recycling. We also provide garbage collection, composting and related waste management services. Our members are self-employed workers.[126]

The union, often referred to as simply Kach, was founded to raise concern for waste-pickers and gain recognition for the types of activities they perform. It has helped waste-pickers get union-based loans, education, and health care.[127] The Pune waste worker organization aimed to make waste work compatible with the requirements of a city and to make workers' claims on valuable waste compatible with middle-class aspirations for an ordered urban setting.

Poornima Chikarmane and Laxmi Narayan recall how the waste workers' movement began in a small upper-class Pune neighborhood.[128]

The challenge that activists and waste-pickers faced was to convince residents about the benefits of segregating waste. For waste-pickers, segregated waste was a boon; it brought "better rates, reduced their hours of work and improved the actual physical conditions of their work."[129] Yet soon after this was achieved, waste-pickers were forced to contend with a local entrepreneur who promised the housing societies a rubbish-free environment. His pitch was attractive: "a doorstep garbage collection service [a motorized vehicle with two laborers] . . . for a fee" and the promise "to rid the area of garbage containers."[130] This appealed to an elite neighborhood, eager to purge anything unsightly, such as waste-pickers delving into wayside skips.

The waste-pickers resisted. Inspired by the celebrated environmental movement the Chipko Andolan, the tree-hugging protesters of the Himalayas, they protested.[131] Instead of embracing trees, as the women of the hills had done to protect their forests, the waste-pickers seized the rubbish bins:

> We protested, first appealing to the entrepreneur and then to the residents. "You are educated and you have capital, why don't you start some other business? We have been doing this for generations. We are not educated and have no money. As it is we live off what you throw. If you take this away what will we eat?" Finally, we did a *bin chipko andolan* [held on to the bins so that they could not be carted away]. The residents relented and discontinued the service, and the entrepreneur withdrew.[132]

A decade later, a study by the International Labour Organization affirmed the contribution of waste-pickers to cleaning the city. The study found that "collectively, scrap collectors salvaged 144 tons of recyclable scrap" each day.[133] Waste-pickers saved the municipal authorities millions of rupees a year by minimizing collection and transportation costs. Further calculations showed that, "by implication, each waste-picker contributed Rs 246 worth of unpaid labour per month to the municipality [and] that the annual contribution of the scrap trade to the total income generated in Pune was about Rs 185 million." Waste-pickers' activities proved environmentally beneficial too. Because less rubbish went to landfills, stress on "the natural resource base" was reduced through "the recycling of paper, plastic, glass, metal, etc."[134] Rather than being surplus labor whose presence polluted the city, waste-pickers made the city work better.

The unions and other civil society bodies, in collaboration with transnational organizations, convinced the authorities of the value of working with existing waste-pickers. Part of the union's success stemmed from its ability to connect with international organizations to promote the cause of waste-pickers. From among waste-pickers themselves, people emerged who were able to speak with feeling born of experience.[135] These women had the skill and confidence to take part in gatherings where women waste handlers from around the world told their stories and deliberated with fellow waste-pickers and advocacy groups.[136]

In Pune most waste-pickers are local Marathi speakers, unlike in New Delhi, where they come from poor states, such as Uttar Pradesh or Bihar; are illegal migrants from Bangladesh; or belong to various Dalit *jatis*.[137] Most are landless Dalits escaping the drought-prone Marathwada region of Maharashtra.[138] The majority are illiterate and have settled in the city to join the army of unskilled labor. Some are second- or even third-generation migrants. The irregularity of work in the informal sector has driven many to work in waste, which is seen as a relatively reliable source of income available for men, women, and children. Waste work, even if seasonally variable and stigmatized, offers marginalized groups possibilities for scratching a living. What distinguishes the KKPKP is its members' similar background—geographical, linguistic, economic, and social. This has advantages, because it means that they share problems they can mobilize around and do not have to overcome differences of language or status. This enables them to claim a modicum of dignity, occupational safety, and economic security. Women are at the forefront of the waste-picking sector.

Women who work in jobs that are totally unregulated experience intimidating difficulties. They earn less than men, even though men are often less reliable workers and contributors to family budgets. Men are prone to abusive behavior often associated with alcohol and gambling.[139] "The husband does not work," writes Bhasha Singh in her book about manual scavengers, "but drinks a lot and beats his wife relentlessly—it is the same story everywhere."[140] The sight of drunken male waste-pickers perpetuates the view that the poor contribute to their own deprivation by wasting their money. Women, even if they engage in hard and repellent labor, are culturally barred from the public drunkenness and brawling associated with men. Women are the primary carer of the household. They face additional disadvantages in waste work. They can be physically intimidated if there are contests over ownership of a particular source of fruitful waste, and they are more easily captured by police if accused of illegally foraging on a municipal dumpsite. When they need to relieve themselves in their workplace, they are more vulnerable to hazards and harassment, including animal bites and predatory men.

Advocacy groups working with women waste handlers attempt to lessen these physical and social dangers. This involves creating crèches and primary schools and providing facilities for small loans. Identification cards provide a little legitimacy, and sometimes gloves, masks, and suitable footwear are available. But these require a willingness to use them and funds to pay for them.

The KKPKP sought a place for waste-pickers in the public-private partnership enthusiasm that became a feature of public policy beginning in the 1990s. The union added "Pro-Poor" to its name and coined the term "Pro-Poor PPP" (PPPPP).[141] In practical terms this meant forming a cooperative, which the union launched in 2007, under the appealing acronym SWaCH (Solid Waste Collection and Handling)—which means "to clean, to cleanse" in Marathi and Hindi. It provided door-to-door collection services funded by user fees. After a successful pilot program, SWaCH signed a five-year agreement with the Pune Municipal Corporation, which at the time was led by a sympathetic commissioner.[142]

SWaCH trained and organized a network of waste-pickers to run a decentralized system "that would be directly accountable to service users as well as . . . comply with statutory and regulatory requirements."[143] Training was a challenge. It was critical that waste-pickers adjust to new routines, especially the fixed working hours demanded by door-to-door collection. The independence associated with waste work also had to be forfeited.[144] This independence, however, should not be glorified. Waste-pickers working on their own often have to work long days before they have enough waste to sell and buy food, and their independence is further curtailed by the demands of their buyers and their own indebtedness. SWaCH provided organization and a system that lone waste-pickers lacked. It set up an administrative structure of supervisors, who worked closely with waste-pickers, and ward and area coordinators, who oversaw wider operations. The organization also collaborated closely with the municipality. With 2,300 members, SWaCH created a waste-management system, primarily via door-to-door collection, that covered 60 to 70 percent of Pune, a city of five million people.

However, even when waste workers altered their habits to suit the demands of the municipality, they encountered difficulties. The habits of middle-class residents in the housing societies were more difficult to change, and the municipal corporation could be unreliable. Aparna Susarla, a SWaCH member, explains: “Households are supposed to be responsible for source segregation of wet and dry waste, but that rarely happens. So they expect SWaCH members to do it. There is also the issue of equipment and protective gear, which is supposed to be supplied by the PMC [Pune Municipal Corporation], but that's often not the case.”[145] There were occasions when the municipal corporation was unable to pay salaries. Similar disruptions occur in other municipalities around the country. In 2013, SWaCH had to cut its outreach and logistics operations by more than two-thirds when expected salaries did not come through. The cooperative continued its core activities but complained about “subsidizing” the local government.[146]

Organizing informal waste-pickers to the point where they can take on contract work is a strategy that has proved suitable in other parts of India. Exnora Green in Pammal near Chennai is an example, as we saw in Chapter 6. A major achievement of such organizations has been to persuade governments to recognize that organized waste-pickers can provide the sustained services that middle-class residents crave and the Solid Waste Management Rules require. However, success requires dedicated leadership and relentless maintenance. For waste-pickers, the benefits can be significant: regular work and payment, access to information and training, pathways to education for their children, and the dignity of recognition.

But creation of these systems has two other consequences. First, the waste business becomes increasingly attractive to contractors and businesses, which may seek contracts from local governments or housing colonies and squeeze out a workers' cooperative. Second, a successful cooperative such as SWaCH may become a closed shop, demanding exclusive access to waste and making it difficult for the poor newly arrived from the countryside to find a foothold.

Private contractors or businesses may try to show that they can do better than the NGO: introduce modern technology, work more cheaply, and do a more thorough job. The experience of a local government near Pune provides an example of the issues and complexity involved when a private contractor pushes out an NGO. Pimpri-Chinchwad Municipal Corporation, with a population in 2011 of 1.7 million, is northwest of Pune on the main road to Mumbai. SWaCH operated the municipality's waste collection. Under an agreement signed in 2010, the cooperative collected and segregated waste, composted wet waste, and sold items of value in the dry waste.[147] Its profits were distributed among members according to how much they collected and also according to their needs.

One of their main collection areas was in the industrial hub of Bhosari. In 2014 about forty women were engaged in waste work when Doron visited. They collected from new office buildings and IT companies and by going door to door of residences. They carried the dry waste to a sorting center under a Bhosari highway overpass, a location given to them by the municipality. The storage site was built specially for the purpose. Unlike other scrap sheds in the vicinity, it was the cooperative's space, and the women felt ownership of it, something no outsider could miss. The women of the cooperative ran the operation. This was in striking contrast to other recycling sheds nearby, where a boss lorded over his workers, many of whom were children.

The narrow entrance to the women's sorting center concealed several chambers beyond, all overflowing with various forms of scrap. A rattling table fan helped circulate air in the stuffy, low-ceilinged rooms. Rubbish bags of all sizes were stacked in heaps, some reaching the ceiling. A large digital scale stood near the open door. A woman sat at a table in the middle of the room, registering the weight and value of scrap and issued receipts. Sari-clad women were coming and going, carrying waste, pouring it out for segregation, and weighing it. Outside, several small trucks were loading waste to be taken to processors elsewhere.

The women in the center were all fee-paying members of Kach, most of whom had worked for the SWaCH co-op for several years. They operated in small teams, collecting waste from company offices or housing societies. They were issued laminated photo ID cards. Some wore Infosys cards that had "rag picker" printed on them. They were contracted by the multinational IT company to remove waste from its premises. They also carried pocket-sized brown notebooks issued by the union, on the back of which membership benefits were listed, including access to loans at reasonable rates and health care insurance. The notebooks carried a careful account, verified and stamped by the union organizer, of the volume of waste its owner had collected.

At the end of the working day more than thirty women congregated in the small rooms, sitting on a floor covered with a carpet of cardboard. They discussed issues of the day pertaining to their work and lives and finished the meeting with an upbeat song (in Marathi):

> Standing tall in front of caste and religious discrimination
> Let the breeze take me
> We play the ceremonial drum of our king
> The government of this country must answer our questions

Many of these "questions" were unanswered. The relationship between the authorities and SWaCH had been strained for some months because of the government's irregular payments and its awarding of waste-collection contracts to private contractors.

The strains were made clear when Doron visited Kavita, a SWaCH member, at her home and learned more about her life as a waste-picker. Kavita's house was in a slum built in the shadow of new housing societies, or gated communities, about forty-five minutes' drive from the scrap center. Kavita's neighbors worked in various domestic jobs, many in the housing societies. The slum colony accommodated various structures, from tent-like shelters made of tarpaulins and waste materials to more permanent shacks of corrugated iron. Some of the lanes

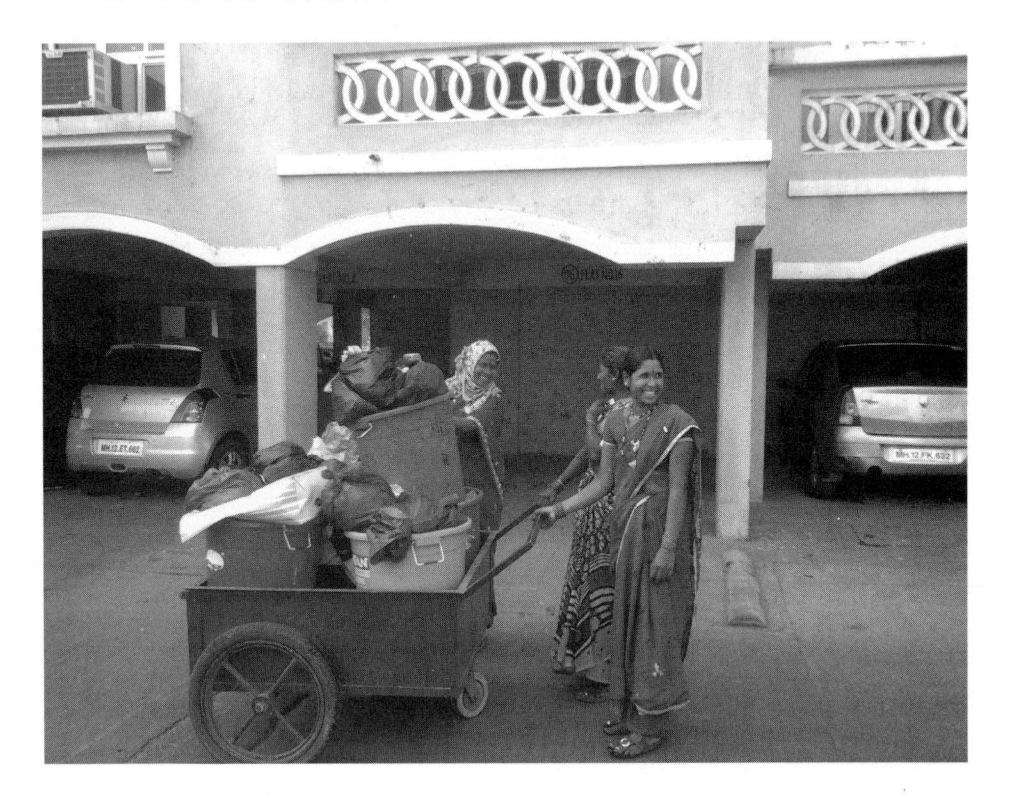

Fig. 7.5 **Orderly recycling: uniformed workers with a sorted load in Pune.** Photo © Assa Doron, 2014.

were paved, others were dirt, and the colony was encircled by vacant land and a patchwork of fences, marking the boundaries of housing societies.

The area was buzzing with activity throughout the day. In the early morning, the vacant land functioned as a toilet for residents of the slum, and for much of the day it served as a parking lot mostly for cars. By the afternoon, the area transformed into a venue for a brisk waste trade. "Many in this locality work in waste," explained Kavita, pointing to piles strewn everywhere.[148] This "wasteland" bordering the slum was anything but monotonous, wild, or unproductive, to invoke some of the terms often associated with such spaces.[149] Rather, economic and social activities went on under the direction of a trader who seemed to manage the interactions efficiently.

Seated in front of a wooden desk, amid piled up bags of scrap, the trader, a well-dressed man in an ironed long-sleeved white shirt, recorded the amounts and details of the scrap brought to him by waste-pickers, who waited patiently in a loosely formed queue. In front of his table, a large digital scale displayed the weight of the scrap as it was weighed. This was a cash-for-trash operation. He employed several locals to segregate and bundle the scrap for the trucks that carried it nightly to a processing destination.

Kavita knew waste work well. She had begun working as a waste-picker a decade earlier, after her husband lost two fingers in an accident at work. He received Rs 1,000 compensation and was fired. She was forced to go out to find employment. Her only option, she said, was scavenging. She explained what waste-picking had meant:

> In the past we had problems, just going around with sacks [*bora leke ghoomta tha*], and people used to throw stones at us, curse us, and set their dogs on us, because they thought we were going to steal something [*ye log chori karega*]. . . . We were in bad shape for ten to fifteen years, and struggled for so long that we thought our lives would never improve [*hum logo ka zindagi nahi sudhrega*]. But in the last three to four years, we have earned a lot. In the past, rich people [*bade-bade log*] would leave rotis on the road for the dogs to eat, and there was no difference between us and the dogs. We used to take those rotis to feed our own children.[150]

Four years earlier Kavita had joined the SWaCH co-op. She was introduced to the organization by Sangita, whom she affectionately referred to as madam. Sangita was an activist and a team member of SWaCH, and she worked with women waste handlers.

After joining the co-op, Kavita's fortunes improved. She was assigned several housing societies from which she collected waste daily. "At the time, madam operated a waste trade shop, just here close by, where we used to sell our dry waste." With the help of SWaCH, the family no longer lived in abject poverty. Like many other Dalit residents of that slum, Kavita and her family were recent converts to Christianity and

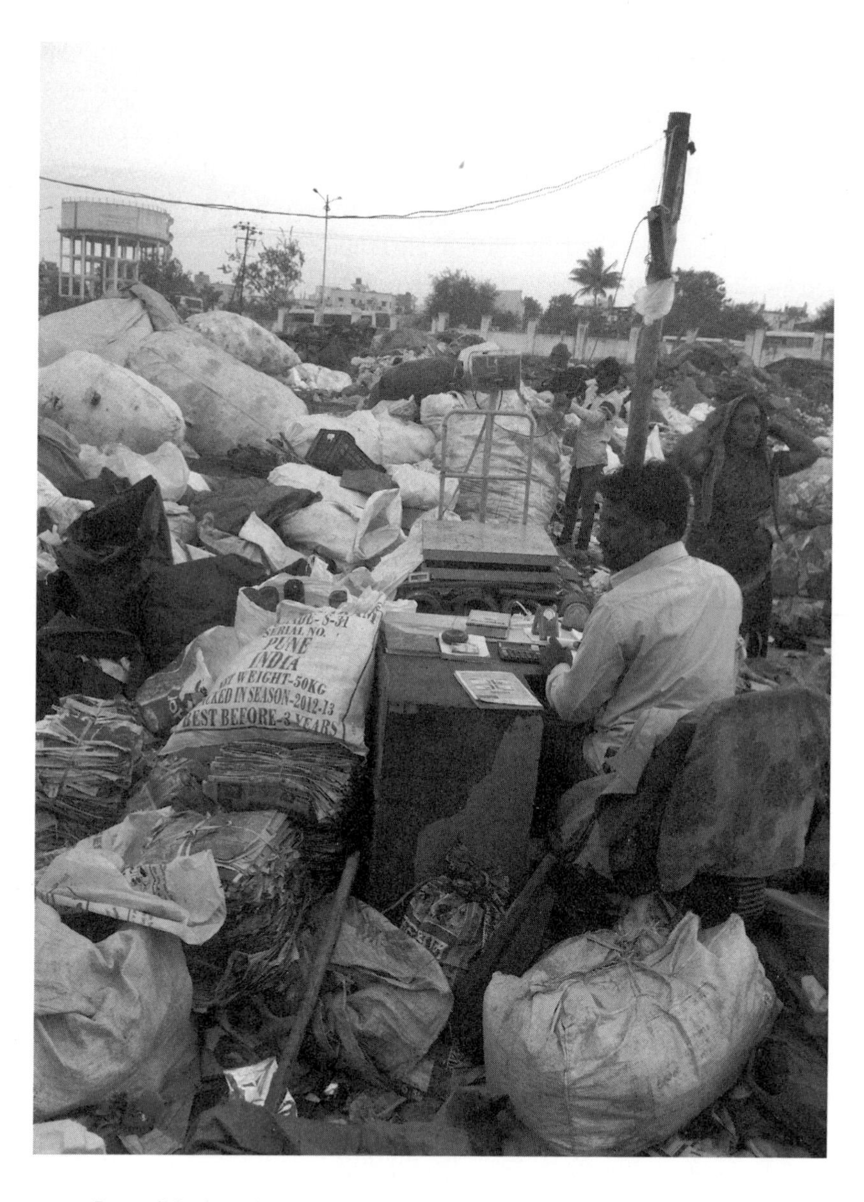

Fig. 7.6 ***Kabaadi*** **presides over payments and acquisitions in Pune.** Photo © Assa Doron, 2014.

went to church regularly. When the family fell on hard times, the church helped them with clothing and food. "But these days, we are doing well and do not require such help."

"Doing well" for Kavita and her family meant that they no longer lived in the same poverty as did many other residents of the slum. Kavita's one-room hut was built of corrugated-iron sheets and had a concrete floor. The interior was painted grassy green, and a large bed occupied a third of the space. The sidewall was fitted with a bench on which a single gas element stood, along with a couple of cupboards with stainless steel pots and utensils. The family had managed to save enough money for a small TV, secured in a glass-paneled cupboard. Recently, the family had installed a large ceiling fan. Nine people lived in this modest house, including three young children. The only signs of the residents were the layers of clothes hanging off the pipes that supported the corrugated-iron walls.

Most residents in the slum had access to electricity twenty-four hours a day, and water was available from a community tap. People went outside (*baahar*) to relieve themselves. There were some community toilets, explained Kavita, but after seeing them, one understood the preference for the outdoors. "If we wanted to have a toilet in our home, we would need to pay Rs 4,000 per month," explained Kavita. The monthly rent for her place was Rs 1,300. For Kavita, joining the co-op had been a boon, but things turned sour: "First, we were told not to segregate the waste . . . near the housing society because residents complained that it was dirty. Then madam's scrap shop was shut down because the government (*sarkaar*) refused to renew her contract." Soon after, the co-op also lost its waste-collection contract to a private contractor. To keep a job, Kavita worked for the new contractor, but the employment conditions were worse.

> When we worked for madam, the people in the housing society used to give us 500 to 600 rupees extra per month, but once the contract with madam was lost [*unka kaam gaya*], the society people don't even give us money for chai. Mahallakshmi [the contractor] tells us that we should just do the work and stop complaining or he'll fire us, and then our children will go

> hungry. He also asks us to do extra work and pick up the garbage on the street side. Now we have to do it with our bare hands, and we get injured because of blades, glass, injections [syringes], and other things. . . . We used to get boots, socks, and gloves from madam, but now we have no equipment and if we want boots we have to buy them ourselves.[151]

Under the new contractor, other benefits were withdrawn, such as increased salary during the monsoon season, holiday leave, and sick leave. "Now if we don't show up for work, he will fire us, or when we are late, we don't get a cart to carry our waste." Kavita continued to work for a daily wage of Rs 110, conducting door-to-door waste collection with her team across five housing societies with more than three thousand homes. The waste was trucked away by the contractors, and other waste-pickers removed what dry waste (largely plastics) they could salvage for sale.

Kavita continued to participate in SWaCH meetings, which she valued, and felt solidarity with the groups of waste-pickers. For waste-pickers like Kavita, job security, relative prosperity, and dignity are elusive goals, but ones that can be achieved with the support of organizations like Kach and SWaCH. Such rights-based associations illustrate the positive effects that institutional arrangements can produce to benefit the urban poor while satisfying middle-class visions of orderly, world-class cities.

Around India, similar organizations grow in ways that respond to distinctive local conditions. In Kolkata, an inquirer into waste and waste workers will find Tiljala Shed; in Thiruvananthapuram, Thanal; in New Delhi, the Safai Karmachari Andolan, Toxics Link, and Chintan; in Pune, the KKPKP; in Mumbai, the Stree Mukti Sanghatana; and in Chennai, Exnora Green.[152] Such a list is anything but exhaustive, but it emphasizes how widespread efforts are to improve public sanitation and the lives of people who live closest to the waste produced every day.

Such collaborative endeavors are difficult, however, to sustain. One explanation relates to the impatience of the growing middle-class and the pace of urban transformation. Cities such as Pune are typical of the surge in population growth over the last decade, largely from migration from nearby towns and rural areas.[153] Throughout India, local governments are called on to manage a rising tide of waste. Local governments, however, are underpowered; their elected councillors lack legal powers and often skills and knowledge; and their senior administrators are rarely in the same job long enough to master its details or take a long-term view. To these administrators, a contractor or a business promising to remove waste quickly and effectively looks to be an expedient way to show results. The alternative seems untidy: a motley array of laborers who are part of what many regard as the existing inefficient, unreliable, and messy informal sector. Local governments respond to well-resourced businesses and articulate householders who want their neighborhoods cleaned up and the urban poor controlled.[154]

NGOs and civil society groups attempt to revise the role of waste workers in the waste chain, alter power imbalances ever so slightly, and help a devalued group become a productive and useful workforce. In making the messy informal labor force of waste workers prominent or at least legible, advocacy groups seek to demonstrate that people who live off waste are a productive and inescapable part of India in the twenty-first century. They deserve protection and respect, and they have the potential to be part of comprehensive responses to India's confrontation with waste. Whether strategies that draw on existing waste workers will prevail over centralized, entrepreneurial models is hard to predict. One thing is sure: when waste has value, a host of powerful interests will be ready to climb on the waste wagon.

❦ ❦ ❦

The four categories of people we construct at the beginning of this chapter are artificial—heuristic devices useful for trying to order and understand the complications of India's confrontation with the detritus of consumer capitalism and growth. The individuals and organizations we focus on exemplify positive stories and modest achievements. It is easy enough to find lazy officials, grasping politicians, unscrupulous capitalists, hard-hearted *kabaadiwalas,* corrupt NGOs, and despicable waste handlers. But these are not where the possibilities for improving India's public sanitation lie.

Those possibilities draw their strength from India's advantages: a long-standing tradition of frugality that has been substantially eroded only for a generation; an existing capacity to extract value from thrown-away things; and large numbers of people eager for decent work who can power the meticulous collection, segregation, and reuse that must play a part in building a cleaner, sustainable, and tolerable society. Today's waste handlers require the organization and dignity that has been patchily achieved around India; they do not want their children to do what they have had to do.

The struggles with waste of course go far beyond households and businesses. They extend to sewage, construction and demolition debris, and hazardous and medical waste. But with all of these, trained and properly paid workers make possible more effective mitigation and reuse. Technology, legislation, and big investment alone are not enough. The possibilities for improvement lie in combining the talents of variously skilled people—professionals, waste handlers, recyclers, and committed facilitators. Where such combinations come together, improvements happen, but turning patchy examples into pervasive practice proves much harder.

CONCLUSION

THIS BOOK BEGAN WITH A QUESTION: "Why is India so filthy?" After reading the book, you may have your own answers. Perhaps you have decided it's the wrong question. "How" questions may be better: How can public sanitation be improved? How can large numbers of people be included? How do attitudes and practices change?

You may also ask, "Will this Clean India campaign work? Will Swachh Bharat succeed?" Much depends on what one means by succeed. In 2017, with the campaign in its third year, Narendra Modi's supporters cheered it and detractors derided it. When targets were met, they were trumpeted; when they were missed, the program was ridiculed. Modi himself warned that "if this [Clean India] is evaluated by a photo-opportunity, then we would be doing a disservice to the nation. We all must come together and do this wherever we can."[1] No previous prime ministers produced such a gallery of photographs of themselves sweeping streets—photographs flashed onto phones everywhere. The large commitment of funds and prime ministerial pressure, coupled with the popularity of "news" received everywhere on mobile phones and social media, meant the campaign's messages were heard, and sometimes acted on, by vast numbers of people in ways that were impossible in the past.

If the Swachh Bharat Mission is to succeed in creating a cleaner India by Gandhi's 150th birth anniversary in 2019, it will involve change to the physical landscape, public culture, and civic consciousness of the country. In what directions would such changes lead? One path might point toward a promised land of development under the banner of a Hindu nationalism aimed at purging India of its unruly elements, including filth. On such a road, there is little room for poor or marginal people, as the slum-clearance and family planning (*nasbandi*) fiascos of Indira Gandhi's 1975–1977 emergency illustrated.[2] A different path to a Swachh Bharat would combine practices of public hygiene with policies calibrated for local conditions and to foster cooperation. Such a Swachh Bharat would rely on a decentralized system endowing local government with powers and resources to ensure that local knowledge and customs informed policy and practice.

If Modi is the architect of Swachh Bharat, then the spirit of Gandhi is the muse. Gandhi's spectacles, the omnipresent logo for the campaign, lend moral force to cleanup projects across the country and telescope past glory into present-day efforts to create a clean nation. Gazing from posters, billboards, and newly minted bank notes, the spectacles inspire, survey, and supervise. (See Figure I.2.) As the master architect, Modi projects a version of Gandhi as an apolitical patron saint—the "Father of the Nation."[3] This vision is captured in the official Swachh Bharat pledge on the government of India website. "Mahatma Gandhi dreamt of an India which was not only free but also clean and developed. Mahatma Gandhi secured freedom for Mother India. Now it is our duty to serve Mother India by keeping the country neat and clean."[4] The Gandhian rhetoric encourages the diaspora, middle classes, and especially children and youth, to fulfill their destiny as model citizens of a future waste-free nation. The website proclaims that nearly two and a half million children and well over five thousand schools have taken the pledge. Members of the public can do so via Twitter and Facebook. Expressing loyalty to the nation, the pledge offers those who take it a sense of purpose and direction—to keep Mother India "neat and clean." The promises are explicit: "I will devote 100 hours per year, that is two hours per week, to voluntarily work for cleanliness. I will neither litter not let others litter. I will initiate the quest for cleanliness with myself, my family, my locality, my village and my work place." The guiding principles are reminiscent of Gandhi's way, an echo of the national struggle and of subsequent movements, sometimes inspired by popular films such as *Lage Raho Munna Bhai*.[5] Celebrating compassionate work carried out for the collective good, this technique of self-improvement provides a stirring call to arms to sweep the nation clean. The pledge continues, "I believe that the countries of the world that appear clean are so because their citizens don't indulge in littering nor do they allow it to happen."

This vision of a clean India highlights a neat, sanitized public space appealing to middle classes and the better-off. But it often excludes the poor. Public shaming of unfortunate transgressors of the Swachh Bharat vision suggest that there may be little tolerance of people unable to fit the description of dutiful citizens committed to the regimen of cleanliness and hygiene. The poor are marginalized not simply for ritual and economic reasons but as deficient citizens.

Civic consciousness and public spiritedness are difficult to imagine or practice for those who live precariously. People who lack secure shelter and workplaces regard public areas as spaces in which they have little investment. At its most threatening, public space is where they encounter police persecution, harassment, and humiliation as scavengers and random defecators. For them, the morally binding contract of the Clean India pledge, let alone its practical application, is meaningless, and they appear left outside the purview of the waste-free nation. Memories of previous slum clearance campaigns bring with them the anxiety that marginalized populations will be swept out of sight along with beggars and stray dogs. The Swachh Bharat campaign suggests a muscular brand of Hindu nationalism. Calls to protect "our mothers, sisters and daughters" from the indignities of open defecation insinuated a patriarchal guardianship (see Appendix). What might seem innocuous action by civil society groups, such as the movement generated by the Ugly Indian, the masked man in the Introduction who asked, "Why is India so filthy?" can lead to aggressive enforcement.[6] New rules imposed on cleaned-up urban spaces may exclude everyday activities of hawkers, peddlers, and street vendors, let alone waste-pickers. The goals of Swachh Bharat mean that governments and their servants are under pressure to produce results and declare yet another area open-defecation-free. Photographing villagers who defecate in the open (regardless of whether they can afford a latrine), blowing whistles like football referees to point out and shame such people, and even physically assaulting them became part of the Swachh Bharat story in 2017.[7]

Magnitude and caste pose challenges that are distinctively Indian, as we have suggested throughout the book. But in other respects, Indian experiences echo those of other places today and in the past. Urbanization, whether in Europe, North America, or Japan, has been ugly and brutal. Thousands of pigs roamed New York streets in the 1890s, and the contents of chamber pots were being thrown into the High Street in Edinburgh a hundred years ago.[8] Conditions in India's worst slums recall, but are no worse than, descriptions of Manchester, Chicago, or Hamburg in the nineteenth century.

In mitigating the effects of feebly regulated consumer capitalism, India can draw on some assets. It has the experience of 150 years of science, technology, and experiments in urban living and public sanitation from around the world. It has a thread in the tapestry of its cultures that commends asceticism, renunciation, and simplicity. Gandhi highlighted that thread during the nationalist movement with his own brand of *swaraj,* based on self-sufficient rural living. It is no accident that Gandhi's metal-rimmed spectacles became the insignia of the Clean India campaign.

There was, too, a time only a generation ago when the volume of waste from all forms of production in India was relatively small, and even in the cities, there was not a lot to throw away. The *kabaadi* tradition—of identifying unwanted things, keeping them, and selling them to a trader—is still alive, and the old *kabaadi* networks have enlarged and coped with new products like plastic and electronics. India's large population, often desperate for work, offers the bare-handed ability to deal more thoroughly and imaginatively with thrown-away things than mere machines can do. These attributes offer the possibility of setting examples of the ways thrown-away things can be captured, reworked, and reborn and the loops of mass production closed.

For each of India's advantages, there is a drawback. Economic growth generates more waste—the manufactured objects, the processes that create them, the packaging that contains them, and the vehicles that move them. The Indian government hopes that gross domestic product, propelled for the near future by pollution-spouting, coal-fired power plants, will grow by at least 7 percent a year over the ten years leading up to 2021. During the same period, India will add 140 million people to its population, even at a very modest growth rate of 1.017 percent a year. At the human level, 140 million additional people mean seven million metric tons of additional feces and 50,000 megaliters (13.2 billion gallons) more urine each year for the environment to account for.[9]

The Ganga and Yamuna Rivers choke on industrial effluent and human excrement. Other rivers, from Kerala to Odisha to Gujarat, are little better. India's capacity to husband its water supplies, whether from the Himalayas or the monsoons, is depleted. Older, more painstaking ways of harvesting and storing water are having to be rediscovered. Small-scale dams and careful irrigation of agriculture hold great promise but are used patchily across the country. Building and maintaining such catchments proves difficult.[10] Engineers, politicians, contractors, and some international agencies have a liking for big dams. Well-off farmers, accustomed to subsidized electricity and water rates, like to flood fields rather than drip feed crops.

India waits for a toilet as cheap, rewarding, and effective as a mobile phone. With today's toilet technology, a toilet alone is not enough, because even in expensive gated communities, beautiful toilets flush into septic tanks, which are often simply cesspits that have to be pumped out by honey-suckers. In theory, the honey-sucker should pay a fee to deliver its cargo to a sewage treatment plant, but that probably won't happen. Sewage treatment plants require large areas, reliable power supplies, and regular maintenance. New York needs fourteen such plants to serve a city of 8.5 million. In 2016, Mumbai had seven sewage treatment plants serving a population of 21 million.[11] The ideal stand-alone toilet will not need connection to a sewerage system. Nor will it need large quantities of water to keep it clean. It will be cheap, compact, easily installed, simple to use, and require no more maintenance than occasional removal of a container of an inoffensive substance, or even an agricultural fertilizer.

Technical and scientific discoveries since the nineteenth century have an important role to play in cleaning up India. But technology needs to be tailored for local circumstances. Big tech and high tech, such as multimillion-dollar complete-combustion incinerators, can be inappropriate white elephants. Effective technologies are sometimes small scale, as simple as providing well-designed equipment for people working with waste. The equipment list of small things is long, beginning with gloves and footwear that fit properly and feel right in India's diverse climates. Suitable equipment and the training to use it instill pride in the wearer and elicit respect from others. The safe costume for working in sewers looks like a space suit, and people who wear it have to be trained. It is not a pink plastic bag put over one's head to protect the hair. Similarly, driving a truck, running a honey-sucker, wearing a smart uniform, or using a well-balanced cart with smooth-moving, roller-blade-like wheels generates teaspoons of respect for the person who does the work.

The ready availability of workers to undertake painstaking recycling tasks may provide favorable opportunities for the containment of waste today, but it carries the depressing possibility that future generations could be condemned to similar work. Today, waste handling is a lifeline for millions. It sustains families and enables even the youngest members to contribute to income and day-to-day survival. But none of the waste handlers we spoke to wanted their children to continue in such work, not even those with government jobs. Why should they? Economies of recycling, as they now operate, reproduce social and economic inequalities.

Those handling waste in most parts of India face economic exploitation, social discrimination, and ill health. Variability of international prices for recyclables is compounded by the creation of the Goods and Services Tax (GST) in 2017, adding another dimension of uncertainty faced by waste pickers. The new tax meant that dealers and wholesalers of all types of recyclables were subject to a far higher tax bracket, which led to a drastic fall in prices, and severely affected ragpickers and their families.[12]

Any celebration of the resourcefulness and self-reliance of the poor lets the state off the hook. Minimal economic security does not remove social stigma. B. R. Ambedkar, the Dalit leader and writer and independent India's first Law Minister, concludes, "The sacred law of the Hindus lays down that a scavenger's progeny shall live by scavenging. Under

Hinduism scavenging was not a matter of choice, it was a matter of force."[13] Ambedkar saw the city as a liberating place, affording anonymity to low-status people who could then take on other occupations. But exclusion and prejudice continue to haunt the underclass of Indian cities.[14] Discrimination works in multiple ways, from spatial segregation to the denial of jobs, social services, and basic sanitation facilities. The drive to eliminate random defecation, a central component of the Clean India campaign, may produce significant results; but they will need to be measured in usage, social attitudes, and long-term public-health outcomes, not solely in achievement of targets for hole digging, cement pouring, and toilet building.

What promotes substantial change? In matters of public sanitation, a binding crisis can be the trigger. A binding crisis, as we suggested earlier, is an event, usually involving a natural disaster or a health panic, that brings a shared sense of menace to both rich and poor. To mitigate the effects in the present and prevent them in the future requires measures that must include the poor. If everyone is not protected, no one is safe is the implicit message widely felt among all classes. In Britain, the Great Stink of the river Thames in 1858, rising under the noses of members of Parliament at Westminster, provoked rapid building of sewers in London that eventually provided a model for British cities. Charles Rosenberg captured the essence of a binding crisis when he quoted in his book *The Cholera Years* a lofty editorial that appeared in New York's *Harper's Weekly* in 1866: "Not the poor and vicious classes alone will fall victims to the coming pestilence, for if the great cholera-fields that now invite epidemics . . . be not closed . . . the poisons which they will breed will infect and kill many persons among the more favoured class."[15] More than a hundred years later, the Surat plague panic of 1994 sent ripples around India at a time when the effects of economic liberalization were increasing the volume of consumer goods. The output of plastic grew, which pleased consumers in many ways but clogged drains and animal intestines and offended the eyes of genteel citizens. "Plague fear spurs BMC [Bombay Municipal Corporation] into garbage collection drive," ran a *Times of India* headline in October 1994. It reported that in Bombay, "facing a crisis," the efficiency of the administration "changed overnight."[16] A binding crisis tends to be localized—London,

New York, Hamburg, and Surat all had them—but the effects can be much wider and longer lasting. More than twenty years later, Sunita Narain, one of India's leading environmentalists and editor of the magazine *Down to Earth,* declared that "the only time urban India was shaken and stirred from its apathy towards filth was when plague hit the city of Surat."[17]

In the United States, citizens' fears about public sanitation led to wider concerns and action. "It was extremely important," the historian Martin Melosi writes, "that refuse came to be perceived as an environmental problem that threatened the entire community." Once this perception was fairly widely held, U.S. towns began to consider "collection and disposal as municipal responsibilities."[18] Confronted inescapably by accumulation of noxious rubbish, people began to see that multiple environmental problems were connected, and a greater sense of the importance of the environment grew.

India has two problems that have some characteristics of a binding crisis. Each offers the potential to heighten consciousness of the environment and provoke change in the actions of individuals and governments. Neither crisis, however, threatens the imminent peril, panic, or publicity of a plague epidemic.

The first is air pollution. Mumbai's notorious Deonar dump bubbles with methane gas that flames into small fires regularly. In January 2016, it grew into a major fire that made the city cough for days. It did it again ten months later.[19] This grotesque marriage of atmospheric pollution and a waste crisis emphasized the immense pressures on the wider environment. Ten Indian cities were in the world's top twenty worst cities for air pollution, according to a World Health Organization report in 2016. Delhi, whose air-pollution traumas gain notoriety because of its size and prominence, ranked number eleven, after the provincial cities of Gwalior, Allahabad, Patna, and Raipur (the capital of Chhattisgarh).[20] Air pollution has one essential characteristic of a binding crisis: it is democratic. It afflicts the rich (although rarely as much as the poor), and it forces itself on individuals by taking them by the throat. They cough, gasp, and sometimes die. Their bodies tell them there is a problem. In the longer term, air pollution leads to higher rates of lung afflictions and cancer. When Delhi was hit by especially high and persistent air pollution in two successive winters (2016–2018), the middle and upper classes, and even parliamentarians, suffered. They could buy air purifiers, wear masks, and ride in cars, but many of their children and they themselves still got sick.[21] There was wide agreement that something must be done.

A concerted campaign against air pollution would do little to help with the taming of garbage and sewage. Indeed, it could prove a distraction. Less than 5 percent of air pollution is estimated to come from the burning of garbage, even including the methane that Deonar and every other dump emit every day. Construction sites in expanding cities produce some of the dust that circulates in polluted air, along with coal-fired power plants and vastly increasing numbers of motor vehicles. The flat dry plains of north India have always produced clouds of dust at particular seasons, and these are now augmented by the effects of farmers burning crop stubble, which mechanized harvesting leaves in the fields.[22] Air pollution is an urban crisis that affects everyone. "Rich or poor," Sunita Narain wrote in 2017, "we live in our airshed."[23] But atmospheric pollution is not something that the poor can do much about. It's a binding crisis with the potential to awaken awareness of the environment and the uncritical use of fossil fuels, but it connects only indirectly with the pollution of land and water.

The other crisis that has potential to change behavior is the alarming level of childhood stunting and infant mortality, strongly related to open defecation. In the north Indian countryside, the children of better-off rural families appear to be as vulnerable to illness and stunting as those of the poor. Flies don't read bank statements, and unwashed fingers that feed children and that toddlers put into their own mouths can belong to rich and poor. Under the Clean India campaign, financial grants make it possible for large numbers of poor, rural people to build toilets, but motivation to use them—for health, convenience, or status—is lacking. If the wealthy were persuaded that building toilets and using them would make their children stronger and healthier, their example of toilet building and usage would increase the desirability of a toilet.

These are long-term changes that can spread only slowly into widespread patterns. Random defecation does not destroy people's dwellings or strike them down with boils and fevers (not, at least, in ways that obviously connect cause and effect). To make the connection between listless, undersized children and feces in fields and lanes requires the skills of imaginative advertisers using all the techniques of the mobile-phone world. And even if rural India had a toilet for every family, who will remove the compost from a pit latrine, and where would the contents of an overflowing septic tank go, and who would deal with it?

India has one further asset in attempts to tame waste—its proliferation of nongovernmental organizations, rights-based organizations, self-help groups, residents' associations, action groups, and the like. Unlike China and other parts of the world, in India such organizations are still allowed to exist and grow, independent of the state. Indeed, it is often the state's deficiencies that generate them. Among the forty thousand such groups that are registered, no doubt some are shady, created to benefit their organizers, as critics sometimes claim.[24] But a great many embody characteristics that make India the vibrant, adaptable place that it is. They often form out of local frustrations, but their reach and influence can be wide. Thanal, the NGO in Kerala, began as a movement to control pesticides and grew to become a vehicle for challenging government methods of managing waste and treating waste handlers. It is now credited with inspiring cleanup strategies in one of India's cleanest states, tiny Sikkim, high in the Himalayas, three thousand kilometers (1,864 miles) away from the steamy southwestern coast. Yishey Yongda, a bureaucrat in the Sikkim government and a public face for the state's sanitation achievements, tells interviewers that she was "introduced to the concept of zero waste by a pioneering non-profit in Kerala, Thanal."[25]

We have stressed throughout this book that important characteristics of waste in India in the twenty-first century are unprecedented but also that some features warrant comparison to other times and places. One of these relates to people. In summing up both the ugliness and the advances of public sanitation in Victorian times in Britain, Anthony Wohl writes, "Fortunately, men and women of compassion and sensitivity do not accept an undesirable *status quo* merely because prior conditions or conditions in other countries are worse."[26] India today shares this much with industrial Britain of long ago: people "of compassion and sensitivity" are to be found at all levels of society. They work in a political framework that still allows groups to organize, governments to be lobbied, and orthodoxy to be questioned. Conditions improve where coalitions—waste handlers, middle-class activists, professionals, officials, politicians—devise approaches to tackle the rising tide of waste.

Such virtuous circles form here and there around the country. It would be unduly optimistic to suggest that they were destined to expand and prosper. Economic liberalization since 1991 has encouraged capitalist activity that seeks to appropriate resources that once seemed available to anyone—such as vacant land and waste. A purely market-driven approach to waste absolves the state of responsibility and leaves many at the bottom of the waste chain to fend for themselves. Socially excluded groups, whether based on caste, ethnicity, or religion, already live in conditions that reinforce exclusion and discrimination.[27] That children of low-status people can be named Mallu (feces) and Kachra (rubbish) at birth underlines the challenges that confront a truly Clean India and Swachh Bharat. The pollution and disease accompanying the uncontrolled waste of an industrializing society ultimately belong to everyone, and as a garbage-truck driver in Kerala told Doron, "The problem with waste is that it doesn't wait for anyone."

APPENDIX

We approached the prime minister's office by email through Jagdish Takkar, public relations officer, with questions about the Swachh Bharat campaign. We received the following reply on March 20, 2017.

Prime Minister Narendra Modi's response to questions about Swachh Bharat submitted through his office

Received 20 March 2017

1. What was the Prime Minister's experience of the so-called "plague outbreak" in Gujarat, particularly Surat, in September and October 1994? Was the Prime Minister, as an RSS worker, part of relief activities? To what extent was the Surat "plague" experience of 1994 memorable for him personally? To what extent did his Surat experience shape his policies towards sanitation in Gujarat and India?

Though I was an RSS worker, I had already joined BJP by the time Surat Plague occurred. I joined BJP in 1988. During the so called Plague, when I reached Surat I found that people were fleeing Surat in large numbers. My first reaction was to stop this exodus and instil confidence in people to stay back and fight. I went around meeting people and encouraging them to stay and not to run away. I told them that there was no need to panic. I tried to remove fear from the minds of the people.

Before Surat incident, I had worked in the post-disaster relief activities as an RSS worker in the aftermath of 1978 Morbi floods in Gujarat. Due to Machhu II Dam breach, which is recorded as one of the worst dam bursts in the Guinness Book of World Records, the entire town of Morbi and the surrounding areas were submerged in water. When the water receded, the town was full of mud and swampy garbage. A huge cleaning up operation was undertaken and I was part of it. We all ensured that the town was restored to pre-disaster levels and an epidemic was averted. So, armed with this experience I motivated the people of Surat to fight back.

In Surat, I went with RSS workers to the places where more plague cases were reported, particularly in the areas where the poor lived. I tried to educate people about the preventive actions to be undertaken. I educated them not only about personal hygiene but also about social hygiene. The Plague incident was a game changer as far as Surat is concerned. People's sensitivity towards hygiene increased. The Municipal Corporation's decision making capacity improved. Encroachments were removed. The crisis was turned into an opportunity. Again in the year 2006 when there was a massive flood in Surat city, as the Chief Minister of the state, I launched a massive drive for post-flood cleaning of the city and prevented the outbreak of an epidemic.

But other cities and villages need not wait for a Surat like crisis. When I became the Chief Minister, I focused on improving the hygiene and sanitation practices in urban as well as rural areas. I declared the year 2005 as the Urban Year in Gujarat. Using this urban year concept, we improved urban sanitation and solid waste management. For the first time solid waste segregation and door to door collection was introduced in many urban areas. Construction of toilets in urban slums was undertaken through the involvement of Civil Society Organizations. In the year 2006, I launched a special mission to make Gujarat Clean and Green, known as the Nirmal Gujarat Mission.

The Nirmal Gujarat Mission aimed at the convergence of activities pertaining to environment and public health in nearly 25 government departments. Construction of toilets in both urban and rural areas, cleaning operations in government offices, disposal of office waste and condemned vehicles and furniture were undertaken. There was a special focus on the construction of toilets in schools, particularly for girls. I knew that one of the important reasons for girl children dropping out from schools was the lack of toilets. Hence, I allotted special funds for construction of toilet blocks in schools on a massive scale. In Gujarat, I launched two special drives to improve the enrolment of children in schools and to improve the quality of education called "Shala Pravesh Utsav" (School enrolment festival) and "Gunotsav" (Quality improvement festival) respectively. On these occasions, all the ministers including myself and senior government officers visited the schools. During these visits one of the key agenda was to inspect the toilets and drinking water facilities in the schools and submit reports.

In the year 2013, I launched Mahatma Gandhi Swachhatha Mission in Gujarat with view to construct toilets in all urban and rural areas to stop open defecation by the year 2019, the year in which India will be celebrating the 150th Birth Anniversary of Mahatma Gandhi. When I became the Prime Minister, I launched the Swachh Bharat. So, Swachh Bharat is the culmination of all the experience I had before I became the PM. It is not a scheme thought overnight, but my dream since my RSS Pracharak days.

2. What were the reasons that the Prime Minister chose to make Swachh Bharat a signature campaign of his new government? He had a remarkable parliamentary majority and striking support throughout the country. Why did he choose to make Swachh Bharat a prime focus?

I believe in focusing on the fundamentals. Only on a strong foundation can a huge building be built. Similarly, if we want to improve the standard of living of the poor, one of the basic things to focus on is improving the sanitation and hygiene practices across the country.

India is a young country with a favourable demographic dividend, and with the ambition and potential to become a global economic superpower. This cannot be achieved without the country achieving freedom from open defecation and unsanitary practices. Swachhata should be a way of life for all Indians.

Various studies have shown that open defecation and unsanitary practices are linked to several diseases, especially among children, which lead to high infant mortality and impairs the growth and development of children. Lack of sanitation is linked to high disease burden, and the bulk of this burden falls on the poor. Therefore, if my Government is dedicated to serving the poor, it is natural that it should place the highest emphasis on cleanliness, and sanitation for all.

Some studies have estimated that globally over 200,000 children die every year due to lack of adequate sanitation and handwashing, of which about 100,000 are in India. This translates to almost 300 children every day, a burden that India cannot carry on with. Other studies suggest that disease which can be linked directly to poor sanitation, presents an average opportunity cost of as much as 7,000 rupees annually for a poor family.

Lack of sanitation and cleanliness leads to physical and cognitive stunting in children, leading to a less productive future workforce. How will we achieve a Skilled India and become a global economic superpower if 40% of our children are not achieving their full potential?

Many reports say that poor children become the victim of unsanitary practices and poor families spend a lot of money towards medical expenses on account of this. When the poor fall ill, it also affects their livelihoods.

Open Defecation is also a serious threat to safety and dignity of millions of women, who are forced to wait till it gets dark to relieve themselves, and have to face the indignity and fear that someone may be watching them. They are also at the risk of contracting infections. Our mothers, sisters and daughters should not be forced to face this indignity every single day.

Poor garbage management also has an adverse effect on tourism, and indirectly impacts the overall health of a city, and impacts India's image on the world stage.

Experience from other countries suggested that the game changer for improved cleanliness and sanitation in a country is when the Chief Executive of the country makes it a national priority and leads it from the front. With the huge mandate that the people of India gave our Government, it was the right time to bring about a paradigm shift in our approach towards cleanliness and sanitation, and by transforming it into a people's movement as a national flagship program in the form of the Swachh Bharat Mission. This Mission is a big step towards giving our children a better future. It is a program that is fundamental to building the India of tomorrow.

Good hygiene and sanitation, and proper disposal of solid and liquid waste will not only help people at the individual level but will also benefit at the collective level. I am sure that it will help in promotion of tourism, reduce expenditure towards curative health, will result in more number of productive working days and contribute to overall GDP.

In 2014, when the new government was formed, over 50% of all Indians, and almost 60% of people in rural India defecated in the open.

Today, block after block; district after district; state after state is working towards achieving Open Defecation Free status. We have succeeded in creating a vibrant people's movement towards cleanliness and sanitation.

By the 150th birth anniversary of Mahatma Gandhi on 2nd October 2019, we strive to achieve his dream of a clean India which practices safe sanitation. Gandhiji valued cleanliness as much as he valued freedom. So, the real tribute which we can pay him is to end open defecation and to celebrate his birthday in a Swachh Bharat.

NOTES

Preface

1. Kaveri Gill, *Of Poverty and Plastic: Scavenging and Scrap Trading Entrepreneurs in India's Urban Informal Economy* (New Delhi: Oxford University Press, 2010); Urvashi Dhamija, *Sustainable Solid Waste Management* (New Delhi: Academic Foundation, 2006); Bhasha Singh, *Unseen: The Truth about India's Manual Scavengers,* trans. Reenu Talwar (Hindi ed., 2012; New Delhi: Penguin, 2014); Dhrubajyoti Ghosh, *The Trash Diggers* (New Delhi: Oxford University Press, 2017); Diane Coffey and Dean Spears, *Where India Goes: Abandoned Toilets, Stunted Development and the Costs of Caste* (New Delhi: HarperCollins India, 2017); Susan E. Chaplin, *The Politics of Sanitation in India*; (Hyderabad: Orient BlackSwan, 2011). Katherine Boo, *Behind the Beautiful Forevers* (New York: Random House, 2012); Sunita Narain and Swati Singh Sambyal, *Not in My Backyard: Solid Waste Management in Indian Cities* (New Delhi: Centre for Science and Environment, 2016); Atul Deulgaonkar, introduction to *In Search of Dignity and Justice: The Untold Story of Conservancy Workers,* written and photographs by Sudharak Olwe (Mumbai: Bharatiya Mahila Federation [Thane Samiti], 2013).

2. For example, see Vinay Gidwani and Bharati Chaturvedi, "Poverty as Geography," in *Urban Navigations: Politics, Space and the City in South Asia,* ed. Jonathan Shapiro Anjaria and Colin McFarlane (New Delhi: Routledge, 2011), 50–78. See also David Arnold, *Colonizing the Body: State Medicine and Epidemic Disease in Nineteenth-Century India* (Berkeley: University of California Press, 1993); Mark Harrison, *Public Health in British India* (Cambridge: Cambridge University Press, 1994); Sandhya L. Polu, *Infectious Disease in India, 1892–1940: Policy-Making and the Perception of Risk* (Houndmills, UK: Palgrave Macmillan, 2012); Mridula Ramana, *Western Medicine and Public Health in Colonial Bombay 1845–1895* (Hyderabad: Orient Longman, 2002); Asher Ghertner, *Rule by Aesthetics: World-Class City Making in Delhi* (New York: Oxford University Press, 2015); and Isher Judge Ahluwalia, Ravi Kanbur, and P. K. Mohanty, eds., *Urbanisation in India: Challenges, Opportunities and the Way Forward* (New Delhi: SAGE, 2014). K. C. Sivaramakrishnan, *Re-visioning Indian Cities* (New Delhi: SAGE, 2011).

Introduction

1. Kachra was also the name of the untouchable man in Aamir Khan's celebrated film *Lagaan* (2001).

2. Gay Hawkins, *The Ethics of Waste: How We Relate to Rubbish* (Lanham, MD: Rowman and Littlefield, 2006), 4.

3. Kelly Alley, "Idioms of Degeneracy: Assessing Ganga's Purity and Pollution," in *Purifying the Earthly Body of God: Religion and Ecology in Hindu India*, ed. Lance E. Nelson (New York: State University of New York Press, 1998), 297–329.

4. Although, as Alley points out, the terms are often interchangeable and overlap. Ibid., 303–309.

5. For the origins of the use of the English word *untouchable* and discussion of its counterparts in Indian languages, see Simon Charsley, "'Untouchable': What Is in a Name?," *Journal of the Royal Anthropological Institute* 2, no. 1 (1996): 1–23.

6. Ugly Indian, "Why Is India So Filthy?," video, 17:33, 27 October 2014, https://www.youtube.com/watch?v=tf1VA5jqmRo. The talk generated over 2.6 million viewings between October 2014 and August 2017.

7. An episode of the popular television program *Satymev Jayate,* "Don't Waste Your Garbage," season 2, episode 3, 2014, presented by the Bollywood film star Aamir Khan, begins with precisely this question; http://www.satyamevjayate.in/dont-waste-your-garbage.aspx.

8. V. S. Naipaul, *An Area of Darkness* (1964; Harmondsworth, UK: Penguin, 1968), esp. 69–71.

9. See the Appendix.

10. Estimates of the economic cost of poor sanitation to India's gross domestic product vary between 5 and 6.5 percent. In 2010 the World Bank suggested a figure of 6.4 percent. Its study broke down costs into health-related impacts and "losses in education, productivity, time, and tourism." India's annual per capita losses were far ahead of other Asian countries examined in the study (e.g., Vietnam, the Philippines, Indonesia). World Bank "Inadequate Sanitation Costs India the Equivalent of 6.4 Per Cent of GDP," press release, 20 December 2010, https://goo.gl/rJmr11.

11. Dipesh Chakrabarty, "Of Garbage, Modernity and the Citizen's Gaze," in *Habitations of Modernity* (Chicago: University of Chicago Press, 2002), 79.

12. Anthony S. Wohl, *Endangered Lives: Public Health in Victorian Britain* (London: J. M. Dent, 1983), 1–2. Recent evidence suggests Prince Albert may have died of Crohn's disease, but it was thought to be typhoid at the time and until about 2011.

13. Hawkins, *Ethics of Waste,* 2. Mary Douglas, *Purity and Danger: An Analysis of the Concepts of Pollution and Taboo* (1966; London: Ark Paperbacks, 1984).

14. Michelle Yates, "The Human-as-Waste, the Labor Theory of Value and Disposability in Contemporary Capitalism," *Antipode* 43, no. 5 (2011): 1680. See also Zigmunt Bauman, *Wasted Lives: Modernity and Its Outcomes* (Cambridge, UK: Polity, 2004).

15. William Rathje and Cullen Murphy, *Rubbish! The Archaeology of Garbage* (Tucson: University of Arizona Press, 2001), 9.

16. "Six Quotes from PM Modi on Swachh Bharat Abhiyan," *India Today*, 2 October 2014, https://goo.gl/xSCmhn.

17. *A Decade of the Total Sanitation Campaign, Rapid Assessment of Processes and Outcomes* (New Delhi: Water and Sanitation Program, 2010), surveys previous programs.

18. Utpal Sandesara and Tom Wooten, *No One Had a Tongue to Speak: The Untold Story of One of History's Deadliest Floods* (Amherst, NY: Prometheus Books, 2011), 245. Modi granted the authors of *No One Had a Tongue* access to government documents on the Morbi dam failure in 2006 (p. 312).

19. See the Appendix. Quotations are from this document.

20. U.S. photos of the trip are celebrated on various websites—e.g., https://goo.gl/BC82rV, preserved, it seems, by G. Kishan Reddy, a BJP leader from Andhra Pradesh and now Telangana, who accompanied Modi. They were guests of the American Council of Young Political Leaders, a bipartisan body founded in 1966 and with an India partnership since 1984. "Trends in Gujarat," *Times of India*, 27 December 1994, p. 14.

21. Robin Jeffrey, "Clean India! Symbols, Policies, Tensions," *South Asia* 38, no. 4 (December 2015): 807–819.

22. See the Appendix.

23. Laurie Garrett, *Betrayal of Trust: The Collapse of Global Public Health* (New York: Hyperion, 2001); Abraham Varghese, "The Mystery Plague," *Esquire* (UK) 5, no. 2 (March 1995): 31–36; Archana Ghosh and S. Sami Ahmad, *Plague in Surat: Crisis in Urban Governance* (New Delhi: Institute of Social Sciences, 1996); Ghanshyam Shah, *Public Health and Urban Development: The Plague in Surat* (New Delhi: SAGE, 1997).

24. Varghese, "Mystery Plague," 31.

25. *Organiser*, 9 October 1994, 1, 2.

26. Shah, *Public Health*, 197, 221. Susan E. Chaplin, *The Politics of Sanitation in India* (Hyderabad: Orient BlackSwan, 2011), 239–240.

27. Varghese, "Mystery Plague," 36, discusses the lack of evidence for plague. *Sydney Morning Herald*, 12 November 1994, using a Reuters story, quotes letters to the British medical publication the *Lancet*.

28. Rahm Emanuel, mayor of Chicago and former adviser in the Barack Obama administration, is sometimes credited with the remark, but it dates from much earlier. Fred Shapiro, “Quotes Uncovered: Who Said No Crisis Should Go to Waste?,” *Freakonomics* (blog), 13 August 2009, https://goo.gl/4R11JB.

29. Ghosh and Ahmad, *Plague in Surat,* vi.

30. *Times of India,* 6 December 1996, A2. Surat, with a population of 4.6 million, ranked third in a survey, after Chandigarh (about 1 million) and Mysore (900,000). It ranked first among India’s ten largest cities. “Rank of Cities on Sanitation, 2009–10,” Ministry of Urban Development, https://goo.gl/orz5Sc.

31. Shobha G. [*sic*], email to R. Jeffrey, 24 February 2017. See also Sunita Narain and Swati Singh Sambyal, *Not in My Backyard: Solid Waste Management in Indian Cities* (New Delhi: Centre for Science and Environment, 2016), 116.

32. Dave Eggers, *Zeitoun* (London: Hamish Hamilton, 2009). Dominique Lapierre and Javier Moro, *Five Past Midnight in Bhopal: The Epic Story of the World’s Deadliest Industrial Disaster* (New York: Warner Books, 2002).

33. “India’s New Rulers,” *Hinduism Today,* November 1999, https://goo.gl/DuqyWY.

34. Richard J. Evans, *Death in Hamburg: Society and Politics in the Cholera Years* (1987; New York: Penguin, 2005), 177, 356, 388.

35. Charles E. Rosenberg, *The Cholera Years: The United States in 1832, 1849 and 1866* (1962; Chicago: University of Chicago Press, 1987), 184.

36. Chaplin, *The Politics of Sanitation in India*, 45.

37. See the Appendix.

38. Telecom Regulatory Authority of India, *The Indian Telecom Services Performance Indicators, October–December 2016* (New Delhi: TRAI, 7 April 2017), ii.

39. See Gay Hawkins, Emily Potter, and Kane Race, *Plastic Water: The Social and Material Life of Bottled Water* (Cambridge, MA: MIT Press, 2015), 126.

40. We use the terms *settlement* and *slum* interchangeably. In north India they are known as *jhuggi-jhopdi* or *basti. Slum* is common in official language to cover a range of legal classifications. A slum is often defined as a congested, unhygienic settlement lacking infrastructure. Scholars have questioned the definition and its implications. Nikhil Anand, *Hydraulic City: Water and the Infrastructures of Citizenship in Mumbai* (Durham, NC: Duke University Press, 2017); Lisa Björkman, *Pipe Politics, Contested Waters: Embedded Infrastructures of Millennial Mumbai* (Durham, NC: Duke University Press, 2015); Lisa Weinstein, *The Durable Slum: Dharavi and the Right to Stay Put in Globalizing Mumbai* (Minneapolis: University of Minnesota Press, 2014); Sanjay Srivastava, *Entangled Urbanism: Slum, Gated Community and Shopping Mall in Delhi and Gurgaon* (New Delhi: Oxford University Press, 2015), 4–5.

41. In her study of class in Madurai, Sarah Dickey identified an increasing use of the category of "middle-class" in popular discussion. But self-identifying groups often fell below objective definitions of middle class. Sarah Dickey, *Living Class in Urban India* (New Brunswick, NJ: Rutgers University Press, 2015), chap. 6. For middle-class activism in Delhi, see Sanjay Srivastava, *Entangled Urbanism*, chap. 4.

42. Sandhya Krishnan and Neeraj Hatekar, "Rise of the New Middle Class in India and Its Changing Structure," *Economic and Political Weekly* 52, no. 22 (3 June 2017): 42, argue that 50 percent of the population is middle class. A different measurement puts "middle income population" at a mere 3 percent. Rakesh Kochar, "A Global Middle Class Is More Promise than Reality," *Global Attitudes and Trends* (Pew Research Center, 8 July 2015), https://goo.gl/QaS6Tj.

43. Telecom Regulatory Authority of India, *Annual Report, 2014–15* (New Delhi: TRAI, 2015), 6. People Research on India's Consumer Economy, "Household Survey on India's Citizen Environmental and Consumer Economy," http://www.ice360.in/en/projects/what-are-ice-360-surveys/upcoming-survey-ice3600-2016; and reported in *LiveMint*, 13 December 2016.

44. Rakesh Shukla quoted in "India's Middle Class to Touch 267 Million in 5 Yrs," *Economic Times*, 6 February 2011.

1. Time and Place

1. David Arnold, *Colonizing the Body: State Medicine and Epidemic Disease in Nineteenth-Century India* (Berkeley: University of California Press, 1993), 65. The mortality figures are difficult to pin down, but Julian Jocelyn, *The History of the Royal and Indian Artillery in the Mutiny of 1857* (London: Naval and Military Press, 1915), app. 3, 444–448, probably has the most accurate estimate. He counts 1,277 European troops killed in action. We are grateful to Peter Stanley for his kindness in tracking this down. Arnold, *Colonizing the Body*, 65, uses the figure of 586 deaths in battle, which comes from the *Report of the Commissioners Appointed to Inquire into the Sanitary State of the Army in India; with Precis of Evidence* (London: Eyre and Spottiswood for Her Majesty's Stationery Office, 1863), 1:xvii.

2. *Sanitary State of the Army.*

3. Ibid., 371.

4. Ibid., 367.

5. David Arnold, "Introduction: Disease, Medicine and Empire," in *Imperial Medicine and Indigenous Societies*, ed. David Arnold (New Delhi: Oxford University Press, 1989), 14.

6. T. E. Dempster, Deputy Inspector-General of Hospitals, *Sanitary State of the Army,* 464.

7. Ibid., 92.

8. Dr. F. J. Mouat, 17 October 1861, *Sanitary State of the Army,* 330.

9. Dr. G. C. Wallich, 17 October 1861, *Sanitary State of the Army,* 336.

10. Addenda submitted by Sir Ranald Martin, *Sanitary State of the Army,* 465.

11. "Observations by Miss Nightingale," 21 November 1862, "Minutes of Evidence," *Sanitary State of the Army,* 347–348.

12. Ibid., 351.

13. Mark Harrison, *Public Health in British India* (Cambridge: Cambridge University Press, 1994), 60, puts it well: the problem was "how to sanitise those elements of the indigenous population which threatened the health of European troops without provoking a backlash which might threaten the stability of British rule."

14. Although Nightingale did not subscribe to germ theory until late in life, she preached cleanliness and hygiene. *Florence Nightingale on Health in India,* ed. Gerard Vallee (Waterloo, ON: Wilfrid Laurier University Press, 2006), 9:863.

15. Richard J. Evans, *Death in Hamburg: Society and Politics in the Cholera Years* (1987; New York: Penguin, 2005), 265–266; Harrison, *Public Health,* 112–116.

16. Evans, *Death in Hamburg,* 287–292.

17. Harrison, *Public Health,* 114.

18. Myron Echenberg, *Plague Ports* (New York: New York University Press, 2007), 70.

19. Florence Nightingale to Lord Stanley, 21 November 1862, *Sanitary State of the Army,* 370.

20. Arnold, *Colonizing the Body,* 167.

21. Ibid., 195.

22. Ibid., 194. Also see Harrison, *Public Health,* 123.

23. Harrison, *Public Health,* 134–137.

24. Ian Catanach, "Plague and the Tensions of Empire: India, 1896–1918," in Arnold, *Imperial Medicine,* 152. See also Arnold, *Colonizing the Body,* 200–239; and Amelia Bonea, *The News of Empire: Telegraphy, Journalism and the Politics of Reporting in Colonial India, c. 1830–1900* (New Delhi: Oxford University Press, 2016), 304–313.

25. Echenberg, *Plague Ports,* 66–68.

26. Sukeshi Kamra, "Law and Radical Rhetoric in British India: The 1897 Trial of Bal Gangadhar Tilak," *South Asia* 39, no. 3 (2016): 546–559.

27. Mahatma Gandhi, *Navajivan*, 30 June 1929, in *Collected Works of Mahatma Gandhi* (New Delhi: Publications Division, Ministry of Information and Broadcasting, 1971), 46:218–219. Also see Hugh Tinker, *The Foundations of Local Self-Government in India, Pakistan and Burma* (London: Athlone Press, 1954), 289, who refers to antivaccination campaigns in a number of districts, especially Gujarat.

28. *Navajivan*, 12 January 1930, *Collected Works of Mahatma Gandhi*, 48:221.

29. Tinker, *Local Self-Government*, 283.

30. Ibid., 292.

31. "The 1848 Public Health Act," U.K. Parliament, accessed 4 September 2017, http://goo.gl/TKCwDo.

32. Anthony S. Wohl, *Endangered Lives: Public Health in Victorian Britain* (London: J. M. Dent, 1983), 147. See also Lee Jackson, *Dirty Old London: The Victorian Fight against Filth* (New Haven, CT: Yale University Press, 2014), 69–79.

33. Edwin Chadwick, *Report on the Sanitary Condition of the Labouring Population and on the Means of Its Improvement* (London, 1842), 22.

34. David Tatham, *Winslow Homer and the Pictorial Press* (Syracuse, NY: Syracuse University Press, 2003), 80.

35. Robin Nagle, *Picking Up: On the Streets and Behind the Trucks with the Sanitation Workers of New York City* (New York: Farrer, Strauss and Giroux, 2013), 97.

36. "How Much Manure Will a Horse Produce?," *Extension*, 29 September 2015, http://articles.extension.org/pages/18868/stall-waste-production-and-management.

37. Martin V. Melosi, *Garbage in the Cities: Refuse, Reform and the Environment*, rev. ed. (Pittsburgh: University of Pittsburgh Press, 2005), 20–21.

38. Prashant A. Pandya, deputy director, Solid Waste Management, Ahmedabad Municipal Corporation, conversation with Jeffrey, Ahmedabad, 16 October 2013.

39. Melosi, *Garbage*, 34–40, quote on p. 48.

40. Ibid., 41. William Rathje and Cullen Murphy, *Rubbish! The Archaeology of Garbage* (Tucson: University of Arizona Press, 2001), 175–176, report that the last compression, or reduction, plant closed in Philadelphia in 1959.

41. Joshua O. Reno, *Waste Away: Working and Living with a North American Landfill* (Berkeley: University of California Press, 2016), 28–32, describes how sanitary landfills are supposed to work.

42. Rathje and Murphy, *Rubbish!*, 86–87.

43. The Energy and Resources Institute (TERI) asserted in 2012 that "there are no sanitary landfills in India." *TERI Energy Data Directory and Yearbook 2011/12* (New Delhi: TERI, 2012), 342, https://goo.gl/SOElZk.

44. D-Waste, *Waste Atlas: The World's 50 Biggest Dumpsites: 2014 Report,* 13, http://goo.gl/5kRbB8.

45. "Hartland Landfill Facility," Capital Regional District, accessed 5 September 2017, https://goo.gl/eLrYba; Carla Wilson, "Victoria House Prices Surge to Another High," *Times-Colonist,* 1 June 2016, http://goo.gl/H2F3Qp. Jeffrey grew up in Victoria, B.C., and toured the Hartland site with friends who worked there.

46. Rathje and Murphy, *Rubbish!,* 3–9; "Fresh Kills Landfill," Wikipedia, updated 27 September 2017, https://goo.gl/1HdJVs.

47. Nagle, *Picking Up,* 33. Elizabeth Royte, *Garbage Land: On the Secret Trail of Trash* (New York: Back Bay Books, 2006), 85–87, did a Freshkills tour with Nagle; and Rathje and Murphy, *Rubbish!,* 3–9, begin their book with an anthropological dig at Freshkills.

48. "The Park Plan," Freshkills Park: The Freshkills Park Alliance, accessed 5 September 2017, http://goo.gl/Foo9y1.

49. Yoshi Silverstein, "The 'Mountain of Crap' Becomes a Park," *The Dirt: Uniting the Built & Natural Environments,* 3 October 2015, https://goo.gl/gVFxnb.

50. See the disturbing film *Good Garbage* (dir. Shosh Shlam and Ada Ushpiz, Israel, 2013) on the garbage dump that serves the Israeli settlements in the Hebron Hills, where poor Palestinians forage to eke out a living.

51. Meera Subramanian, "The Burning Garbage Heap That Choked Mumbai," *New Yorker,* 29 February 2016, http://goo.gl/9gghyH.

52. "Largest Landfills, Waste Sites, and Trash Dumps in the World," World Atlas, updated 25 April 2017, http://goo.gl/fWVSma. The authors of this collection combined four of Delhi's dispersed landfills to bring Delhi in at number seven.

53. D-Waste, *Waste Atlas,* 16–72.

54. Chris Mills, "The Worlds [*sic*] Largest Landfills with Photos and Stats," Owlcation, 9 March 2016, http://goo.gl/xnzfMx.

55. Jennifer Robinson, "Apex Landfill: There's No Place like Home for Las Vegas Garbage," *Las Vegas Review-Journal,* 21 April 2013, https://goo.gl/FPTYHm. "Republic Services, Inc.," 2014 Fortune 500, updated 31 March 2014, http://fortune-500.silk.co/page/Republic-Services—Inc.

56. Christopher Helman, "America's Biggest Landfills," *Forbes,* 13 October 2010, https://goo.gl/HkYa35.

57. "Shanghai Laogang Engineered Sanitary Landfill Phase IV," Veolia, accessed 5 September 2017, http://goo.gl/2h7fvz. "The Survivor," *Economist,* 20 May 2017, p. 54.

58. "Public Private Partnerships in India," Ministry of Finance, updated 30 August 2017, http://www.pppinindia.com/. Four of India's more prominent waste-management companies were A2Z (based in Gurgaon), Essel (Mumbai), IL&FS (Mumbai), and Ramky (Hyderabad).

59. J. Ayee and R. Crook, "Toilet Wars: Urban Sanitation Services and the Politics of Public-Private Partnerships in Ghana" (working paper, Institute of Development Studies, Brighton, UK, 2003), 4.

60. "Providing Safe and Sustainable Water for All," Veolia, accessed 28 September 2017, https://veolia.in/about-us/about-us/history.

61. Emilio Godoy, "The Waste Mountain Engulfing Mexico City," *Guardian,* 9 January 2012, http://goo.gl/KTuFvy.

62. Mills, "The Worlds Largest Landfills."

63. Eugenio M. Gonzales, "From Wastes to Assets: The Scavengers of Payatas," International Conference on Natural Assets, Tagatay City, 8–11 January 2003, paper revised December 2003, http://www.peri.umass.edu/fileadmin/pdf/conference_papers/CDP7.pdf. Carmilita Morante, "Electioneering in the Promised Land: Payatas Dumpsite, 2016," University of Nottingham Blogs, 6 May 2016, https://goo.gl/PaC1Pp.

64. Muchemi Wachira, "Heaps of Garbage Chokes [*sic*] Nairobi City," *Daily Nation,* 29 December 2015, http://goo.gl/yQHzWu. "Environmental Pollution and Impacts on Public Health: Implications of the Dandora Municipal Dumping Site in Nairobi, Kenya" (Nairobi: United Nations Environment Program, c. 2010), accessed 28 September 2017 via http://www.habitants.org/news/inhabitants_of_africas/dandora_dumping_site_the_biggest_human_rights_violation_in_kenya.

65. *Project Information Document (Concept Stage)—Cairo Municipal Solid Waste Management Project—P152961* (Washington, DC: World Bank Group, 2014), https://goo.gl/Akol4u. Patrick Kingsley, "Waste Not: Egypt's Refuse Collectors Regain Role at Heart of Cairo Society," *Guardian,* 28 March 2014, https://goo.gl/qIXvrY.

66. "The Malagrotta Landfill and Speculation in the Galeria Valley," Ejolt, fact sheet 22, 20 July 2015, http://goo.gl/uehYwD. Massimiliano Di Giogio, "Italy's Woeful Waste Management on Trial with Il Supremo Trash King," Reuters, 25 May 2014, http://goo.gl/JJXRC1.

67. Harold Crooks, *Giants of Garbage: The Rise of the Global Waste Industry and the Politics of Pollution Control* (Toronto: James Lorimer, 1993), 5; and Harold Crooks, *Dirty Business* (Toronto: James Lorimer, 1983), 9–10.

68. Maurice D. Hinchey, "Organized Crime's Involvement in the Waste Hauling Industry," The American Mafia: The History of Organized Crime in the United States, 24 July 1986, http://mafiahistory.us/maf-hinc.html.

69. Royte, *Garbage Land,* 72. See also Hinchey, "Organized Crime's Involvement."

70. Lata Mishra and Kunal Guha, "Stench of Money," *Mumbai Mirror,* 7 February 2016, https://goo.gl/8eiy2x. Doron, conversations with locals in Deonar, 19 March 2016.

71. R. N. Bhaskar, "Policy Watch: Converting Waste into Energy Can Spell End of Garbage Mafia," *DNA*, 11 August 2014, https://goo.gl/zd66Bh.

72. "Kerala Waste Time-Bomb Ticks Away in Kovai," *New Indian Express*, 17 July 2016, https://goo.gl/vh2SA8.

73. Mohammed Iqbal, "The Case of Delhi's Missing Dustbins," *Hindu*, 4 December 2014, https://goo.gl/p6qfXb; Aravind Gowda, "Bengaluru Garbage Mafia Issues Threat to Residents," *India Today*, 5 December 2015, https://goo.gl/sQCbKd.

74. Di Giogio, "Italy's Woeful Waste Management."

75. Gopal Guru, "Introduction: Theorizing Humiliation," *Humiliation: Claims and Context*, ed. Gopal Guru (New Delhi: Oxford University Press, 2011), 13.

76. Josy Joseph, *A Feast of Vultures: The Hidden Business of Democracy in India* (New Delhi: HarperCollins, 2016), 18–19, provides recent examples.

77. Jairam Ramesh, "A Toilet for Everyone," *India Today*, 6 June 2014, https://goo.gl/vNKSdW.

78. *The Laws of Manu*, trans. Wendy Doniger and Brian K. Smith (New Delhi: Penguin, 1991), 242 (verses 51–55).

79. Premchand, *Deliverance and Other Stories*, trans. David Rubin (1931; New Delhi: Penguin, 1988); Mulk Raj Anand, *Untouchable* (1935; Harmondsworth: Penguin, 1988). See also Hazari, *Untouchable: The Autobiography of an Indian Outcaste* (London: Praeger, 1971), 4–5, 83; and the Marathi-language award-winning film *Court* (dir. C. Tamhane, India, 2014), which revolves around the death of a municipal sanitation worker.

80. "After Una Atrocity, Dalits Protest and Refuse to Dispose of Carcasses in Gujarat," *Hindu*, 30 July 2016, https://goo.gl/EP8VUx. The boycott of carcass disposal was difficult for poor people to maintain. Hiral Dave, "Despite Dalit Protests, Cow Carcass Disposal on Track in Gujarat," *Hindustan Times*, 21 August 2016, https://goo.gl/C7NMLc.

81. J. C. Molony, *A Book of South India* (London: Methuen & Co., 1926), 144.

82. Ibid., 144–145.

83. Arjun Appadurai, "Deep Democracy: Urban Governmentality and the Horizon of Politics," *Public Culture* 14, no. 1 (2002): 21–47.

84. Chadwick, *Report*, 29.

85. Roger-Henri Guerrand, "Private Spaces," in *A History of Private Life*, vol. 4, *From the Fires of Revolution to the Great War*, ed. Michelle Perrot (Cambridge, MA: Harvard University Press, 1990), 172.

86. Chadwick, *Report*, 14 (italics in the original).

87. *Sanitary State of the Army*, 472.

88. There are a few examples of human waste being collected for agriculture. Farmers around Delhi in the 1890s bought night soil and drain effluent from the local

government. Vijay Prashad, "The Technology of Sanitation in Colonial Delhi," *Modern Asian Studies* 35, no. 1 (2001): 140–141.

89. Yong Xue, "'Treasure Nightsoil as If It Were Gold': Economic and Ecological Links between Urban and Rural Areas in Late Imperial Jiangnan," *Late Imperial China* 26, no. 1 (2005): 41–71; Yamin Xu, "Policing Civility on the Streets: Encounters with Litterbugs, 'Nightsoil Lords,' and Street Corner Urinators in Republican Beijing," *Twentieth-Century China* 3, no. 2 (2005): 28–71.

90. Susan B. Hanley, "Urban Sanitation in Preindustrial Japan," *Journal of Interdisciplinary History* 18, no. 1 (1987): 9.

91. Ibid., 10.

92. Yu Xinzhong, "The Treatment of Night Soil and Waste in Modern China," in *Health and Hygiene in Chinese East Asia*, ed. Angea Ki Che Leung and Charlotte Furth (Durham, NC: Duke University Press, 2010), 54–55.

93. Ibid.

94. Ibid., 56, citing Wilhelm Wagner's book on Chinese agriculture, *Die Chinesische Landwirtschaft* (Berlin: Parcy, 1926), 926.

95. Yu, "Treatment," 66.

96. Timothy D. Amos, *Embodying Difference: The Making of Burakumin in Modern Japan* (Honolulu: University of Hawaii Press, 2011), 30.

97. Amos, *Embodying Difference*, 22 (italics in the original).

98. Rosalind Fredericks, "Vital Infrastructures of Trash in Dakar," *Comparative Studies of South Asia, Africa and the Middle East* 34, no. 3 (2014): 539.

99. Sjaak van der Geest, "Akan Shit: Getting Rid of Dirt in Ghana," *Anthropology Today* 14, no. 3 (1998): 9–10.

100. Shannon Deery, "Melbourne Water Fined after Worker Drowns in Sewerage Channel," *Herald Sun*, 27 February 2014, http://goo.gl/qP4QJt.

101. Rose George, *The Big Necessity: The Unmentionable World of Human Waste and Why It Matters* (New York: Holt Paperback, 2009), 15.

102. Ibid., 18.

103. Bhasha Singh, *Unseen: The Truth about India's Manual Scavengers*, trans. Reenu Talwar (New Delhi: Penguin, 2014), xxvi–xxvii.

104. Atul Deulgaonkar, Introduction, *In Search of Dignity and Justice: The Untold Story of Conservancy Workers*, by Sudharak Olwe (Mumbai: Bharatiya Mahila Federation [Thane Samiti], 2013), 9–11.

105. See Olwe, *In Search of Dignity and Justice*, especially the cover and the photos on pp. 45–61. Many of these photos are at http://www.sudharakolwe.com/insearch.html.

106. “Hundreds of Sanitation Workers Carrying Bodies of 4 Colleagues Storm Collectorate,” *Nagpur Today,* 16 March 2016, http://goo.gl/ZvAolg; Vivek Narayanan, “Four Die of Asphyxiation in Restaurant Septic Tank at Chennai Hotel,” *Hindu,* 20 January 2016, https://goo.gl/Tfp2ml. See also Tamhane, *Court.*

107. *Times of India,* 22 June 1853, p. 1183, digesting the *Prabhakar* account. *Prabhakar* was one of the earliest newspapers in the Marathi language and was published for twenty-five years. J. Natarajan, *History of Indian Journalism* (New Delhi: Publications Division, Ministry of Information and Broadcasting, 1955), 57.

108. Chandra Bhan Prasad, “Markets and Manu: Economic Reforms and Its Impact on Caste in India” (working paper no. 08-01, Center for the Advanced Study of India, University of Pennsylvania, 2008), 29.

109. The common term for Muslim manual scavengers is *halalkhor,* which is also used in some states, such as Maharashtra, as an official designation.

110. Assa Doron, “The Intoxicated Poor: Alcohol, Morality and Power among the Boatmen of Banaras,” *South Asian History and Culture* 1, no. 2 (2010): 294.

111. Kaveri Gill, *Of Poverty and Plastic: Scavenging and Scrap Trading Entrepreneurs in India's Urban Informal Economy* (New Delhi: Oxford University Press, 2010), 92, and see 113, 155.

112. Evans, *Death in Hamburg,* 110.

2. Growth and Garbage

1. World Bank, “Population Density (people per sq. km of land area),” http://goo.gl/s3c6aL.

2. U.S. Environmental Protection Agency, *Municipal Solid Waste Generation, Recycling, and Disposal in the United States: Facts and Figures for 2012,* accessed 30 September 2017, https://goo.gl/D7tzNh.

3. If 320 million Americans generate 250 million metric tons of waste a year, that is an average of 780 kilograms (1,720 pounds) of waste per person. If 1.27 billion Indians generate 65 million metric tons of waste, that is an average of 5 kilograms (11 pounds) per person. The Organization for Economic Cooperation and Development estimates that U.S. waste generation per capita in 2011 was 730 kilograms (1,610 pounds). “Environment at a Glance 2013,” OECD iLibrary, http://goo.gl/8gxz8S.

4. These raw comparisons make no allowance, of course, for mountains and deserts or climates that make human habitation difficult.

5. *Chandigarh Master Plan—2031,* accessed 30 September 2017, http://chandigarh.gov.in/cmp_2031.htm.

6. Rishi Rana, Rajiv Ganguly, and Ashok Kumar Gupta, "An Assessment of Solid Waste Management System in Chandigarh City, India," *EJGE* 20, no. 6 (2015): 1547–1572. The average Chandigarh resident, by these figures, generated about 13 kilograms (29 pounds) of waste a year, not surprising given that it is one of India's most privileged cities.

7. Ibid., 1551.

8. In Jerry Pinto and Rahul Srivastava, eds., *Talk of the Town* (New Delhi: Penguin, 2008), 29.

9. Sushila Raja, conversation with Doron, Delhi, 23 January 2015.

10. Dietmar Rothermund, *An Economic History of India* (London: Routledge, 1993), 133.

11. Dharma Kumar, and Meghnad Desai, *Cambridge Economic History of India,* vol. 2, *c. 1751–c. 1970* (Cambridge: Cambridge University Press, 1983), 489.

12. Paul R. Ehrlich, *The Population Bomb* (New York: Ballantine Books, 1968), xi. The book has gone through many printings and revisions.

13. Ibid., 15, and many more pages that referred to the threat posed by India's population growth.

14. M. K. Gandhi, "Some Mussooree Reminiscences," *Harijan,* 23 June 1946, p. 198.

15. The Khadi and Village Industries Commission also has offshoots in a number of states; see http://www.kvic.org.in/kvicres/index.html.

16. K. C. Sivaramakrishnan, "Revisiting the 74th Constitutional Amendment for Better Metropolitan Governance," *Economic and Political Weekly* 48, no. 13 (20 March 2013): 87.

17. Ashish Rajadhyaksha and Paul Willemen, *Encyclopaedia of Indian Cinema,* rev. ed. (New Delhi: Oxford University Press, 1999), 344.

18. K. C. Sivaramakrishnan, *Re-visioning Indian Cities: The Urban Renewal Mission* (New Delhi: SAGE, 2011), 8.

19. Quoted in Rafiq Dossani, *India Arriving* (New York: American Management Association, 2008), 49.

20. *9th Five Year Plan,* vol. 1, chap. 6, para 6.47, and also vol. 1, chap. 1, para 1.38, 10, http://planningcommission.nic.in/plans/planrel/fiveyr/9th/default.htm.

21. For the push and pull factors underpinning migration to towns and cities and for a view of work in India's informal sector, see Vinay Gidwani, "The Work of Waste: Inside India's Infra-economy," *Transactions* 40 (2015): 578.

22. William Rathje and Cullen Murphy, *Rubbish! The Archaeology of Garbage* (Tucson: University of Arizona Press, 2001), 66–67.

23. See S. Subramanian, "The Poverty Line: Getting It Wrong Again . . . and Again," *Economic and Political Weekly* 49, no. 47 (22 November 2014): 66–70, for a digest of disputes about how to set the poverty line.

24. Stuart Corbridge, John Harriss, and Craig Jeffrey, *India Today: Economy, Politics and Society* (Cambridge, UK: Polity, 2013), 124–128; "Budget 1991: What Manmohan Singh Promised and What Was Delivered," *Economic Times*, 24 July 2011, updated 15 September 2011, http://goo.gl/reBXHF.

25. Tapas Piplai, "Automobile Industry: Shifting Strategic Focus," *Economic and Political Weekly*, 36, no. 30 (28 July 2001): 2892–2897.

26. Charles E. Rosenberg, *The Cholera Years: The United States in 1832, 1849 and 1866* (1962; Chicago: University of Chicago Press, 1987), 227.

27. *Times of India*, 7 January 1884, p. 3, reported that "2 packages toothpaste" arrived on the SS *Govino* in Mumbai.

28. *Times of India*, 16 July 1902, p. 13.

29. *Times of India*, 7 November 1923, p. 16.

30. Shelley Moore, "About Toothpaste Tubes Made of Metal," eHow, accessed 5 September 2017, https://goo.gl/Do3M8A.

31. Amy Wu, "Good Product, Bad Package," *Guardian*, 18 July 2014, http://goo.gl/Yhsq5a.

32. *Times of India*, 16 July 1902, advertising pots of "Tooth Paste" for four annas (approximately 10 cents).

33. A. Hooda, M. Rathee, and J. Singh, "Chewing Sticks in the Era of Toothbrush: A Review," *Internet Journal of Family Practice* 9, no 2 (2009): 2, http://print.ispub.com/api/o/ispub-article/4968.

34. "Toothpaste Industry: An Overview," Allprojectreports.com, accessed 5 September 2017, http://goo.gl/AlI8jK.

35. Mativathani Karunanathan, "Toothbrush and Toothpaste Use in Australia" (master's thesis, University of Sydney, 1987), iii.

36. *Sunday Observer*, 17 July 1988, p. 16; *Business India*, 3–16 October 1988, p. 113; *Hindu International Edition*, 21 May 1988, p. 13.

37. *Advertising and Marketing*, 15 October 1994, p. 67, reported two-thirds of Indians were nonusers. *Sunday Observer*, 17 July 1994, p. 16, reported 85 percent were nonusers.

38. Katherine Ashenburg, *Clean: An Unsanitized History of Washing* (London: Profile Books, 2009), 246. Profits from Listerine hit $8 million in 1928, up from $115,000 in 1921.

39. These findings came from a Massachusetts Institute of Technology survey, reported on a Manchester Unity website. "Reason to Smile," http://goo.gl

/gWPQFD. Of 1,500 respondents, 41 percent nominated the toothbrush; 37 percent, the car.

40. See Nita Kumar's examination of changing patterns of leisure and concepts of time and space in Varanasi, where she looks at the male practice of going to the other side of the river for the ritualized consumption of *bhang,* washing clothes, and defecation. Nita Kumar, *The Artisans of Banaras: Popular Culture and Identity, 1880–1986* (Princeton, NJ: Princeton University Press, 1988).

41. "Colgate-Palmolive (India) Gains after Gujarat Unit Starts Producing Toothpaste," *Business Standard,* 23 May 2014, http://goo.gl/RttxFO.

42. "Toothpaste Market in India to 2017," *Wattpad,* 17 June 2014, https://goo.gl/Bw9GWa.

43. World Bank, "Motor Vehicles (per 1,000 people)," citing data for 2009–2013 (site discontinued but available at the Internet Wayback Machine, accessed 5 September 2017, https://goo.gl/hB3Nzf).

44. N. S. Mohan Ram, "Recycling End of Life Vehicles," *Seminar,* no. 690 (February 2017): 47.

45. "Junk Old Car, Get 50% Excise Cut on New?," *Times of India,* 18 January 2016, http://goo.gl/KPVKgI.

46. "Number of Vehicles Scrapped in the U.S. from 2002 to 2014 (in million units)," *Statista,* 2016, http://goo.gl/92H53V.

47. "Make Your Own Car at Meerut Auto Scrapyard in Just 4 Weeks," *Economic Times,* 20 May 2011, http://goo.gl/oCcwPn.

48. "Cops Take On Auto Mafia, Raid Godown in Sotiganj," *Times of India,* 31 January 2015, http://goo.gl/p4yKma.

49. Ben Messenger, "First Integrated End-of-Life Vehicle Recycling Facility for India by 2018," *Waste Management World,* 11 August 2016, https://goo.gl/zjzhPM.

50. Adam Minter, *Junkyard Planet: Travels in the Billion-Dollar Trash Trade* (New York: Bloomsbury, 2013, 161–163.

51. *India 1959: Annual Review* (London: Information Service of India, 1959), 81–82.

52. *Mass Media in India 1980–81* (New Delhi: Publications Division, Ministry of Information and Broadcasting, 1982), 99, 193.

53. *Census of India, 2011,* "Houselisting and Housing Census, 2011. Table HH-14: Percentage of Households to Total Households by Amenities and Assets," http://goo.gl/of7rrA. Also see Nalin Mehta, *India on Television* (New Delhi: HarperCollins, 2008), 42–44.

54. "Jayalalithaa Govt Scraps Free TV Scheme in Tamil Nadu," *Daily News and Analysis,* 10 June 2011, http://goo.gl/MivZPl.

55. "Ewaste Up as More Dump Old Television Sets for Flat Screen," *Times of India,* 13 June 2014, http://goo.gl/gNSH1c.

56. Vance Packard, *The Waste Makers* (1960; Brooklyn, NY: Ig Publishing, 1988), esp. chaps. 6 and 7. For a history, see Giles Slade, *Made to Break: Technology and Obsolescence in America.* (Cambridge, MA: Harvard University Press, 2006).

57. Assa Doron and Robin Jeffrey, *The Great Indian Phone Book* (Cambridge, MA: Harvard University Press, 2013), 213–215.

58. Tania Goklany, "How Karma Recycling Is Giving Life to E-waste," NDTV, 23 September 2015, http://goo.gl/A2oPXX; "Ewaste Up," *Times of India,* 13 June 2014, http://goo.gl/gNSH1c.

59. Elizabeth Royte, *Garbage Land: On the Secret Trail of Trash* (New York: Back Bay Books, 2006), 282.

60. "Hazardous Wastes (Management and Handling) Rules, 1989," Ministry of Environment and Forests, 28 July 1989, http://envfor.nic.in/divisions/hsmd/notif.html.

61. "Status Report on Management of Hazardous Waste in India," 15 March 1990, p. 4, https://goo.gl/N6hBI3.

62. "Environment Ministry Announces New Rules for Disposal of Hazardous Waste," *Economic Times,* 3 April 2016, http://goo.gl/UTlyEB, reported 7.46 million metric tons from 44,000 industrial units in India. An earlier report from Gujarat gave a figure of 7.9 million metric tons from 42,000 units. Anita S. Ahuja and Sachin D. Abda, "Industrial Hazardous Waste Management by Government of Gujarat," *RHIMRJ* 2, no. 5 (May 2015), 1, http://oaji.net/articles/2015/1250-1434252379.pdf. The U.S. Environmental Protection Agency calculated U.S. hazardous waste at 35 million metric tons in 2013. Environmental Protection Agency, *Report on the Environment: Hazardous Waste,* accessed 6 November 2017, https://cfpub.epa.gov/roe/indicator.cfm?i=54.

63. Central Pollution Control Board, "National Inventory of Hazardous Wastes Generating Industries and Hazardous Waste Management in India," 2009, 6, http://goo.gl/1I3Wt8.

64. "Hazardous Waste Management," West Bengal Pollution Control Board, accessed 5 September 2017, http://www.wbpcb.gov.in/pages/display/36-hazardous-waste-management.

65. Snehangshu Chakraborty, group coordinator eastern zone, Ramky Enviro Engineers, conversation with Jeffrey, Haldia, 19 March 2015.

66. See Sarah Hodges, "Chennai's Biotrash Chronicles: Chasing the Neoliberal Syringe" (working paper no. 44/08, GARNET, May 2008) 1–28, https://goo.gl/ksMnTp. We thank Sarah Hodges for permission to quote from her working paper.

67. Narendra K. Arora et al., "Biomedical Waste Management: Situational Analysis and Predictors of Performance in 25 Districts across 20 Indian States," *Indian Journal of Medical Research* 139, no. 4 (2014): 141, 151, http://goo.gl/xx2rjr.

68. Ibid., 147.

69. Central Pollution Control Board, "State-wise Status of Common Bio-medical Waste Treatment Facilities (CBWTFs)," 2008, http://cpcb.nic.in/wast/biomedicalwast/CBWTF_Status_2008.pdf.

70. Corporate hospitals often sold medical waste in the informal, unregulated market while appearing to comply with international standards. Hodges, "Chennai's Biotrash Chronicles," 12, 23.

71. "Growth Graph," 2003–13, IMAGE (Indian Medical Association Goes Eco-friendly), http://www.imageima.org/growth_graph.

72. For background, see Alex Broom, Katherine Kenny, Emma Kirby, and Mahati Chittem, "Improvisation, Therapeutic Brokerage and Antibiotic (Mis)use in India" (unpublished, 2017).

73. Chandra Bhushan, Amit Khurana, Rajeshwari Sinha, and Mouna Nagaraju, *Antibiotic Resistance in Poultry Environment: Spread of Resistance from Poultry Farm to Agricultural Field* (New Delhi: Centre for Science and Environment, 2017), 17.

74. See Ramanan Laxminarayan and Ranjit Roy Chaudhury, "Antibiotic Resistance in India: Drivers and Opportunities for Action," *PLOS Medicine* 13, no. 3 (2016): 1–7.

75. Sally Davies, "Antimicrobial Resistance: The End of Modern Medicine?," public lecture, Royal Institution, London, 8 March 2017, accessed 11 October 2017, https://youtu.be/2H_Ox1vVnTc.

76. Government of India, *National Action Plan on Antimicrobial Resistance,* April 2017, https://goo.gl/T7iCqw. See also Maryn McKenna, "NDM-1 in India: Drug Resistance, Political Resistance," *Wired,* 16 October 2012, https://goo.gl/oENeBM.

77. Central Pollution Control Board, "Waste Generation and Composition," 2004–2005, http://goo.gl/Bhv7ZI.

78. Sunita Narain and Swati Singh Sambyal, *Not in My Backyard: Solid Waste Management in India Cities* (New Delhi: Centre for Science and Environment, 2016), 14, detail the difficulties of measurement.

79. Ranjith Kharvel Annepu, "Sustainable Solid Waste Management in India" (master's thesis, Columbia University, 2012), 38.

80. This comparison does not claim mathematical precision. A Toyota Corolla is 4.6 meters (15 feet) long by 1.8 meters (6 feet) wide—8.3 square meters (90 square feet). There are 1 million square meters in a square kilometer. One could therefore park 120,482 theoretical Corollas in a square kilometer, each one weighing 1.7 metric tons. If India's annual waste accumulation is 65 million metric tons, that is equal to 38,235,294 Corollas, which require 317 square kilometers (122 square miles) to park. The area of Goa is 3,700 square kilometers (1,429 square miles), so Goans could breathe easy for twelve years, not ten.

81. K. C. Sivaramakrishnan, *Governance of Megacities: Fractured Thinking, Fragmented Setup* (New Delhi: Oxford University Press, 2015), xxiv, quoted in Sahil

Gandhi and Vaidehi Tandel, "What Urbanisation Reforms Owe to K. C. Sivaramakrishnan," *Economic and Political Weekly* 52, no. 22 (3 June 2017): 27.

3. Sewage and Society

1. Dholavira is an Indus valley civilization site 370 kilometers (230 miles) northwest of Ahmedabad. Archaeologists date Dholavira from about 2600 BCE; Rome, from about 750 BCE.

2. For a fascinating study of Western civilization's ambivalence toward waste, especially human waste, see Dominique Laporte, *History of Shit* (Cambridge, MA: MIT Press, 1993).

3. Rose George, *The Big Necessity: The Unmentionable World of Human Waste and Why It Matters* (New York: Holt Paperback, 2009), 24.

4. Nikhila Henry, "Research Scholar Hangs Self after Expulsion from Central University," *Hindu,* 17 January 2016, https://goo.gl/d5SSIJ. In the aftermath, BJP groups have contended that the dead youth was not a Dalit, although his mother was a Dalit and he identified as a Dalit. The aim of questioning his status appears to be to obscure that the origins of his expulsion related to censorship, intimidation, and violence.

5. Vivek Narayanan, "Four Die of Asphyxiation as They Enter Septic Tank at Chennai Hotel," *Hindu,* 19 January 2016, http://goo.gl/boU9pp.

6. Ghanshyam Shah, Harsh Mander, Sukhadeo Thorat, Satish Deshpande, and Amita Baviskar, *Untouchability in Rural India* (New Delhi: SAGE, 2006).

7. Ibid., 81.

8. Ibid., 94–95.

9. Ibid., 106.

10. See Bhasha Singh, *Unseen: The Truth about India's Manual Scavengers,* trans. R. Talwar (New Delhi: Penguin, 2014), 250–258, for a list of names given to manual-scavenging subcastes in different parts of India.

11. Bezwada Wilson, foreword to Bhasha Singh, *Unseen,* xii.

12. Bhasha Singh, *Unseen,* 38.

13. *Scavenging Conditions Enquiry Committee* (New Delhi: Ministry of Home Affairs, Central Advisory Board for Harijan Welfare, 1960), chap. 11, "Customary Rights," 79–84. The committee was chaired by N. R. Malkani (1890–1974), who was a devotee of Mahatma Gandhi. His brother was K. R. Malkani (1921–2003), a stalwart of the Jana Sangh political party, one of the roots of the BJP.

14. See the Safai Karmachari Andolan website, accessed 5 September 2017, http://safaikarmachariandolan.org/index.html. Bezwada Wilson, interview by Jeffrey, New Delhi, 30 April 2014.

15. Wilson interview.

16. Divya Trivedi, "A Blot upon the Nation," *Hindu,* 30 March 2012, https://goo.gl/frMklW.

17. Satish Nandgaonkar, "Photo Essay Led to Tata's Mission Dignity," *Hindu,* 22 January 2105, http://goo.gl/6JtAsE.

18. "BJP's Next Mission: End Manual Scavenging," *Hindu,* 3 April 2015, http://goo.gl/TzTjZi.

19. "Bhim Yatra," Safai Karmachari Andolan, 10 December 2015, http://www.safaikarmachariandolan.org/Bhim-Yatra.html.

20. *Census of India, 2011,* "Houselisting and Housing Census, 2011. Table HH-14: Percentage of Households to Total Households by Amenities and Assets," column 98. Susan E. Chaplin, *The Politics of Sanitation in India: Cities, Services and the State* (Hyderabad: Orient BlackSwan, 2011), 175–176, has a table listing more than twenty measures intended to eliminate manual scavenging—and failing—between 1952 and 2005.

21. Bhasha Singh, *Unseen,* 168.

22. Ibid., 168–169.

23. Takashi Shinoda speaks of two types of such customary rights: the first and more common is the "right to clean dry latrines," and less common is the "right to dispose and sell the human waste collected." Takashi Shinoda, *Marginalization in the Midst of Modernization: A Study of Sweepers in Western India* (New Delhi: Manohar, 2005), 52.

24. "Bhim-Yatra."

25. Quoted in Tulasi Srinivas, "Flush with Success: Bathing, Defecation, Worship, and Social Change in South India," *Space and Culture* 5, no. 4 (2002): 370–371.

26. Craig Jeffrey, Patricia Jeffery, and Roger Jeffery, *Degrees without Freedom? Education, Masculinities and Unemployment in North India* (Stanford, CA: Stanford University Press, 2008), 135.

27. Weston Bate, *Essential but Unplanned: The Story of Melbourne's Lanes* (Melbourne, Australia: State Library of Victoria / City of Melbourne, 1994), 88. The caste name Bhangi has related terms in different regions. "Halalkhor" is used for Muslim manual scavengers in Bihar and Uttar Pradesh. K. S. Singh, *People of India: The Scheduled Castes* (Delhi: Oxford University Press for Anthropological Survey of India, 1993), 2:235–243.

28. Reginald Craufuird Sterndale, *Municipal Work in India; Hints on Sanitation, General Conservancy and Improvement in Municipalities, Towns, and Villages* (Calcutta: Thacker, Spink, 1881), 122.

29. *Scavenging Conditions,* 4.

30. *Report of the Working Group on Urban and Industrial Water Supply and Sanitation for 12th Five Year Plan 2012–2017* (New Delhi: Planning Commission, 2011), 8.

31. "Status of Sewage Treatment in India" (New Delhi: Central Pollution Control Board, 2005), Table B, 2, accessed 6 October 2017, http://cpcb.nic.in/newitems/12.pdf.

32. "Lok Sabha Unstarred Question No. 1478," 8 December 2015, citing Central Pollution Control Board figures from March 2015, http://www.indiaenvironmentportal.org.in/files/file/Capacity%20of%20Sewage%20Treatment%20Plants.pdf.

33. Lee Jackson, *Dirty Old London: The Victorian Fight against Filth* (New Haven, CT: Yale University Press, 2014), 97, quoting *Saturday Review,* 19 June 1858, p. 631.

34. *Times* (London), 21 July 1858, quoted in Jackson, *Dirty Old London,* 98.

35. *Times* (London), 5 April 1865, p. 9, quoted in Jackson, *Dirty Old London,* 99.

36. *Times* (London), 5 April 1865, p. 5.

37. C. Carkeet James, *Drainage Problems of the East: Being a Revised and Enlarged Edition of "Oriental Drainage"* (Bombay: Times of India, 1906), xxvii.

38. Ibid., 241.

39. Ibid., 264.

40. Maharashtra Pollution Control Board, *Annual Report, 2012–13* (Mumbai: Maharashtra Pollution Control Board, n.d. [c. 2013]), 20, http://goo.gl/pRMdct. Maharashtra's 26 municipal corporations had a total population of about thirty-six million people; its 230 municipal councils had about ten million people. The Maharashtra Pollution Control Board estimated that these urban areas generated nine thousand megaliters of effluent a day.

41. James, *Drainage Problems,* 234, 105, 109, 145, 235.

42. *India: A Reference Annual* (New Delhi: Ministry of Information and Broadcasting, 1953), 283.

43. Ravi Sundaram, *Pirate Modernity: Delhi's Media Urbanism* (London: Routledge, 2010), 19–20.

44. *Rural-Urban Relationship Committee* (New Delhi: Government of India, Ministry of Health and Family Planning, 1966), 3:238. *Rural-Urban Relationship* is quoted in Virendra Kumar, ed., *Committees and Commissions in India, 1947–73* (New Delhi: Concept Publishing, 1988), 11:172. For analysis of the reports, policies, and their implementation, see Shinoda, *Marginalization in the Midst of Modernization.*

45. *Annual Report, 2013–14* (New Delhi: Ministry of Drinking Water and Sanitation, 2014), 54.

46. Maharashtra, *Annual Report,* 20.

47. Ibid., 20.

48. M. Suchitra, "Stench in My Backyard," *Down to Earth,* 15 September 2012, http://www.downtoearth.org.in/coverage/stench-in-my—backyard-38970.

49. For a concise description, see "The Septic Tank," Department of Health, Australian Government, updated November 2010, http://goo.gl/bxi8TN.

50. *Census of India, 2011,* "Availability and Type of Latrine Facility. Houses, Household Amenities and Assets," https://goo.gl/Ux7c2g.

51. See Srinivas, "Flush with Success," 369.

52. Elisabeth Kvarnström et al., "Honey-Suckers: Sanitation Systems without Pipes. Eco-san at work?," c. 2011, accessed 5 September 2017, http://goo.gl/c1X2Xz.

53. For example, "Slurry Dumping Leading to Destruction of Mangrove," *Hindu,* 14 December 2015, http://goo.gl/uPWXOe.

54. Suchitra, "Stench in My Backyard."

55. The estimate comes from Vishwanath Srikantaiah, a Bengaluru activist involved in the initial work of linking honey-suckers with manure production. Email to Jeffrey, 20 January 2016.

56. "Eliminating Manual Scavenging—The Honey-Sucker Approach," *Rainwaterharvesting* (blog), 10 November 2011, https://goo.gl/vHdMEg.

57. Sydney Harbor contains about five hundred gigaliters of water. If 260 million households flushed ten liters six times a day, that comes to about sixteen gigaliters a day.

58. Maharashtra, *Annual Report,* 20. "Sewage Treatment in Pune Region Gives State the Jitters," *Times of India,* 17 October 2015, https://goo.gl/htUqRd.

59. Yashpal Prabhakar, deputy city engineer, and Prashant A. Pandya, deputy director, Solid Waste Management, Ahmedabad Municipal Corporation, interviews by Jeffrey, 16 October 2013. Ahmedabad Municipal Corporation, "India's First Largest STP," c. 2011, brochure given to R. Jeffrey, 16 October 2013, Enviro Control Associates (I) Pvt. Ltd., 6, http://goo.gl/K5Rcqd.

60. For estimates, see David Waltner-Toews, *The Origin of Feces* (Toronto: ECW Press, 2013), 22; George, *Big Necessity,* 19; and Giulia Enders, *Gut* (Vancouver, BC: Greystone Books, 2015), 68–77.

61. Diane Coffey and Dean Spears, *Where India Goes: Abandoned Toilets, Stunted Development and the Costs of Caste* (New Delhi: HarperCollins India, 2017), especially chapter 5.

62. Martin Bloem, "The 2006 WHO Child Growth Standards," *British Medical Journal,* 7 April 2007, 705–706. UNICEF, "Nearly One Third of Children under Five in Developing Countries Are Stunted," Progress for Children, December 2007, https://goo.gl/SQi5eB.

63. Stuart Gillespie, "Myths and Realities of Child Nutrition," *Economic and Political Weekly* 48, no. 34 (24 August 2013): 66. Gillespie was replying to Arvind Panagarhiya, "Does India Really Suffer from Worse Child Malnutrition than Sub-Saharan Africa?," *Economic and Political Weekly* 48, no. 10 (4 May 2013): 98–111, who attempted to argue that India's high proportion of shorter children was the result of Indian genetics and that the WHO methodology was flawed.

64. Andrew J. Prendergast and Jean H. Humphrey, "The Stunting Syndrome in Developing Countries," *Paediatrics and International Child Health* vol. 34, no. 4 (2014): 257–258.

65. For example, see Mark D. Niehau et al., "Early Childhood Diarrhea Is Associated with Diminished Cognitive Function 4 to 7 Years Later in Children in a Northeast Brazilian Shantytown," *American Journal of Tropical Medicine and Hygiene* 66, no. 5 (2002): 590–593; and Eugene M. Lewit and Nancy Kerrebock, "Population-Based Growth Stunting," *Children and Poverty* 7, no. 2 (Summer / Fall 1997): 149–156.

66. Joe Brown, Sandy Cairncross, and Jeroen H. J. Ensink, "Water, Sanitation, Hygiene and Enteric Infections in Children," *Archives of Diseases in Childhood* 98 (2013): 629.

67. Gillespie, "Myths," 67.

68. Dean Spears, "How Much International Variation in Child Height Can Sanitation Explain?" (working paper, Princeton Research Program in Development Studies, 2013), quoted in Diane Coffey et al., "Stunting among Children: Facts and Implications," *Economic and Political Weekly* 48, no. 34 (24 August 2013): 69.

69. "How Did Bangladesh Reduce Stunting So Rapidly?," Global Nutrition Report, 2014, http://goo.gl/jUHnQ4.

70. Nitin Dhaktode, "Freedom from Open Defecation," *Economic and Political Weekly* 49, no. 20 (17 May 2014): 28–30.

71. *Census of India, 2011,* "Percentage of Households to Total Households by Amenities and Assets. Number of Households Not Having Latrine Facility within the Premises," http://goo.gl/rIhkYG. "Child Health and Nutrition," *Child Line 1098,* accessed 5 September 2017, http://goo.gl/bmUblc.

72. "Rate of Stunting Dropping Fast," *Daily Star,* 4 November 2015, http://www.thedailystar.net/frontpage/rate-stunting-dropping-fast-166978. Rockli Kim et al., "Relative Importance of 13 Correlates of Child Stunting in South Asia: Insights from Nationally Representative Data from Afghanistan, Bangladesh, India, Nepal, and Pakistan," *Social Science and Medicine* 187 (2017): 144–154.

73. Gardiner Harris, "Starving, but Not from the Lack of Food," *International New York Times,* 12–13 July 2014, pp. 1, 6.

74. Nicholas Kristof, "Half the Kids in This Part of India Are Stunted," *New York Times,* 15 October 2015, http://goo.gl/IpGfuP.

75. Harris, "Starving, but Not from the Lack of Food," 6. See also Dean Spears and Sneha Lamba, "Effects of Early-Life Exposure to Sanitation on Childhood Cognitive Skills: Evidence from India's Total Sanitation Campaign," *Journal of Human Resources* 51, no. 2 (2016): 316.

76. Hippolyte Marié-Davy, *De l'évacuation des vidanges,* 69, quoted in Alain Corbin, *The Foul and the Fragrant: Odour and the French Social Imagination* (London: Picador 1994), 226–227.

77. Sneha Lamba and Dean Spears "Caste, 'Cleanliness' and Cash: Effects of Caste-Based Political Reservations in Rajasthan on a Sanitation Prize," *Journal of Development Studies* 49, no. 11 (2013): 1592–1606.

78. Brian Larkin, "The Politics and Poetics of Infrastructure," *Annual Review of Anthropology* 42 (2013): 327–343.

79. Kathleen O'Reilly, Richa Dhanju, and Elizabeth Louis, "Subjected to Sanitation: Caste Relations and Sanitation Adoption in Rural Tamil Nadu," *Journal of Development Studies,* 1 November 2016, http://dx.doi.org/10.1080/00220388.2016.1241385, 2. See also Diane Coffey, Aashish Gupta, Payal Hathi, Nidhi Khurana, Dean Spears, Nikhil Srivastav, and Sangita Vyas. "Revealed Preference for Open Defecation: Evidence from a New Survey in Rural North India," *Economic and Political Weekly* 49, no. 38 (20 September 2014): 43–55.

80. "Infant, Child and Maternal Mortality Rate" (Delhi: Press Information Bureau, Government of India, Ministry of Health and Family Welfare, 11 July 2014), http://goo.gl/sLZSxc. Among the populous north Indian states—Gujarat, Rajasthan, Haryana, Uttar Pradesh, Madhya Pradesh, and Jharkhand—the lowest infant mortality rate was forty-two in Haryana, the state that touches Delhi on three sides.

81. Paul Gertler et al., "How Does Health Promotion Work? Evidence from the Dirty Business of Eliminating Open Defecation" (working paper 20997, National Bureau of Economic Research, Cambridge, MA, 2015), 5–6, 20–21.

82. Valerie A. Curtis, Nana Garbrah-Aidoo, and Beth Scott, "Masters of Marketing: Bringing Private Sector Skills to Public Health Partnerships," *American Journal of Public Health* 97, no. 4 (April 2007): 636.

83. Ibid., 637. A similar campaign was offered to Kerala, but it was rejected by the state government. Ibid., 635.

84. Jeffrey S. Hammer et al., "Hygiene and Health: An Evaluation of the Total Sanitation Campaign in Maharashtra" (working paper, 2007), cited in Spears and Lamba, "Effects of Early-Life Exposure," 304.

85. "Rs 94 Crore Spent on Ads of Swachh Bharat Mission in 1 year," *Economic Times,* 8 July 2015, http://goo.gl/4XGVwk.

86. "Jairam Ramesh's Remark on Toilets and Temples Stirs Controversy," *NDTV,* 12 October 2012, https://goo.gl/6KIyMz.

87. "UNICEF Total Sanitation TVC 1 Priyanka Bharti Featuring Vidya Balan," Youtube, accessed 6 October 2017, www.youtube.com/watch?v=aa1S1ZzkD9Y. "Vidya Balan Campaigns for Sanitation in UP, Bihar," *Indian Express,* 26 August 2015, https://goo.gl/zT9EkV.

88. A month later the film aired on the national channel *Door Darshan,* accompanied by a social media campaign and an offical Tweet posted on 17 September 2017 with a text "WATCH NOW! #ToiletEkPremKatha on @DDNational—Clean toilet Must for health. Let's give PM @narendramodi #SwatchBharat as birthday present!"

89. Shilpa Phadke, Sameera Khan, and Shilpa Ranade, *Why Loiter? Women and Risk on Mumbai Streets* (New Delhi: Penguin, 2011), 79.

90. Gender prejudice and violence feature in the powerful film *Q2P* (dir. Paromita Vohra, 2006), https://www.youtube.com/watch?v=hsJh_BamKgo. On the gendered ramifications of poor infrastructure and long toilet queues, see Renu Desai, Colin McFarlane, and Stephen Graham, "The Politics of Open Defecation: Informality, Body, and Infrastructure in Mumbai," *Antipode* 47, no. 1 (2015): 108–109.

91. "2014 Badaun gang rape allegations," Wikipedia, accessed 6 October 2017, https://en.wikipedia.org/wiki/2014_Badaun_gang_rape_allegations, summarizes this widely reported and disputed event.

92. For a detailed examination of gender and sanitation, see Assa Doron and Ira Raja, "The Cultural Politics of Shit: Class, Gender and Public Space in India," *Journal of Postcolonial Studies* 18, no. 2 (2015): 189–207.

93. See Kathleen O'Reilly, Richa Dhanju, and Abhineety Goel, "Exploring 'The Remote' and 'The Rural': Open Defecation and Latrine Use in Uttarakhand, India," *World Development* 93 (2017): 193–205; and O'Reilly, Dhanju, and Louis, "Subjected to Sanitation," 7.

94. Assa Doron and Robin Jeffrey, "Notes on Open Defecation in India," *Economic and Political Weekly* 49, no. 49 (6 December 2014): 72–78, review obstacles to elimination of open defecation.

95. See Colin McFarlane, "Sanitation in Mumbai's Informal Settlements: State, 'Slum,' and Infrastructure," *Environment and Planning A* 40, no. 1 (2008): 98.

96. For NGO-driven sanitation programs that promote traditional gender roles, see Sapna Doshi, "The Politics of the Evicted: Redevelopment, Subjectivity, and Difference in Mumbai's Slum Frontier," *Antipode* 45, no. 4 (2012): 856–857.

97. "Lok Sabha Unstarred Question No. 1478."

98. Vijay Jagannathan, "Cleaning the Ganga River," *Economic and Political Weekly,* 49, no. 37 (13 September 2014): 24–26, reviews Ganga cleanups.

99. Raghu Dayal, "Dirty Flows the Ganga," *Economic and Political Weekly* 51, no. 25 (18 June 2016): 56.

100. Ibid.

101. Ruhi Kandhari, "Drinking Sewage in Varanasi," *Thethirdpole.net*, 12 October 2015, https://goo.gl/mDCxXg.

102. "Indian Rail Is World's Largest 'Open Toilet': Jairam Ramesh," *NDTV*, 27 July 2012, https://goo.gl/BAHWpm.

103. Lata Jinsu, "Modi's Ganga Sutra and the Politics of Varanasi," *Down to Earth*, 12 May 2014, https://goo.gl/Mxavmd.

104. Ibid.

105. For a more detailed account of the Ganga Action Plan in Varanasi, see Assa Doron, *Life on the Ganga: Boatmen and the Ritual Economy of Banaras* (New Delhi: Cambridge University Press, 2013), 68–79. Kelly Alley, *On the Banks of the Ganga* (Ann Arbor: University of Michigan Press, 2002), analyzes the Ganga Action Plan.

4. Recycling and Value

1. *Raddiwala* is another common term used to describe the door-to-door collector who purchases paper and various broken items from households in north India.

2. Apeetha Arunagiri, email to Surjeet Dhanji, University of Melbourne, 22 June 2016. Quoted with permission.

3. For an obituary of Nek Chand, see *Economist*, 27 June 2015, p. 78. For information and images, see "Ned Chand Foundation," accessed 5 September 2017, http://nekchand.com/.

4. William Rathje and Cullen Murphy, *Rubbish! The Archaeology of Garbage* (Tucson: University of Arizona Press, 2001), 64.

5. Da Zhu et al., *Improving Municipal Solid Waste Management in India: A Sourcebook for Policy Makers and Practitioners* (Washington, DC: World Bank Group, 2008), 130–131. Rajkumar Joshi and Sirajuddin Ahmed, "Status and Challenges of Municipal Solid Waste Management in India: A Review," *Cogent Environmental Science* 2 (2016): 5.

6. Rathje and Murphy, *Rubbish!*, 45–46.

7. "The ship recycling yard Alang-Sosiya is not the graveyard of ageing ships, but it is worthwhile naming this yard as the Re-incarnation of these vessels." *Alang: A Green Re-incarnation* (Bhavnagar, India: Ship Recycling Industries Association, no. 1 (March 2013): 1.

8. "Number of Ships in the World Merchant Fleet as of January 1, 2015, by Type," *Statista*, http://goo.gl/CwP4v6.

9. Haresh Parmar, Chintan Kalthia, and Rohit Agarwal, Ship Recycling Industries Association, conversations with Jeffrey, Bhavnagar, 12 October 2013. See also

"Ship Recyclers," Ship Recycling Industries Association (India), accessed 5 September 2017, http://goo.gl/VP1Qab.

10. For links to eight *Baltimore Sun* articles written in December 1997, see http://goo.gl/wBe3lU. Manish Tiwari, "Titanic Junkyard," *Down to Earth,* 15 March 2008, http://archive.ban.org/library/down_to_earth.html.

11. William Langewiesche, "The Shipbreakers," *Atlantic* 286, no. 2 (August 2000): 31–49.

12. Parmar, Kalthia, and Agarwal, conversations with Jeffrey.

13. *Alang: A Green Re-incarnation,* 1.

14. "Alang Yard Dismantles Record Ships in 2011–12," *Business Standard,* 9 April 2012, http://goo.gl/z1VjB3.

15. Adam Minter, *Junkyard Planet: Travels in the Billion-Dollar Trash Trade* (New York: Bloomsbury, 2013), 135. The price of copper the day Minter visited a recycling business in China was $3.12.

16. Geetanjoy Sahu, "Workers of Alang-Sosiya: A Survey of Working Conditions in a Ship-Breaking Yard, 1983–2013," *Economic and Political Weekly* 49, no. 50 (13 December 2014): 52–59.

17. R. Jeffrey, anonymous conversations at Alang, 12 October 2013.

18. For Europe, see Zsuzsa Gille, *From the Cult of Waste to the Trash Heap of History: The Politics of Waste in Socialist and Postsocialist Hungary* (Bloomington: Indiana University Press, 2007).

19. "CRISIL Reaffirms BB-/P4+Ratings on Atam Manohar Ship Breakers' Bank Facilities," *Daily Brief,* 9 February 2011, https://goo.gl/hoOZg7.

20. Mary Douglas, *Purity and Danger* (London: Ark Paperbacks, 1984), 2. See also Zigmunt Bauman, *Wasted Lives: Modernity and Its Outcomes* (Cambridge, UK: Polity, 2004), 21–22.

21. Emma Tarlo, *Entanglement: The Secret Lives of Hair* (London: Oneworld, 2016), see especially chap. 4, "Tonsure," for temple hair.

22. Documentaries on the temple hair industry include "The Rapunzel Machine," *Foreign Correspondent,* Australian Broadcasting Corporation, video, 01:07:00, 25 June 2015, http://www.dailymotion.com/video/x2vdw61; "Witness - Hair India," Al Jazeera English, video, 45:09, 31 January 2010, https://goo.gl/zsccr3; and the comedian Chris Rock's feature film *Good Hair* (for a trailer, see "Good Hair ft. Chris Rock," video, 02:32, 31 July 2009, https://goo.gl/DTKJdd).

23. For example, see Patrick Olivelle "Hair and Society: Social Significance of Hair in South Asia Traditions" in *Hair: Its Power and Meaning in Asian Cultures,* ed. Alf Hiltebeitel and Barbara D. Miller (New York: State University of New York Press, 1998), 11–50.

24. Eliuned Edwards, “Hair, Devotion and Trade in India,” in *Hair: Styling, Culture and Fashion,* ed. Geraldine Biddle-Perry and Sarah Cheang (London: Bloomsbury, 2008), 157.

25. Neeta Lal, “Hair for the Gods at Tirumala Temple,” *Star* (Malaysia), 18 November 2011, https://goo.gl/LKjY11, reports a “daily average of 800 kg of hair,” and this “easily crosses 1,000 kg” during peaks. The temple, “one of the richest religious pilgrimage sites in the world,” uses the Scrap Metal Association’s experience to e-auction hair to ensure transparency and higher prices.

26. “Tirupati Temple Earns Rs 5.7 Crore through Hair Auction,” *Times of India,* 15 June 2016, http://goo.gl/Iu7zkQ.

27. Widows of Orthodox families, condemned to a life of renunciation, are expected to abandon bright clothing and adornments and to shave their heads.

28. The institution of *pheriya,* door-to-door trading characterized by bartering with villagers, is not confined to hair, as Lucy Norris shows in relation to clothing. Lucy Norris, *Recycling Indian Clothing: Global Contexts of Reuse and Value* (Bloomington: Indiana University Press, 2010), 136.

29. Mr. A. Khan, conversation with Doron, Varanasi, 28 January 2015.

30. Mr. Ashok, conversation with Doron, New Delhi, 25 November 2015.

31. Ibid.

32. Khatiiks are classified as Scheduled Castes, or Dalits. Kaveri Gill discusses their role in the New Delhi waste trade in *Of Poverty and Plastic: Scavenging and Scrap Trading Entrepreneurs in India’s Urban Informal Economy* (New Delhi: Oxford University Press, 2010), 154–183.

33. Mr. Sonu, conversation with Doron, New Delhi, 26 November 2015.

34. Ibid.

35. *DCS International Company,* brochure, 2015, http://dcshairsinternational.com/brochure.pdf and https://www.youtube.com/watch?v=AhipZFpEnvs. The claim of sixty metric tons a month is made in the company’s promotional brochure. D. C. Solanki, conversation with Doron, New Delhi, 27 November 2015.

36. D. C. Solanki, conversation with Doron, New Delhi, 27 November 2015. Tarlo observes that the majority of Indian-sourced hair ends up in Chinese factories for processing before export as hair extensions and wigs to markets across the globe. Tarlo, *Entanglement,* 178, 210.

37. Daniel J. Wakin, “Rabbis’ Rules and Indian Wigs Stir Crisis in Orthodox Brooklyn,” *New York Times,* 14 May 2004, https://goo.gl/uYimN7.

38. Tarlo, *Entanglement,* 85. She describes what came to be known as “Sheitelgate,” which sent many Jewish wig manufacturers out of business with losses estimated up to a billion dollars.

39. Nicky Gregson and Mike Crang "From Waste to Resource: The Trade in Wastes and Global Recycling Economies," *Annual Review of Environment and Resources* 40 (2015): 155.

40. "Ship Breaking in Bangladesh," Young Power in Social Action, accessed 5 September 2017, https://goo.gl/pnvDaq. Nicky Gregson, Helen Watkins, and Melania Calestani, "Inextinguishable Fibres: Demolition and the Vital Materialisms of Asbestos," *Environment and Planning A* 42 (2010): 1065–1083.

41. Abhijit Dasgupta, "From Dust to Gold," *India Today,* 23 November 2009, https://goo.gl/Vg5uPQ.

42. R. V. Russell, *Tribes and Castes of the Central Provinces* (London: Macmillan, 1916), 1:394.

43. M. Rochan, "India's Short Gold Supply Forces Families to Melt Down Heirlooms to Recycle for Weddings," *International Business Times,* 29 November 2013 (updated 1 July 2014), https://goo.gl/ZnJRvf.

44. Dasgupta, "From Dust to Gold."

45. On Kolkata's gold panners, see Taniya Dutta's photographic report, "Desperate Fathers and Sons Scour the Dirt for Any Treasure That They Can Sell Back to Factories," *Daily Mail,* 2 December 2014, https://goo.gl/1eng5E; and "Gold Panning," *Welcome to India,* BBC Two, which follows the daily life of Niarewalas (Newaras), http://www.bbc.co.uk/programmes/p00z4cc6.

46. Mr. Kumar, conversation with Doron, Varanasi, 30 January 2016.

47. In our previous book on mobile phones we detailed the prevalence of dynamic and innovative reuse and repair economies, sustained through an intricate network of shopkeepers, shops, roadside stalls, repairers, and second-hand dealers, largely operating in the informal sector. See Assa Doron and Robin Jeffrey, *The Great Indian Phone Book* (Cambridge, MA: Harvard University Press, 2013), especially chap. 4.

48. "Delhi-NCR Likely to Generate 95,000 MT E-wastes by 2017: ASSOCHAM," ASSOCham website, 7 August 2014, http://assocham.org/newsdetail.php?id=4633.

49. Dumping of e-waste from developed nations to the developing ones is illegal according to the Basel Convention. Local officials were keen to conceal any illicit activities.

50. Mr. Sharma, owner of a recycling factory in Dharavi, conversation with Doron, Mumbai, 19 March 2016.

51. Ghazala Jamil, "The Capitalist Logic of Spatial Segregation," *Economic and Political Weekly* 49, no. 3 (18 January 2014): 54.

52. *Recommendations to Address the Issues of Informal Sector Involved in E-waste Handling, Moradabad, Uttar Pradesh* (New Delhi: Centre for Science and Environment, 2015), 3, https://goo.gl/QMRDSG.

53. Ibid., 5.

54. For an account of the global e-waste industry, see Abdul Khaliq et al., "Metal Extraction Processes for Electronic Waste and Existing Industrial Routes: A Review and Australian Perspective," *Resources* 3 (2014): 152–179. PCBs are 40 percent metal, 30 percent plastic, and 30 percent ceramic, and "coated with base metals . . . (tin, silver or copper) to make them conductive" (154).

55. *Recommendations to Address*, 7–9.

56. Malika Rodrigues, "Sachet Up the Ramp," *Economic Times*, 13 March 2002, https://goo.gl/WertbV.

57. *Recommendations to Address*, 4.

58. Ibid., 10.

59. Anna L. Tsing, *The Mushroom at the End of the World: On the Possibility of Life in Capitalist Ruins* (Princeton, NJ: Princeton University Press, 2015).

60. Ibid., 63.

61. Recent figures speak of fifty thousand metric tons dumped in India in 2012. Zhaohua Wang, Bin Zhang, and Dabo Guan, "Take Responsibility for Electronic-Waste Disposal," *Nature*, 3 August 2016, https://goo.gl/mPTf8q.

62. I. Rucevska et al., *Waste Crime—Waste Risks: Gaps in Meeting the Global Waste Challenge; a Rapid Response Assessment* (Nairobi, Kenya: UN Environment Program and GRID, 2015), 22–23, https://goo.gl/iwGMRG; David N. Pellow, *Resisting Global Toxics: Transnational Movements for Environmental Justice* (Cambridge, MA: MIT Press, 2007), chap. 6 focuses on illegal e-waste flows, including in India.

63. See Lucy Norris, "The Limits of Ethicality in International Markets: Imported Second-hand Clothing in India," *Geoforum* 67 (2015): 185. For ethnographic studies that examine the global trade in waste, see Catherine Alexander and Joshua Reno, eds., *Economies of Recycling: The Global Transformation of Materials, Values and Social Relations* (London: Zed Books, 2012).

64. Vinay Gidwani and Julia Corwin argue that the updated Solid Waste Management Rules of 2016 fail to recognize the complexity of e-waste recycling and privilege ill-equipped private companies over informal workers who are further marginalized. Gidwani and Corwin, "Governance of Waste," *Economic and Political Weekly* 52, no. 31 (5 August 2017): 52.

65. In China, Xin Tong and Jici Wang argue that e-waste flows are driven by local demand for raw materials and the need to create employment for unskilled workers. Xin Tong and Jici Wang, "The Shadow of the Global Network: E-waste Flows to China," in Alexander and Reno, *Economies of Recycling*, 103.

66. "Government Notifies Plastic Waste Management Rules, 2016" (New Delhi: Press Information Bureau, Ministry of Environment and Forests, 18 March 2016),

https://goo.gl/OKEWfy. *Study on Plastic Waste Disposal through "Plasma Pyrolysis Technology"* (New Delhi: Central Pollution Control Board, October 2016), 4, https://goo.gl/dYd9r3.

67. Rathje and Murphy, *Rubbish!*, 206. "Plastics" (Washington, DC: Environmental Protection Agency, March 2015), 2, https://goo.gl/QsDZ1a.

68. *Plastics: In a New Mould* (Mumbai: Plastics Promotions Council, 2013), 2.

69. *Organiser*, 25 September 1994, p. 4.

70. "Delhi Warned of Ecological Disaster," *Times of India*, 31 October 1994, p. 3.

71. *Times of India*, 14 February 1996, p. A1.

72. Gill, *Of Poverty and Plastic*, 161.

73. For the invention of PET bottles and transformation of packaging, see Gay Hawkins, Emily Potter, Kane Race, *Plastic Water: The Social and Material Life of Bottled Water* (Cambridge, MA: MIT Press, 2015).

74. *Plastic Management from Source to Resource: Engineer's Day 2011* (Ahmedabad: School of Building Science and Technology, CEPT University, 2011), 22–23.

75. Jeffrey visited sites in Kolkata with Aftabuddin Ahmed of Tiljala Shed, an NGO, on 17 and 18 March 2015. Minter, *Junkyard Planet*, 147, reports that in China, too, visitors are not welcome where small-scale plastic recycling goes on.

76. *Plastic Management*, 25.

77. Vinay Gidwani, "Remaindered Things and Remaindered Lives: Travelling with Delhi's Waste," in *Finding Delhi: Loss and Renewal in the Megacity*, ed. Bharati Chaturvedi (New Delhi: Penguin Viking, 2010), 38.

78. Jamie Furniss describes similar processes in his study of the PET plastic industry in Egypt. Jamie Furniss, "Alternative Framings of Transnational Waste Flows: Reflections Based on the Egypt–China Pet Plastic Trade," *Area* 47, no. 1 (2015): 24–30.

79. Kamla Mankekar, *Breaking News: A Woman in a Man's World* (New Delhi: Rupa, 2014), 222.

80. Jogarao Bhamidipati, divisional head (Commercial), ITC, Paperboards and Specialty Papers Division, conversation with Jeffrey, Hyderabad, 10 March 2015. "Import and Export of Paper and Cardboard, an International Comparison in 2015," *Statista*, https://goo.gl/RNtqHB.

81. See Rathje and Murphy, *Rubbish!*, 115–119, for colorful examples of the survival of paper in landfills.

82. K. K. Sruthijith, "Newsprint Price Hikes Forcing Publishing Cos to Rejig Practices," *LiveMint*, 12 March 2008, https://goo.gl/lVZsyI. Karolina Tomczyk, "Paper

Prices Remain Soft Despite Supply Cuts," *Spend Matters,* 28 July 2016, http://spendmatters.com/2016/07/28/95660/.

83. "The Letsrecycle.com Prices Section," Letsrecycle.com, accessed 22 November 2016, http://www.letsrecycle.com/prices. The quoted price range for glass was £0–£35; for mixed plastic, £35–£100.

84. Katherine Boo, *Behind the Beautiful Forevers* (New York: Random House, 2012), 190. Waste paper in India in 2015 fetched between four and eight rupees a kilogram. Bhamidipati, conversation with Jeffrey.

85. See Norris, "The Limits of Ethicality," and its bibliography for her other publications.

86. Ibid., 186.

87. Ibid., 183. Such blurring of boundaries between formal and informal sectors is sometimes referred to as a hybrid. Gidwani, and Corwin, "Governance of Waste," 47.

88. Furniss, who examines the recycling economies in Egypt, cautions against overemphasizing the amount of first-world dumping, which he argues tends to overlook the intricacies of waste flows across boundaries. Local agency, national tariffs, and market dynamics also shape the value-adding processes driving global economies of recycling. Furniss, "Alternative Framings," 28–29.

89. Boyan Slat et al., *How the Oceans Can Clean Themselves: A Feasibility Study* (Delft, Netherlands: Ocean Cleanup, 2014). James Temperton, "Toxic Time Bomb: Here's the Science That Explains Why Microbeads Are a Disaster," *Wired,* 25 August 2016, https://goo.gl/Pt1olU.

90. Rathje and Murphy, *Rubbish!,* 202.

91. Chennai City Municipal Corporation Act, 1919 (Tamil Nadu Act 4 of 1919), section 199, https://goo.gl/guBStB.

92. Vinay Gidwani and Amita Baviskar, "Urban Commons," *Economic and Political Weekly* 46, no. 50 (10 December 2011): 42. We should not overstate ideas of the commons. Exchange relations and social rules outside state control have also structured access to resources, as the notion of *haq* (right; privilege, duty) indicates.

93. Soutik Biswas, "Do India's Stray Dogs Kill More People than Terror Attacks?," *BBC News,* 6 May 2016, https://goo.gl/8SZJc2. "Humane Dog Population Management Guidance," *International Companion Animal Management Coalition,* p. 10, 2007, https://goo.gl/rmr2ir.

94. "Humane Dog Population Management Guidance," 10.

95. Gill, *Of Poverty and Plastic,* 28–30, notes some of the recipes for better methods of collection and recycling.

96. For an overview, see Gidwani, and Corwin, "Governance of Waste," 49–50.

97. Tulika Tripathi, "Safai Karmi Scheme of Uttar Pradesh: Caste Dominance Continues," *Economic and Political Weekly* 47, no. 37 (15 September 2012): 28.

5. Technology and Imperfection

1. "Before the National Green Tribunal Southern Zonal Bench, Chennai, Application No. 247 of 2014," 30 September 2015, http://goo.gl/SoHwxc.

2. Shibhu Nair, "Mobile Stupidity," video, 3:30, 8 November 2012, https://www.youtube.com/watch?v=4fJ6QZ24lug.

3. G. Mahadevan, "Mobile Incinerator Brought to Trivandrum Remains Inoperational," *Hindu,* 10 December 2012, http://goo.gl/RHTyIe.

4. T. P. Nijish and Aswin J. Kumar, "Mobile Incinerator Deal Heads for a Legal Fight," *Times of India,* 9 October 2013, http://goo.gl/I4O8xq.

5. "'Tony' Projects: Council in Firing Line," *Times of India,* 16 January 2016, http://goo.gl/wWYofE.

6. Conversations with Doron, Varanasi, 6–12 September 2017.

7. Krishna Pokharel, "Why Narendra Modi's E-boats on Ganges Aren't So Popular with Boatmen," *Wall Street Journal,* 17 May 2016, https://goo.gl/4EQjmW.

8. For a review of the "wicked problem" as a concept in public policy, see Angi English, "Ten Properties of Wicked Problems," Center for Homeland Defense and Security for Radical Homeland Security Experimentation: Homeland Security, accessed 7 September 2017, https://goo.gl/9egxOF.

9. Louis E. Garrick, "A Historical Context of Municipal Solid Waste Management in the United States," *Waste Management and Research* 22, no. 4 (2004): 306–322.

10. L. W. Michael (compiler), *The History of the Municipal Corporation of the City of Bombay* (Bombay: Union Press, 1902), 258–259.

11. Ibid., 269.

12. Greater Chennai Municipal Corporation, "Solid Waste Management," accessed 17 October 2017, https://goo.gl/2b7HLn.

13. Jeffrey and Mumbai friends climbed Deonar on 9 May 2014. Doron found it more difficult to get access two years later (March 2016), although he managed to enter the site. It was then on fire and full of smoke.

14. William Rathje and Cullen Murphy, *Rubbish! The Archaeology of Garbage* (Tucson: University of Arizona Press, 2001), 111–115.

15. Dhrubajyoti Ghosh, *The Trash Diggers* (New Delhi: Oxford University Press, 2017), focuses on Dhapa.

16. Ministry of Environment, Forest and Climate Change, "Solid Waste Management Rules, 2016," 65, https://goo.gl/DEFaPo.

17. HDPE, high-density polyethylene, is the material that containers bearing the code number two are made from.

18. Daniel P. Duffy, "Landfill Economics: Getting Down to Business—Part 2," Forester Network, 16 March 2016, first published in 2005, http://goo.gl/t8anvh. Koride Mahesh, "Waste Management Project: Greater Hyderabad Civic Body in Dilemma as Workers Oppose Move," *Times of India,* 13 February 2014. https://goo.gl/o1l21T.

19. *Consolidated Annual Review Report on Implementation of Municipal Solid Wastes (Management and Handling) Rules, 2000. Annual Review Report: 2013–14* (Delhi: Central Pollution Control Board, 6 February 2015), annex 3, 51–52.

20. When Jeffrey visited the Jawahar Nagar site in Hyderabad in May 2015, it had characteristics of a model landfill. Later, a *Times of India* reporter saw a different side. See Siddharth Tadepalli, "The Filthy Tale of Jawahar Nagar," *Times of India,* 1 October 2015, https://goo.gl/8Gjhxy; *Deccan Chronicle,* 18 May 2016.

21. Ministry of Environment, Forest and Climate Change Notification, New Delhi, 8 April 2016, "Solid Waste Management Rules, 2016," 55, https://goo.gl/DEFaPo.

22. Michael, *History of the Municipal Corporation of the City of Bombay,* 257–258, 261–262, 269.

23. *Mumbai Mirror,* 14 April 2016, https://goo.gl/P9OlyZ. The eight thousand bags of collected waste were, according to a railway spokesman, "dumped . . . into the creeks."

24. Khader Sahib, former joint director Andhra Pradesh Administrative Service, conversation with Jeffrey, Hyderabad, 10 March 2015.

25. Jeffrey walked round the plant at Arcot, Tamil Nadu, with S. Parijatham, municipal commissioner, on 14 November 2013.

26. Jeffrey visited the plant on 26 November 2015 accompanied by Dr. B. Veerabhadrappa, joint commissioner, Raha Rajeshwarrinagar, Bengaluru.

27. "Solid Waste Management Rules, 2016," 58.

28. "Mafia Obstructing Scientific Disposal of Garbage in City," *Deccan Herald,* 14 August 2012, https://goo.gl/cS7ZPc.

29. Natasha Cornea, Renne Veron, and Anne Zimmer, "Clean City Politics: An Urban Political Ecology of Solid Waste in West Bengal, India," *Environment and Planning A* 49, no. 4 (2017): 728–744.

30. Martin V. Melosi, *Garbage in the Cities: Refuse, Reform and the Environment,* rev. ed. (Pittsburgh: University of Pittsburgh Press, 2005), 39.

31. Michael, *History of the Municipal Corporation of the City of Bombay,* 261.

32. Edward J. Walsh and Rex Warland, *Don't Burn It Here: Grassroots Challenges to Trash Incinerators* (University Park, PA: Penn State University Press, 1997), 2.

33. Ibid., 3–4.

34. "Trash to Cash: Norway Leads the Way in Turning Waste into Energy," *Guardian,* 15 June 2013, http://goo.glTkejaG. Phoenix Energy, "Kwinana Waste to Energy Project. Public Environmental Review. MHIEC Global WtE Plant Delivery Record," 2013, http://goo.gl/ESoJbU.

35. http://www.towmcl.com.

36. Kedar Nagarajan, "Delhi: Waste-to-Energy Plants Face Opposition from People in Vicinity," *Indian Express,* 30 May 2016, https://goo.gl/MMsym3.

37. Ibid., and Gaurav Vivek Bhatnagar, "Okhla Waste-to-Energy Plant Using Experimental Chinese Technology Back in Limelight," *The Wire,* 26 April 2016, https://goo.gl/Z4iFpu.

38. Joydeep Thakur, "Today It Is Ghazipur, Tomorrow It Can Be Bhalswa or Okhla in Delhi, Say Experts," *Hindustan Times,* 1 Sept 2017, https://goo.gl/ReE7cQ.

39. Annie Leonard, *The Story of Stuff* (New York: Free Press, 2010), 212–217.

40. "Controversial Durham Energy-from-Waste Incinerator a Year Behind Schedule," *Star* (Toronto), 5 January 2016, http://goo.gl/tHKEST.

41. Eliza Laschon, "Contract Inked for $400m Kwinana Thermal Waste Facility in WA," ABC (Australian Broadcasting Corporation) News, 16 February 2016, http://goo.gl/qBXQZA.

42. "Tuas South Incineration Plant," Singapore, brochure with data for 2013. Jeffrey toured the Tuas South plant with Chong Kuek On, general manager, 13 August 2014.

43. Henri Dwyer and Nickolas J. Themelis, "Inventory of U.S. 2012 Dioxin Emissions to Atmosphere," *Waste Management* 46 (December 2015): 242–246. We are grateful to Professor Ian Rae of the University of Melbourne for helping us compose this paragraph in ways that both a chemist and Doron and Jeffrey can understand.

44. See Global Alliance for Incinerator Alternatives / Global Anti-Incinerator Alliance website, accessed 5 September 2017, http://www.no-burn.org/.

45. Chong Kuek On, general manager, Tuas South Incineration, National Environment Agency, Singapore, conversation with Jeffrey, Singapore, 14 August 2014. The plant has a theoretical capacity to generate eighty megawatts of electricity. http://www.nea.gov.sg/docs/default-source/energy-waste/waste-management/tsip-brochure.pdf. Singapore in 2014 had electricity consumption of more than twelve thousand megawatts.

46. See "Can Incinerators Help Manage India's Growing Waste Management Problem?," *Economic Times,* 9 September 2015, for a discussion of the Okhla plant and other incineration attempts.

47. Rough calculations suggest the engine of a ten-metric-ton truck making a twenty-two kilometer (fourteen-mile) journey at eighty kilometers (fifty miles) an hour uses about seven liters (1.8 gallons) of fuel. For three hundred round-trip journeys of that distance each day, fuel consumption would be more than four thousand liters (1,057 gallons). "The Fuel Efficient Truck Drivers' Handbook" (London: Department of Transport, Her Majesty's Stationery Office, 2009), 9, https://goo.gl/Fsg1ai.

48. "Stench Welcomes Them at Work," *Times of India,* 22 July 2016, https://goo.gl/7pzHQx.

49. *Report of the Working Group on Urban and Industrial Water Supply and Sanitation for 12th Five Year Plan (2012–2017)* (New Delhi: Planning Commission, 2011), 8. The vice president estimated that 80 percent of wastewater escaped treatment. "Sewage Disposal Most Flawed Part of Urban Planning in India," *Times of India,* 5 March 2013.

50. Prakash Javadekar, minister of Information and Broadcasting, quoted in "70% of Indian Sewage Treatment Plants Dysfunctional: Javadekar," *Times of India,* 21 November 2014. https://goo.gl/CL5Oe6.

51. "Capital Regional District Approves Victoria-Area Sewage Treatment Plant," CBC (Canadian Broadcasting Corporation) News, 14 September 2016, https://goo.gl/wqnaCv.

52. Anil Padkar, conversation with Doron, Mumbai, 24 March 2016.

53. Ibid.

54. David Sedlak, *Water 4.0: The Past, Present and Future of the World's Most Vital Resource* (New Haven, CT: Yale University Press, 2014), 55.

55. Sedlak, *Water 4.0,* 121, explains "combined sewers," which use only one set of pipes to collect sewage and storm water, and why they "are no longer being built in most parts of the world."

56. For a fine sequence of illustrations that clarify the subterranean complications, see S. Sarkar, "Sewers and Sewer Networks," 28 August 2015, https://goo.gl/szmIHc. Also see Sedlak, *Water 4.0,* 129; and Rashmi Tiwari and Sanatan Nayak, "Drinking Water, Sanitation and Waterborne Diseases," *Economic and Political Weekly* 52, no. 23 (10 June 2017): 137–138.

57. Conversations with sewer divers, Doron, Varanasi, March 2016.

58. Sedlak, *Water 4.0,* 55.

59. "NEWater," PUB: Singapore's National Water Agency, https://goo.gl/a752xI.

60. "Activated Sludge Treatment Process," World Bank, http://siteresources.worldbank.org/INTTOPSANHYG/Resources/1923125-1186000305809/Infrastructure_All_073107.pdf.

61. *Hindu*, 18 March 2016, https://goo.gl/ZySgES.

62. E. H. Pathan, executive engineer, Drainage and Solid Waste Management, Surat Municipal Corporation, conversation with Jeffrey, Surat, 9 October 2013. *Integrated Waste Management Practices* (brochure) (Surat: Surat Municipal Corporation, n.d. [c. 2013]), 4–5. Black Rock, a moderately sized sewage treatment plant serving much of the western part of the state of Victoria in Australia, occupies about ninety hectares.

63. *Water Supply and Sanitation*, 7.

64. Ibid., 5.

65. Vinay Kumar Srivastava, "On Sanitation: A Memory Ethnography," *Social Change* 44, no. 2 (2014): 277.

66. S. Chaplin, email to Jeffrey, 3 August 2016. Also see Susan E. Chaplin, *The Politics of Sanitation in India* (Hyderabad: Orient BlackSwan, 2011).

67. Kathleen O'Reilly, Richa Dhanju, and Elizabeth Louis, "Subjected to Sanitation: Caste Relations and Sanitation Adoption in Rural Tamil Nadu," *Journal of Development Studies*, November 1, 2016, 2, 8.

68. "Two-Pit System," Sulabh International Social Service Organisation, https://goo.gl/EYi1T9.

69. One study suggests that, to understand open defecation in rural India, we must consider "beliefs, values, and norms about purity, pollution, caste, and untouchability that cause people to reject affordable latrines." Coffey et al., "Understanding Exceptionally Poor Sanitation in Rural India: Purity, Pollution, and Untouchability," *Economic and Political Weekly* 52, no. 1 (7 January 2017): 59.

70. Rose George, *The Big Necessity: The Unmentionable World of Human Waste and Why It Matters* (New York: Holt Paperback, 2009), 216.

71. David Waltner-Toews points to potential problems in treated manure, depending on the diets of the people or animals doing the excreting. *The Origin of Feces* (Toronto: ECW Press, 2016), 118–120.

72. Maggie Black and Ben Fawcett, *The Last Taboo* (London: Earthscan, 2008) quoted in Sarah Jewitt, "Poo Gurus? Researching the Threats and Opportunities Presented by Human Waste," *Applied Geography* 31 (2011): 765–766.

73. Tulasi Srinivas points out that for Bengaluru's Hindu middle class, bathrooms have become spaces for displaying wealth. Tulasi Srinivas, "Flush with Success: Bathing, Defecation, Worship, and Social Change in South India," *Space and Culture*

5, no. 4 (2002): 379. For an illustrated history, see Barbara Penner, *Bathroom* (London: Reaktion Books, 2013).

74. C. C. James, *Notes on Disposal of Sewage at the Matunga Leper Asylum* (Bombay: Times of India Press, 1901).

75. "Terra Preta Toilets," Sustainable Sanitation and Water Management, accessed 5 September 2017, https://goo.gl/vB51cJ.

76. O'Reilly, Dhanju, and Louis, "Subjected," 8.

77. Jewitt, "Poo Gurus?," 765.

78. For simple explanations, see "Yellow Is the New Green," *Treehugger,* 11 April 2014, https://goo.gl/Z84xjh.

79. "How Does Clivus Multrum Work?," accessed 5 September 2017, http://www.clivusmultrum.eu/compostingprocess.php.

80. Ernest Tiedt, Ecosan, Pretoria, South Pretoria, email to Jeffrey, 1 February 2016; and see http://www.ecosan.co.za/contact.html.

81. "Railway Minister Prabhu to Launch First Discharge Free Rail Corridor on Sunday," *Indian Express,* 23 July 2016.

82. Indian Railways, Centre for Advanced Maintenance Technology, "Presentation on IR-DRDO Bio-Toilet System," 3 May 2016, slides 11 and 117, http://iced.cag.gov.in/wp-content/uploads/2016-17/NTP%2003/RK.pdf.

83. "Bio Toilets," CBS Technologies, http://www.cbsenergy.com/FRP-bio-toilet.php#. Sushmita Sengupta, "On Green Track," *Down to Earth,* 15 November 2013, https://goo.gl/91JviS.

84. "The Nano Membrane Toilet," accessed 5 September 2017, http://www.nanomembranetoilet.org/.

85. "Peepoople," accessed 5 September 2017, http://www.peepoople.com.

86. "Peepoo, a Bag That Could Solve India's Toilet Woes," *Deccan Herald,* 11 March 2010, https://goo.gl/NYtaOa.

87. "Swachh Bharat Mission (Gramin)—At a Glance," 17 June 2017, http://sbm.gov.in/sbm/.

88. Smaller-scale sewage treatment technologies are at production stage, but whether they will be capable of being expanded and put into wide use remains to be seen. The Israeli company Emefcy, which recently merged with RWL Water to become Fluence, is one example. "About Us," accessed 29 September 2017, https://www.fluencecorp.com.

89. Peter Redfield, "Bioexpectations: Life Technologies as Humanitarian Goods," *Public Culture* 24, no. 1 (2015): 158.

6. Local Governments and Limitations

1. Emily Cockayne, *Hubbub: Filth, Noise and Stench in England, 1600–1770* (New Haven, CT: Yale University Press, 2007), 186, along with other juicy examples.

2. David Arnold, *Colonizing the Body: State Medicine and Epidemic Disease in Nineteenth-Century India* (Berkeley: University of California Press, 1993), 88–90.

3. Tom Crewe, "The Strange Death of Municipal England," *London Review of Books* 38, no. 24 (2016): 6.

4. For insights into urban change, see Douglas E. Haynes and Nikhil Rao, "Beyond the Colonial City: Re-evaluating the Urban History of India, ca. 1920–1970," *South Asia* 36, no. 3 (2013): 317–335, and other articles in the issue.

5. Sahil Gandhi and Vaidehi Tandel, "What Urbanisation Reforms Owe K. C. Sivaramakrishnan," *Economic and Political Weekly* 52, no. 22 (3 June 2017): 27.

6. Tim Edensor, "The Culture of the Indian Street," in *Images of the Street: Planning, Identity and Control of Public Space,* ed. Nicholas Fyfe (London: Routledge, 1998), 204.

7. Ibid.

8. A. B. Keith, *A Constitutional History of India, 1600–1935,* 2nd ed. (Allahabad: Central Book Depot, 1961), 11–12.

9. Harold A. Gould, "Local Government Roots of Contemporary Indian Politics," *Economic and Political Weekly* 6, no. 7 (13 February 1971): 458. S. Gopal, *The Viceroyalty of Lord Ripon 1880–1884* (London: Oxford University Press, 1953), 1–4, 171.

10. "Memorandum on the Policy of the Government of India in Regard to Local Self-Government," 26 December 1882, quoted in S. R. Mehrotra, *The Emergence of the Indian National Congress* (New Delhi: Vikas, 1971), 305.

11. Evelyn Baring to Louis Mallet, 25 September 1882, quoted in Gopal, *The Viceroyalty of Lord Ripon,* 95.

12. Arnold, *Colonizing the Body,* 204, 274–276.

13. For Ahmedabad and Vallabhbhai Patel as its Mayor, see Abigail McGowan, "Ahmedabad's Home Remedies: Housing in the Re-making of an Industrial City, 1920–1960," *South Asia* 36, no. 3 (2013): 400–409.

14. Stanley Reed and S. T. Sheppard, eds., *Indian Year Book 1930* (Bombay: Bennett Coleman, 1930), 370.

15. Abul Fazl Allami, *The Ain i Akbari of Abul Fazl Allami,* trans. H. S. Jarrett (Calcutta: Asiatic Society of Bengal, 1891), 2:42.

16. Philip Oldenburg, *Big City Government in India: Councillor, Administrator and Citizen in Delhi* (Tucson: University of Arizona Press for the Association for Asian Studies, 1976), 42.

17. Constitution of 1950, part 4, directive principles of state policy, article 40, "Organization of Village Panchayats." Articles 42 and 51 deal with motherhood and peace.

18. Girish Kumar, *Local Democracy in India* (New Delhi: SAGE, 2006), 16–17.

19. Balvantray (Balwantrai) G. Mehta, *Report of the Team for the Study of Community Projects and National Extension Service,* 1957, esp. para. 2.8, http://goo.gl/CrJStl.

20. Michael Tharakan, "Gandhian and Marxist Approaches to Decentralised Governance in India: Points of Similarity," *Social Scientist* 40, nos. 9 / 10 (2012): 53.

21. *Third Five-Year Plan, 1961–6,* chap. 33, para. 33, http://goo.gl/MEKTVk.

22. Rodney W. Jones, *Urban Politics in India* (Berkeley: University of California Press, 1974), 20.

23. V. Nath, "Urbanisation in India: Review and Prospects," *Economic and Political Weekly* 28, no. 8 (22 February 1986): 339–352.

24. Lisa Björkman, *Pipe Politics, Contested Waters: Embedded Infrastructures of Millennial Mumbai* (Durham, NC: Duke University Press, 2015), 1–3.

25. Lisa Weinstein, *The Durable Slum: Dharavi and the Right to Stay Put in Globalizing Mumbai* (Minneapolis: University of Minnesota Press, 2014), 104–114.

26. T. M. Thomas Isaac and Richard W. Franke, *Local Democracy and Development: People's Campaign for Decentralized Planning in Kerala* (New Delhi: LeftWord, 2000), 19–21. Kerala is an exception to much of this discussion.

27. For digests of the inquiries into local government, see Bibek Debroy and P. D. Kaushik, *Energising Rural Development through "Panchayats"* (New Delhi: Academic Foundation, 2005), 82; and S. R. Maheshwari, *Indian Administration,* 6th ed. (Bombay: Orient Longmans, 2001), 544–545.

28. Seventy-Fourth Amendment, part 9A, para. 243q (a).

29. Simanti Bandyopadhyay, "Municipal Finance in India: Some Critical Issues" (working paper, no. 11, International Centre for Public Policy, Atlanta, Georgia State University, 2014), 11.

30. *Bengaluru: Way Forward—Expert Committee; BBMP Restructuring, June 2015* (Bengaluru: Government of Karnataka, 2015), 10–12, 42–43. The Bruhat Bengaluru Mahanagara Palike (the name given to the local government of Bengaluru) in 2007 grew from about 210 square kilometers (81 square miles) to more than 700 square kilometers (270 square miles).

31. D. Narayana, "Local Governance without Capacity Building: Ten Years of Panchayati Raj," *Economic and Political Weekly* 40, no. 26 (25 June 2005): 2822.

32. A broader geographical definition of Chennai pushes it into semirural areas that include more than two hundred village panchayats. See "Chennai Metropolitan Area," Wikipedia, updated 1 September 2015, https://goo.gl/KqiJxo.

33. *Census of India, 2011.*

34. *Inspiring Progress: Learning from Exnora Green Lammapuram's Solid Waste Management Partnerships in South Localities* (Chennai: Exnora Green, 2010), 11. Bharat Dahiya, "Hard Struggle and Soft Gains: Environmental Management, Civil Society and Governance in Lammapuram, South India," *Environment and Urbanization* 15, no. 1 (April 2003): 95–96.

35. *Inspiring Progress,* 11; Dahiya, "Hard Struggle," 95–96.

36. *Inspiring Progress,* 11.

37. Dr. Mangalam Balasubramanian, managing director, Exnora Green Pammal, conversation with Jeffrey, Pammal, 15 November 2013.

38. Dahiya, "Hard Struggle," 97.

39. Balasubramanian, conversation with Jeffrey.

40. *Inspiring Progress,* 11.

41. Exnora Green Pammal, *Annual Report, 2012–13* (Pammal: Exnora Green, 2013), 9–14, 32–34.

42. "About Us," Municipal Administration and Water Supply, Government of Tamil Nadu, http://www.tn.gov.in/maws/about_us.htm.

43. Balasubramanian, conversation with Jeffrey.

44. *Census of India, 2011,* "C-1 Population by Religious Community—2011," http://goo.gl/ZHfO2z.

45. "Mandate," Ministry of Urban Development, http://moud.gov.in/cms/mandate.php.

46. Senior official, South Delhi Municipal Corporation, interview with Jeffrey, New Delhi, 1 May 2014.

47. Ibid.

48. Douglas Haynes, *Rhetoric and Ritual in Colonial India,* (Berkeley: University of California Press, 1991), 113.

49. *Hindu,* 14 March 2015, p. 3.

50. "GHMC Tries to Wriggle Out of 'Dustbin' Mess," *Indian Express* (Hyderabad ed.), 12 March 2015, p. 3.

51. Chetan Vaidya and Brad Johnson, "Ahmedabad Municipal Bond," *Economic and Political Weekly* 36, no. 30 (28 July 2001): 2885.

52. Kiran Sandhu, "Between Hype and Veracity: An Analysis of Privatization of Solid Waste Management Services, Amritsar City, India," paper presented at the 5th International Conference on Solid Waste Management, Bengaluru, November 2015.

53. Om Prakash Mathur, Debdulal Thakur, and Nilesh Rajadhyaksha, *Urban Property Tax Potential in India* (New Delhi: National Institute of Public Finance and Policy, 2009), ix, https://goo.gl/wjAaUi.

54. Ibid., 17, 21, 60.

55. Rumi Aijaz, *Challenges for Urban Local Government in India* (working paper no. 19, London School of Economics, August 2007), 18, 20, 26, https://goo.gl/9XnVxh.

56. "Prime Minister's Speech on JNNURM, 3 December 2005, New Delhi," in K. C. Sivaramakrishnan, *Re-visioning Indian Cities: The Urban Renewal Mission* (New Delhi: SAGE, 2011), 227–232.

57. "President's Speech to the Parliament, 4 June 2009, New Delhi," in Sivaramakrishnan, *Re-visioning Indian Cities,* 235.

58. M. Venkaiah Naidu, "The Rediscovery of Urban India," *Hindu,* 3 January 2017, https://goo.gl/9AbPdo. For an analysis of the Smart Cities program of the BJP government, see Kristian Hoelscher, "The Evolution of the Smart Cities Agenda in India," *International Asia Studies Review* 19, no. 1 (2016): 39. For the Smart Cities program, see "Smart Cities Mission," Ministry of Housing and Urban Affairs, http://smartcities.gov.in/.

59. Naidu, "The Rediscovery of Urban India."

60. Vaidya and Johnson, "Ahmedabad Municipal Bond," 2884–2891, tell the story in detail.

61. Surojit Gupta, "Time Indian Cities Woke Up to Municipal Bonds," *Times of India,* 20 July 2013, https://goo.gl/aNkm5I. *Hindu,* 8 September 2016, https://goo.gl/XBdIRz. See Bandyopadhyay, "Municipal Finance," for a valuable summary.

62. "20 Years Down the Line What Ails the Urban Local Bodies," *Down to Earth,* 1 June 2012, https://goo.gl/fcLDio.

63. "Observations by Miss Nightingale," 370. "The Sanitary Commissioner with the Government of India," *British Medical Journal,* 11 November 1911, pp. 1294–1295.

64. Arnold, *Colonizing the Body,* 275–276.

65. Hugh Tinker, *The Foundations of Local Self-Government in India, Pakistan and Burma* (London: Athlone Press, 1954), 72.

66. *Third Five-Year Plan.*

67. *Approach towards Establishing Municipal Cadres in India* (New Delhi: Ministry of Urban Development and the World Bank, 2014), 10, https://goo.gl/Srz2f5.

68. Local government is the theme of the Australian and the U.S. television comedy series *Grass Roots* and *Parks and Recreation.*

69. Clay Lucas and Aisha Dow, "Town Hall Troubles," *Age* (Melbourne), 20 October 2016, p. 13.

70. Björkman, *Pipe Politics,* 29.

71. Ibid., 25–30.

72. Sunali Rohra and Barnik Maitra, "The Urban Capacity Conundrum," *Financial Express,* 20 May 2015, https://goo.gl/FxfwKr.

73. *Orissa State Level: Background Paper* (Bhubaneshwar: KIIT School of Rural Management, 2011), 49, http://urk.tiss.edu/images/pdf/Orissa-State-level-Background-Paper.pdf.

74. Narayana, "Local Governance," 2825.

75. Ibid., 2824.

76. Ibid., 2832.

77. Kuldeep Mathur, *Panchayati Raj* (New Delhi: Oxford University Press, 2013), 89.

78. *B.PAC 2nd Anniversary Special* (Bengaluru: B.PAC, 2014), 1, statement from Kiran Shaw-Mazumdar, B.PAC president.

79. Revathy Ashok, chief executive officer, B.PAC, conversation with Jeffrey, Bengaluru, 25 November 2015.

80. http://www.ssampathkumar.com, accessed 5 January 2017 (site discontinued).

81. N. S. Ramakanth, B.PAC, conversation with Jeffrey, Bengaluru, 25 November 2015.

82. Meeta Rajivlochan, principal secretary, government of Maharashtra, "Swachh Bharat's Success Lies in Trusting the Town Councils," *Hindustan Times,* 9 December 2015, https://goo.gl/FJrtQf.

83. T. M. Thomas Isaac quoted in Shaju Philip, "'Clean Home, Clean City': Alappuzha Municipality Shows the Way," *Indian Express,* 6 October 2014, https://goo.gl/fMqsZc.

84. "CSE's Clean City Awards Conferred on Three Indian Cties," Centre for Science and Environment, 11 July 2016, https://goo.gl/XuxDku. For an elegant essay on waste management in Alappuzha and Kerala, see Kushanava Choudhury, "Raising a Stink: How People Power Forced a Waste-Management Revolution in Kerala," *Caravan,* 1 May 2017, https://goo.gl/yCcas4.

85. Natasha Cornea, Renne Veron, and Anne Zimmer, "Clean City Politics: An Urban Political Ecology of Solid Waste in West Bengal, India," *Environment and Planning A* 49, no. 4 (2017): 735.

86. Philip, "Clean Home, Clean City."

87. *Hindu,* 4 September 2005, 21 February 2010 and 12 February 2014, record changes of Raichur's municipal commissioner.

88. "Six Officers, Contractor Booking for Irregularities," *Hindu,* 12 February 2014. "Daily Wagers in Raichur to Get 9 Months' Arrears," *Indian Express,* 21 February 2010. "Lokayukta Serves Notice on CMC President, Three Others," *Hindu,* 4 September 2005. *India: North Karnataka Urban Sector Investment Program, Tranche 1* (Asian Development Bank, August 2015), https://www.adb.org/sites/default/files/evaluation-document/189851/files/pvr-451.pdf, 5, 10.

89. The state of Telangana was created out of Andhra Pradesh in 2014.

90. Much of the plan is embraced in the case studies in *Urban Solid Waste Management in Indian Cities* (New Delhi: National Institute of Urban Affairs, 2015), https://goo.gl/yIYsbn. Khader Saheb was a member of the peer review group.

91. The Centre for Ash Utilisation Technology and Environment Conservation was no typical NGO. It had been supported with expertise and equipment by the coal-fired power station in cooperation with the Indo-Norwegian Environment Program, "Cashing In on Fly Ash," *Hindu BusinessLine*, 4 August 2006, https://goo.gl/IIZMxH.

92. Jeffrey joined this walk on 13 March 2015. Although the councillor no doubt knew where he would find sympathetic territory, he heard grievances as well as satisfaction.

93. District commissioner, conversation with Jeffrey, 13 March 2015.

94. Kumar Burradikatti, "Waste Management Is Better in Raichur than Bengaluru: Supreme Court Panel," *Hindu*, 19 October 2015, http://goo.gl/UZszYf. Raichur dump site supervisor, conversation with Jeffrey, Bengaluru, 27 November 2015. Rukesh Doddamani, the supervisor, later reported that he had left Raichur in dejection at deteriorating waste-management practices and started his own waste-management business in Bengaluru in January 2017.

95. Vidhee Kiran Avashiha and Amit Garg, "Urban Infrastructure and Governance Mission under JNNURM," *Economic and Political Weekly* 51, no. 2 (9 January 2016): 57.

7. Occupations and Possibilities

1. Katherine Boo, *Behind the Beautiful Forevers* (New York: Random House, 2012).

2. Avalok Langer, "From Rags to Ditches," *Tehelka*, 23 April 2011, https://goo.gl/tSYfHW. Swati Singh Sambyal, "Trashing the Ragpicker," *Down to Earth*, 30 April 2016, p. 17.

3. Taking the low-end New Delhi estimates of 200,000 waste-pickers in a city of 16 million as a basis, a city of 1 million would have 12,500 waste-pickers. The average population of India's 465 cities with between 100,000 and 1 million is 270,000, which would translate to about 3,400 waste-pickers in each such city.

4. Shiv Kumar, sewer diver, conversation with Doron, Varanasi, 29 March 2016.

5. In Pakistan, the sewer people belong to the lowest castes. Some of these have converted to Christianity but cannot shake the stigma associated with their previous caste background. See Alice Albinia's poignant travelogue, *Empires of the Indus: The Story of a River* (London: John Murray, 2008), 29.

6. Chandra Bhan Prasad, interview with S. Anand, *Outlook*, 16 April 2016, https://goo.gl/4MzaeZ/.

7. Adam Minter, *Junkyard Planet: Travels in the Billion-Dollar Trash Trade* (New York: Bloomsbury, 2013).

8. People saw great promise in action groups in the 1980s, but the upscaling to national influence did not happen. For examples, see Robin Jeffrey, *What's Happening to India?* (London: Macmillan, 1986), 201–205.

9. For more on the uneven effects of NGOs, see Colin McFarlane, "Sanitation in Mumbai's Informal Settlements: State, "Slum," and Infrastructure." *Environment and Planning A* 40, no. (1): 88–107; Sapna Doshi, "The Politics of the Evicted: Redevelopment, Subjectivity, and Difference in Mumbai's Slum Frontier," *Antipode* 45, no. 4 (2012): 844–865; and Mukul Sharma, "Brahmanical Activism As Eco-Casteism: Reading the Life Narratives of Bindeshwar Pathak, Sulabh International, and 'Liberated' Dalits," *Biography* 40, no. 1 (2017): 199–221.

10. C. Carkeet James, *Drainage Problems of the East: Being a Revised and Enlarged Edition of "Oriental Drainage"* (Bombay: Times of India Press, 1906). *Report of the Commissioners Appointed to Inquire into the Sanitary State of the Army in India; with Precis of Evidence* (London: Eyre and Spottiswood for Her Majesty's Stationery Office, 1863). *Scavenging Conditions Enquiry Committee* (New Delhi: Ministry of Home Affairs, Central Advisory Board for Harijan Welfare, 1960). Ministry of Environment, Forest and Climate Change, "Solid Waste Management Rules, 2016," https://goo.gl/DEFaPo. "Six Quotes from PM Modi on Swachh Bharat Abhiyan," *India Today*, 2 October 2014, https://goo.gl/xSCmhn.

11. C. Carkeet James, *Oriental Drainage: A Guide to the Collection, Removal and Disposal of Sewage in Eastern Cities* (Bombay: Times of India Press, 1902); C. Carkeet James, *Further Notes on Sewage Disposal* (Bombay: Times of India Press, n.d. [c. 1900]); C. Carkeet James, *Notes on Disposal of Sewage at the Matunga Leper Asylum* (Bombay: Times of India Press, 1901).

12. Nomination and Admission, Institute of Civil Engineers, No. 6655, 6 December 1887. A note is added to this document in red ink that, from August 1887, James's address was c / o Indian Midland Railway, Gwalior. Jeffrey is grateful to Debra Francis of the Institute of Civil Engineers in the UK for providing this material (26 September 2016).

13. Quote from Martin V. Melosi, *Garbage in the Cities: Refuse, Reform and the Environment*, rev. ed. (Pittsburgh: University of Pittsburgh Press, 2005), 43. Elizabeth Royte, *Garbage Land: On the Secret Trail of Trash* (New York: Back Bay Books, 2006), 22–23.

14. Dr. S. S. Pandya, conversation with Doron, Matunga, 18 March 2016.

15. *Times of India*, 20 February 1902, p. 4; and *Times of India*, 11 June 1902, p. 3.

16. *Plastic Management from Source to Resource. Engineer's Day 2011* (Ahmedabad: School of Building Science and Technology, CEPT University, 2011), 8.

17. Sandy, conversation with Jeffrey, Ahmedabad, 16 April 2013. Interview, deputy director, solid waste management, Ahmedabad Municipal Corporation, with Jeffrey, Ahmedabad, 16 April 2013.

18. *Environmental Impact Assessment Study: Common Municipal Solid Waste Management Facility, Doddabidirakallu, Bengaluru* (Gurgaon: AECOM India, 2015), http://kspcb.gov.in/PH/Final%20EIA%20Doddabidarakallu_23062015.pdf; "Solid Waste Management Overview," Bruhat Bengaluru Mahanagara Palike, n.d. (c. 2015) https://goo.gl/eXqfRv. Prince Devasagayam, conversation with Jeffrey, Thippenahalli, 26 November 2015.

19. Bengaluru has six administrative zones: North, South, West, East, Central, and Northeastern.

20. Prince Devasagayam, conversation with Jeffrey, Thippenahalli, 26 November 2015.

21. M. Suchitra, "Stench in My Backyard," *Down to Earth,* September 15, 2012, http://www.downtoearth.org.in/coverage/stench-in-my—backyard-38970; Kushanava Choudhury, "Raising a Stink: How People Power Forced a Waste-Management Revolution in Kerala," *Caravan,* 1 May 2017, https://goo.gl/yCcas4.

22. S. Panicker, conversation with Doron, Vilappilsala, 22 December 2014.

23. Suresh Jangir, "Garbage Wars: Villages Stand Firm against Bengaluru," *First .in,* 12 April 2016, http://goo.gl/hdsb2U.

24. Prince Devasagayam, conversation with Jeffrey, Thippenahalli, 26 November 2015.

25. G. P. Mohapatra, Ahmedabad Municipal Commissioner, conversation with Jeffrey, Ahmedabad, 16 October 2013. Mohapatra was appointed chairman of the Airports Authority of India in 2016. "Surtis Elated over Mohapatra's Appointment as AAI chairman," *Times of India,* 15 July 2016, http://goo.gl/OK9JSg.

26. Mohapatra, conversation with Jeffrey.

27. E. H. Pathan, conversation with Jeffrey, Surat, 10 October 2013.

28. This is unlike the IAS, in which a member of a state's cadre may come from a different part of India.

29. Khader Saheb, conversation with Jeffrey, Hyderabad, 10 March 2015.

30. Ibid.

31. Ibid.

32. *Down to Earth,* 15 June 2016, p. 48.

33. Sunita Narain and Swati Singh Sambyal, *Not in My Backyard: Solid Waste Management in Indian Cities* (New Delhi: Centre for Science and Environment, 2016), 86, 128.

34. Almitra Patel, "Waste Management Miracle in Warangal, Oct 2012," n.d. (c. 2013), accessed 10 October 2017, http://goo.gl/MKJXEU. Some scholars have argued that such judicial activism perpetuated the marginalization of the poor. See Asher Ghertner, *Rule by Aesthetics: World-Class City Making in Delhi* (New York: Oxford University Press, 2015), 104–107; and Vinay Gidwani, "Value Struggles: Waste Work and Urban Ecology in Delhi," in *Ecologies of Urbanism in India: Metropolitan Civility and Sustainability,* ed. Anne Rademacher and K. Sivaramkrishnan (Hong Kong: Hong Kong University Press, 2013), 184–189.

35. Keya Acharya, "Trash Driving," *Hindu,* 24 November 2012, http://goo.gl/i8wzrR.

36. Ibid.

37. "Clean Cities Championship Campaign," Warangal Municipal Corporation, accessed 5 September 2017, http://gwmc.gov.in/clean/About.aspx.

38. Engineers of the Greater Hyderabad Municipal Corporation stressed the difficulties faced by big cities in interviews with Jeffrey in Hyderabad, 12 March 2015.

39. "Garbage Piles Up across City as Sanitation Workers Continue Strike," *New Indian Express,* 12 July 2015, http://goo.gl/LWWNUo.

40. Jogarao Bhamidipati, divisional head (Commercial), ITC, conversation with Jeffrey, Hyderabad, 10 March 2015. Bhamidipati's figures don't agree precisely with "Paper and Paperboard Production and Consumption for India," Pulp and Paper Resources and Information Site, accessed 8 October 2017, http://www.paperonweb.com/India.htm, but they are roughly similar.

41. Preeti Mehra, "Want That Waste Paper!," *Hindu,* 1 January 2012, updated 25 July 2016, https://goo.gl/CrRiap.

42. For an evaluation of CSR after two years, see Oliver Balch, "Indian Law Requires Companies to Give 2% of Profits to Charity. Is It Working?," *Guardian,* 5 April 2016, https://goo.gl/uxOPBj. ITC ranked seventh in a list of CSR performance of one hundred companies in 2016. "India's Top Companies for Sustainability and CSR 2016," *futurescape,* accessed 8 October 2017, https://goo.gl/ozWPY6.

43. See the "About Us" webpages for Republic Services (https://www.republicservices.com/about-us) and Waste Management (http://www.wm.com/about/index.jsp).

44. "Companies Located in India and Involved in Sewage and Refuse Disposal, Sanitation and Similar Activities," Zauba Corp, accessed 7 November 2017, https://www.zaubacorp.com/company-list/nic-900-company.html. A similar search on 14 September 2016 showed 761 such companies, 69 of which were public.

45. Ibid. Four Ramky representatives were directors of Delhi MSW Solutions and West Bengal Waste Management. Two of the four were directors of Hyderabad Integrated MSW.

46. "Ramky Enviro Engineers," Ramky Group, accessed 5 September 2017, http://ramkyenviroengineers.com/.

47. "Richie Rich of Seemandhra," *Hindu,* 17 April 2014, https://goo.gl/YLg5Zv. Running as a candidate of an Andhra Pradesh party founded by the son of deceased chief minister, he lost by about thirty-five thousand votes.

48. "Company Overview of Ramky Infrastructure Limited," *Bloomberg,* accessed 16 September 2016, https://goo.gl/8TVAVD.

49. "India's Worlds of Waste," workshop, Institute of South Asian Studies, Singapore, 27–28 July 2015; Robin Jeffrey, *India's Worlds of Waste,* Institute of South Asian Studies Special Report, no. 28 (Singapore: ISAS), 17 September 2015.

50. M. S. Goutham Reddy, director, Ramky Group, conversation with Jeffrey, Hyderabad, 14 March 2015.

51. Ibid.

52. Ibid.

53. The first Apollo hospital of Dr. Prathap Reddy, whose group is often credited as being the pioneer of for-profit hospitals in India, opened in Chennai in 1983. One well-informed source in 2014 refers to "the recent trend of using disposables." INCLEN Program Evaluation Network (IPEN) Study Group, New Delhi, India, "Bio-medical Waste Management: Situational Analysis & Predictors of Performance in 25 Districts across 20 Indian States," *Indian Journal of Medical Research* 139 (2014): 141–153. See also Sarah Hodges. "Medical Garbage and the Making of Neo-liberalism in India," *Economic and Political Weekly* 48, no. 48 (30 November 2013): 112–119.

54. "India Releases New Rules for Biomedical Waste Management," *International Business Times,* 28 March 2016, https://goo.gl/oabfOV. A survey in 2008 found about 170 such centers, none of them operated by Ramky. Central Pollution Control Board, "State-wise Status of Common Biomedical Waste Treatment Facilities (CBWTFs)," 2008, http://cpcb.nic.in/wast/bioimedicalwast/CBWTF_Status_2008.pdf.

55. Goutham Reddy, conversation with Jeffrey, 14 March 2015.

56. IPEN Study Group, "Bio-medical Waste Management," 141.

57. The English scholar Sarah Hodges tracks the journey of a disposal syringe from a corporate hospital in Chennai through the informal sector and to its reentry into the market with a gleaming new look. See Hodges, "Chennai's Biotrash Chronicles: Chasing the Neo-liberal Syringe" (working paper 44/08, GARNET, 2008), 1–28, accessed 18 October 2017, https://goo.gl/ksMnTp.

58. http://www.greentribunal.gov.in/, accessed 10 October 2017.

59. *Hindu*, 21 August 2016, https://goo.gl/sGGt7w. Sarah Hodges follows the illegal and profitable trade in medical waste in Chennai in "Medical Garbage and the Making of Neo-liberalism in India."

60. "Environment Ministry Announces New Rules for Disposal of Hazardous Waste," *Economic Times*, 3 April 2016, http://goo.gl/UTlyEB. The U.S. Environmental Protection Agency calculated that the United States produced 28.8 million tons of hazardous waste in 2011. "EPA's Report on the Environment (ROE): Hazardous Waste," accessed October 18, 2017, https://cfpub.epa.gov/roe/indicator.cfm?i=54.

61. Goutham Reddy, conversation with Jeffrey, 14 March 2015.

62. "Hazardous Waste Management," Ramky Enviro Engineers, accessed 5 September 2017, https://goo.gl/rXoCy2.

63. Snehangshu Chakraborty, Ramky eastern zone coordinator, conversation with Jeffrey, Haldia, 19 March 2015.

64. Ibid.

65. "National Inventory of Hazardous Wastes Generating Industries and Hazardous Waste Management in India" (New Delhi: Central Pollution Control Board, 2009), 11, accessed 5 October 2017, https://goo.gl/GRsEbj, reported 13,645 registered industries in West Bengal.

66. "Mumbai Waste Management Ltd.," Ramky Group, accessed 5 September 2017, http://www.mumbaiwastemanagement.com/incineration-plant.htm.

67. Chakraborty, conversation with Jeffrey.

68. "Ragpickers Battle Toxic Fumes and Hunger as Deonar Fire Smolders" *Times of India*, 2 February 2016, http://bit.ly/2e7k82u.

69. Waste-pickers must contend with multiple dangers when venturing out to relieve themselves in Deonar. Renu Desai, Colin McFarlane, and Stephen Graham, "The Politics of Open Defecation: Informality, Body, and Infrastructure in Mumbai," *Antipode* 47, no. 1 (2015): 113–115.

70. Shiv Sunny, "Delhi's Ghazipur Landfill Collapse: 2 Dead as Mountain of Trash Sweeps Many into Nearby Canal," *Hindustan Times*, 2 September 2017, https://goo.gl/PvdxXZ.

71. "18 Stories High and Still Burning, Fire at Landfill Exposes India's Growing Trash Crisis," *Los Angeles Times*, 23 March 2016, http://lat.ms/22Ji1SJ.

72. "Ragpickers Battle Toxic Fumes."

73. Economists are familiar with value chains in trade relations among countries. Countries can get stuck in the low-value-extraction and basic-preparation stages of production, just as waste handlers can be trapped with no possibility of adding value and improving lives. Kevin Cheng et al., *Reaping the Benefits from Global Value*

Chains (working paper 15/204, International Monetary Fund, September 2015), https://goo.gl/fntW5a. We are grateful to Deeparghya Mukherjee for the reference and basic education.

74. A photo-essay powerfully captures the conditions ragpickers in the Okhla landfill in Delhi work in. William Brown, "Delhi's Dilemma: What to Do with Its Tonnes of Waste?," *Aljazeera,* 29 November 2016, https://goo.gl/fKdqki.

75. Ujwala Samarth, "The Occupational Health of Waste Pickers in Pune: KKPKP and SWaCH Members Push for Health Rights" (Manchester, UK: Women in Informal Employment: Globalizing and Organizing, March 2014), 6, http://bit.ly/2e4hCc5.

76. Boo's *Behind the Beautiful Forevers,* especially 247–254, pays tribute to the gutsy survival of the waste-pickers she got to know. For an anthropologist's account of life on a big Asian dump, see Cindy Bryson's prize-winning thesis and photographs, "A Valuable Life: Seeing Transformative Practice among Phnom Penh's Waste Pickers" (PhD diss., Australian National University, Canberra, 2014).

77. Protection from the police is a concern for *kabaadiwalas.* Kaveri Gill, "Interlinked Contracts and Social Power: Patronage and Exploitation in India's Waste Recovery Market," *Journal of Development Studies* 43, no. 8 (2007): 1456.

78. Santosh, conversation with Doron, Delhi, 25 November 2015.

79. Ibid.

80. Frank Korom, "On the Ethics and Aesthetics of Recycling in India," in *Purifying the Earthly Body of God: Religion and Ecology in Hindu India,* ed. Lance E. Nelson (Albany: State University of New York Press, 1998), 197–223.

81. Jo Beall, "Thoughts on Poverty from a South Asian Rubbish Dump," *IDF Bulletin* 28, no. 3 (1997): 73–90.

82. Joshua Reno, *Waste Away: Working and Living with a North American Landfill* (Berkeley: University of California Press, 2016), 67.

83. Rose George, *The Big Necessity: The Unmentionable World of Human Waste and Why It Matters* (New York: Holt Paperback, 2009), 15.

84. Ibid.

85. Sumit Kumar, conversation, with Doron, Varanasi, 29 March 2014.

86. James, *Drainage Problems,* 313.

87. "Bhim Yatra," Safai Karmachari Andolan, 10 December 2015, http://www.safaikarmachariandolan.org/Bhim-Yatra.html. See "Sewer Gas Guide," North Dakota Department of Health, accessed 5 September 2017, https://www.ndhealth.gov/aq/iaq/Biological/Sewer%20gas%20guide%20final.pdf.

88. Nikhil Srivastav, "Why Open Defecation in India Will End Only with the Annihilation of Caste," *Scroll.in,* 11 September 2016, https://goo.gl/qkbTgg.

89. Piyush Garud, "Dirt of a Nation!," 19 January 2013, https://goo.gl/1Bcq09.

90. Ibid.

91. For more of Olwe's work, which was recognized when he was awarded one of India's highest decorations in 2016, see "Sudharak Olwe," accessed 5 September 2017, http://sudharakolwe.com/index.html.

92. Dhasu Chandrakant, conversation with Doron, 21 March 2016.

93. Ajaz Ashraf, "It's Safer Being a Soldier Fighting in Kashmir Than a Sewer Worker. What Does That Say About India?," Scroll.in, 11 September 2017, https://goo.gl/mzWf9C.

94. Robin Nagle, *Picking Up: On the Streets and Behind the Trucks with the Sanitation Workers of New York City* (New York: Farrer, Straus and Giroux, 2013), 227, 162.

95. Ibid., 162.

96. Garud, "Dirt of a Nation!"

97. P. S. Vivek, "Scavengers: Mumbai's Neglected Workers," *Economic and Political Weekly* 35, no. 42 (14 October 2000): 3723. See also P. S. Vivek, *The Scavengers: Exploited Class of City Professionals* (Mumbai: Himalaya Publishing House, 1998).

98. *Hindu,* 21 January 2016, https://goo.gl/SF4X99.

99. Gill, "Interlinked Contracts," 1466.

100. Tire dealer, conversation with Doron, 24 December 2014.

101. "Kerala Waste Time-Bomb Ticks Away in Kovai," *New Indian Express,* 17 July 2016.

102. Devaraj, conversation with Doron, Thiruvananthapuram, 20 December 2014.

103. "US Toxic Waste Dumped at Indian Port," *Times of India,* 11 June 2008, http://bit.ly/2e4kt4N.

104. See Kaveri Gill, *Of Poverty and Plastic: Scavenging and Scrap Trading Entrepreneurs in India's Urban Informal Economy* (New Delhi: Oxford University Press, 2010), 83–122.

105. Devaraj, conversation with Doron.

106. Mr. Raman, conversation with Doron, Thiruvananthapuram, 20 December 2014.

107. The Bihari man probably had collaborators in the hotel. The Indian government mandated that bottles and caps of premium imported liquor be destroyed to avoid counterfeiting. Empty bottles were, however, sold to waste traders and came back into the market with local bootlegged liquor.

108. "Introduction," Tamilnadu Small Industries Development Corporation Ltd, accessed 5 September 2017, http://www.sidco.tn.nic.in.

109. In contrast, see, for example, "Environmental, Health, and Safety Guidelines for Foundries," (International Finance Corporation, World Bank Group, 30 April 2007), http://bit.ly/2dtD8qD.

110. Md Alamgir, Tiljala Shed, conversations with Jeffrey, Kolkata, 17 and 18 March 2015.

111. Sanjay Sharma, conversation with Doron, Varanasi, 31 March 2014.

112. Robin Jeffrey, *Politics, Women and Well-Being: How Kerala Became "a Model,"* 3rd ed. (New Delhi: Oxford University Press, 2010).

113. Usha, conversation with Doron, 7 December 2013.

114. Tamil Nadu had qualities Kerala lacked: flexible regulation, cheap labor, and space. See "Kerala Waste Time-Bomb."

115. For the U.S. ban on feeding unsterilized slops to pigs, see Melosi, *Garbage in the Cities*, 187–188. Also see William Rathje and Cullen Murphy, *Rubbish! The Archaeology of Garbage* (Tucson: University of Arizona Press, 2001), 35, 37.

116. "Welcome to Chintan!," Chintan Environmental Research and Action Group, accessed 5 September 2017, http://www.chintan-india.org.

117. "Welcome to Safai Sena," Safai Sena, accessed 5 September 2017, http://www.safaisena.net.

118. David Mosse, "The Anthropology of International Development," *Annual Review of Anthropology* 42 (2013): 229.

119. Tania M. Li, *The Will to Improve: Governmentality, Development, and the Practice of Politics* (Durham, NC: Duke University Press, 2007), 7.

120. On the "politics of visibility," see Arjun Appadurai, "Deep Democracy: Urban Governmentality and the Horizon of Politics," *Public Culture* 14, no. 1 (2002): 21–47.

121. During BJP rule in the late 1990s, the "presence of Bengali-speaking Muslims (assumed to be from Bangladesh) was used to strip all Muslims of their right to vote, in a context where there is no firm proof of national identity." Amita Baviskar, "Between Violence and Desire: Space, Power, Identity in the Making of Metropolitan Delhi," *International Social Science Journal* 55, no. 175 (2003): 96.

122. Bharati Chaturvedi, conversation with Doron, 23 January 2015.

123. In Chennai, this was made clear as early as 1919 in the Chennai City Municipal Cooperation Act, 1919, clause 199, https://goo.gl/guBStB.

124. Chaturvedi, conversation with Doron, 23 January 2015.

125. Jan Breman, "The Informal Sector," in *The Oxford India Companion to Sociology and Social Anthropology*, ed. V. Das (New Delhi: Oxford University Press, 2003), 1307.

126. "About Us," KKPKP, accessed 5 September 2017, http://www.kkpkp-pune.org/about-us.html.

127. Anjor Bhaskar and Poornima Chikarmane, "The Story of Waste and Its Reclaimers: Organising Waste Collectors for Better Lives and Livelihoods," *Indian Journal of Labour Economics* 55, no. 4 (2012): 600.

128. Poornima Chikarmane and Laxmi Narayan, "Organising the Unorganised: A Case Study of the Kagad Kach Patra Kashtakari Panchayat (Trade Union of Waste-Pickers)," accessed 5 September 2017, http://swachcoop.com/pdf/casestudy-kagadkachpatrackashtakari.pdf.

129. Ibid., 1.

130. Ibid.

131. Thomas Weber, *Hugging the Trees: The Story of the Chipko Movement* (New Delhi: Viking, 1988).

132. Chikarmane and Narayan, "Organising the Unorganised," 1.

133. Ibid., 13–14.

134. Samarth, "Occupational Health of Waste Pickers in Pune."

135. See *Satyamev Jayate,* "Don't Waste Your Garbage," season 2, episode 3, 2014, http://www.satyamevjayate.in/dont-waste-your-garbage.aspx.

136. For example, see the report from the "First Global Strategic Workshop of Waste Pickers: Inclusive Solid Waste Management" (Pune, 27–29 April 2012), https://goo.gl/JBwnCE.

137. Gill, "Interlinked Contracts," 1452–1453.

138. See "Profile of Scrap Collectors," KKPKP, accessed 5 September 2017, http://www.kkpkp-pune.org/profile-of-scrap-collectors.html.

139. Cultural associations between the money earned from polluting labor (such as dealing with corpses or waste) foster belief that such earnings are best spent on polluting practices, such as drinking alcohol, gambling, or prostitution. Assa Doron, "The Intoxicated Poor: Alcohol, Morality and Power among the Boatmen of Banaras," *South Asian History and Culture* 1, no. 2 (2010): 282–300.

140. Bhasha Singh, *Unseen: The Truth about India's Manual Scavengers,* trans. R. Talwar (New Delhi: Penguin, 2014), 248.

141. "Salient Features of the PMC-SWaCH Partnership," Women in Informal Employment: Globalizing and Organizing, accessed 5 September 2017, http://wiego.org/sites/wiego.org/files/swach%20fact%20sheet.pdf.

142. Aparna Susarala, conversation with Doron, Pune, 18 January 2014.

143. Bhaskar and Chikarmane, "The Story of Waste," 611.

144. For a critique, see Jan Breman, *Footloose Labour: Working in India's Informal Economy* (Cambridge: Cambridge University Press, 1996), and Barbara Harriss-White,

"Inequality at Work in the Informal Economy: Key Issues and Illustrations," *International Labour Review* 142, no. 4 (2003): 459–469.

145. Aparna Susarla, conversation with Doron, Pune, 18 January 2014.

146. Laxmi, "Waste Pickers to Stop Subsidizing the Pune Municipal Cooperation!," Global Alliance of Waste Pickers, 24 January 2014, http://globalrec.org/2014/01/24/waste-pickers-to-stop-subsidising-the-pune-municipal-corporation/.

147. The memorandum of understanding of 28 October 2010 is on the SWaCH website, http://www.swachcoop.com/pdf/SWACH-PCMC%20MOU.pdf.

148. Kavita, conversation with Doron, 17 January 2014.

149. Vinay Gidwani, "'Waste' and the Permanent Settlement in Bengal," *Economic and Political Weekly* 27, no. 4 (25 January 1992): 41.

150. Kavita, conversation.

151. Ibid.

152. See these organizations' websites at http://thanal.co.in/; http://tished.org/; http://toxicslink.org/; http://www.chintan-india.org/; www.streemuktisanghatana.org; http://www.safaikarmachariandolan.org/; http://www.greenpammal.in/.

153. Dipankar Gupta, "The Importance of Being 'Rurban': Tracking Changes in a Traditional Setting, *Economic and Political Weekly* 50, no. 24 (13 June 2015): 40.

154. For Delhi, see Ghertner, *Rule by Aesthetics,* and Sanjay Srivastava, *Entangled Urbanism: Slum, Gated Community and Shopping Mall in Delhi and Gurgaon* (New Delhi: Oxford University Press, 2015); and for Mumbai, see Lisa Weinstein, *The Durable Slum: Dharavi and the Right to Stay Put in Globalizing Mumbai* (Minneapolis: University of Minnesota Press, 2014). For long-term effects of a slum relocation project in Chennai, see Karen Coelho, T. Venkat, and R. Chandrika, "The Spatial Reproduction of Urban Poverty: Labour and Livelihoods in a Slum Resettlement Colony," *Economic and Political Weekly* 47, nos. 47 and 48 (1 December 2012): 53–63.

Conclusion

1. "Six Quotes from PM Modi on Swachh Bharat Abhiyan," *India Today,* 2 October 2014, https://goo.gl/xSCmhn.

2. On the intimidation and forceful measures across India related to achieving Swatch Bharat targets, see Sushmita Sengupta, Snigdha Das, and Rashmi Verma, "Mission Madness," *Down to Earth,* 24 July 2017, https://goo.gl/ysaUjb.

3. Ashis Nandy, "Gandhi after Gandhi after Gandhi," *Little Magazine,* accessed 5 September 2017, http://www.littlemag.com/nandy.htm.

4. "Take A Pledge," accessed 11 October 2017, https://swachhbharat.mygov.in/basic-page/take-pledge.

5. In *Lage Raho Munna Bhai* (dir. Rajkumar Hirani, India, 2006), a small-time Mumbai gangster goes straight and gets the girl after he starts seeing visions of Gandhi. The term *Gandhigiri*—Gandhi's way—is used in the film.

6. For the authoritarian populism implicit in such youth mobilization, see Assa Doron, "Unclean, Unseen: Social Media, Civic Action and Urban Hygiene in India," *South Asia* 39, no. 4 (2016): 715–739.

7. "'Saw Father Die in Front of My Eyes,' says Daughter of Man Lynched in Rajasthan," *Indian Express,* 17 June 2017; "CPI(ML) Activist Lynched for Objecting to Rajasthan Officials Taking Photos of Women Defecating," *The Wire,* 17 June 2017, https://goo.gl/ZVQ5tR. For techniques to eliminate open defecation, see Salvi Manish, "Fine, Public Shaming and Training: India Finds Ways to Stop Open Defecation," *SBS,* 17 January 2017, https://goo.gl/6hmZhV.

8. "Garday loo!" (perhaps a corruption of the French "look out for the water") was shouted before emptying a chamber pot into the street. Wiktionary tells us that the phrase and practice still existed in the 1930s and 1940s. "Gardyloo," Wiktionary, updated 30 August 2017, http://goo.gl/3NKu5E. Jeffrey's father, who grew up in Edinburgh, 1900–1916, told similar stories.

9. Rose George, *The Big Necessity: The Unmentionable World of Human Waste and Why It Matters* (New York: Holt Paperback, 2009), 19; and David Waltner-Toews, *The Origin of Feces* (Toronto: ECW Press, 2013), 22, have roughly similar estimates of annual production of urine and feces by an average person.

10. Priyanka Kadokari, "Only 12% Potential of Maharashtra's 70,000 Small Dams used," *Times of India,* 15 April 2015, https://goo.gl/x83mtA.

11. *Indian Express,* 11 February 2016, https://goo.gl/GfQuVN.

12. For an overview, see "The GST Is Taking Away Ragpickers' Already-Meagre Income," *The Wire,* 13 September 2017, https://goo.gl/aozwy7.

13. B. R. Ambedkar, *What Congress and Gandhi Have Done to the Untouchables* (Bombay: Gautam Book Centre, 1945), 280.

14. Durgesh Solanki, "Cast(e)ing Life: The Experience of Living in Peripheral Caste Quarters," in *Peripheral Visions in the Globalizing Present: Space, Mobility and Aesthetics,* ed. Esther Pareen, Hanneke Stuit, and Astrid Van Weyenberg (Leiden, Netherlands: Brill, 2016), 109–125.

15. Charles Rosenberg, *The Cholera Years: The United States in 1832, 1849 and 1866* (1962; Chicago: University of Chicago Press, 1987), 189.

16. *Times of India,* 8 October 1994, p. 5.

17. Sunita Narain, "Twice Bitten Not Yet Shy," *Down to Earth,* 15 October 2016, p. 3.

18. Martin Melosi, *Garbage in the Cities: Refuse, Reform and the Environment,* rev. ed. (Pittsburgh: University of Pittsburgh Press, 2005), 230.

19. "Second Fire at Mumbai's Deonar Dump in a Week," *Hindustan Times,* 29 October 2016, https://goo.gl/On67Pd.

20. Mallica Joshi, "Half of World's 20 Most Polluted Cities in India, Delhi in 11th Position, *Hindustan Times,* 4 June 2016, https://goo.gl/e9VWAv, reports on Global Urban Ambient Air Pollution Database released by the World Health Organization. "Gwalior Is the Most Polluted Indian City, Not Delhi: WHO Report," *Indian Express,* 27 September 2016, https://goo.gl/wLbfSX.

21. See *Down to Earth,* 30 November 2016, pp. 18–44, for a detailed account of Delhi's condition.

22. Ibid., 23; "'Change Policy to Stop Crop Fire,'" *Times of India,* 13 April 2017; "'Full Ban on Stubble Burning Hard,'" *Times of India,* 26 July 2017.

23. Sunita Narain, "The Undisclosed Air Pollutants," *Down to Earth,* 31 January 2017, p. 3. See also "Runners Exposed to High Pollution Levels during Delhi Marathon," *Down to Earth,* 30 November 2016, pp. 18–44. See also Dinesh Mohan, "Transport and Health: Clearing the Air," *Economic and Political Weekly* 51, no 9 (27 February 2016): 29–31.

24. See Yatish Yadav, "Over 42,000 NGOs Under Government Scanner," *New Indian Express,* 26 April 2015, https://goo.gl/lKpftm, for an account of the Government of India targeting NGOs that received donations from outside India. Indian governments, suspicious of NGOs that lobby effectively, have often pointed to meddling by foreign hands.

25. *Down to Earth,* 31 May 2014, https://goo.gl/I5oQyt.

26. Anthony S. Wohl, *Endangered Lives: Public Health in Victorian Britain* (London: J. M. Dent, 1983), 341.

27. Amartya Sen, "Social Exclusion: Concept, Application and Scrutiny" (Social Development paper no. 1, Asian Development Bank, Manila, June 2000), 1–54. Sukhadeo Thorat, "On Economic Exclusion and Inclusive Policy," *Little Magazine* 6, nos. 4–5: 8–17.

GLOSSARY

achhuut Untouchable

aerobic Using air or oxygen

anaerobic Not using or requiring air

apavitra Impure (in religious context)

ashuddha Polluted, impure, unclean

aswatchhta Uncleanliness; filthiness

burakumin Japanese low-status community associated with impure tasks such as work in slaughterhouses, tanneries, or preparation of corpses

chhataai The thing that is sorted; the act of sorting

Chintan A Delhi-based NGO whose name means "contemplation"

daatuun Neem twig used for cleaning teeth

Dalit Scheduled Caste; so-called untouchable in former times

dhalao Local dustbin, or garbage collection point, usually owned by the municipality

dhoti Untailored lower cloth worn by men

Diwali Major Hindu festival in October or November

Dumpster North American term for what British and Australians call a skip; bin; metal container ranging in size from five to three cubic meters

gandagi Filth, litter

geela kachra Wet waste as opposed to dry waste (*suukha kachra*)

ghat Steps leading down to a river or tank

godown Shed; warehouse

henna Reddish-brown, plant-based dye used on the hair and skin

honey-sucker A vacuum truck; vehicle with equipment capable of sucking liquid out of a tank and transferring it to the truck

jati A subcaste, usually endogamous

jhuggi-jhopdis Hut; slums, settlement; also *bastis*

juutha Touched, or having come into contact with someone's mouth or saliva, hence polluted

kabaad Dry, segregated, inorganic waste; all recyclable

kabaadi/kabaadiwala Itinerant buyer of low-value scrap and dry waste

kaccha Uncooked, untreated, raw, crude, rough

kachra Mixed trash (dry and wet), sweepings, rubbish

Kagad Kach Patra Kashtakari Panchayat (KKPKP) Paper, Glass, and Metal Workers Association

kuuda kachra Mixed rubbish; unsegregated waste, garbage, muck

kuuda khaana Public rubbish dump

leachate The effluent seeping from a rubbish dump

mal Feces

naala Drain, water channel

paan masala Mouth freshener with tobacco, usually sold in small containers

panchayat A unit of rural local government

panchayati raj The system of rural local government

pheriwala Itinerant trader, hawker (usually with a cart or bicycle)

raddi Scrap, discarded paper, or cloth

raddiwala Waste-picker or buyer (often interchangeable with *kabaadiwala,* depending on the area)

redi Cart; also called a *thela*

Scheduled Caste Dalit; so-called untouchable in former times

sewer The channels and pipes that carry away wastewater

sewerage The system of channels and pipes that carry away wastewater

sheitel (Yiddish) A wig worn by Orthodox Jewish women after marriage

skip *See* "Dumpster"

***swachh* (or *swatch*)** Clean

thali A round metal plate used in restaurants and homes

tziniut Covering hair as a mark of modesty by Orthodox Jewish women

untouchable Term that gained currency in the early twentieth century to describe people of the lowest-status *jatis,* subject to harsh discrimination; Dalit is today's term; Scheduled Caste is the bureaucratic term

ward A geographically defined electoral unit of a municipality or municipal corporation

wet waste Biodegradable waste, food scraps and agricultural by-products

windrow A long line of biodegradable material exposed to the air for composting

zabaleen Coptic Christian waste-pickers of Cairo

BIBLIOGRAPHY

Reports, Official Publications, and Annual Compendiums

"Activated Sludge Treatment Process." World Bank. http://siteresources.worldbank.org/INTTOPSANHYG/Resources/1923125-1186000305809/Infrastructure_All_073107.pdf.

Alang: A Green Re-incarnation. Bhavnagar: Ship Recycling Industries Association (India), no. 1, March 2013.

Almitra H. Patel vs. Union of India, Original Application No. 199 of 2014, National Green Tribunal, Annexure VI, "Consolidated Annual Review Report on Implementation of Municipal Solid Wastes (Management and Handling) Rules, 2000. Annual Review Report: 2013–14. State-Wise Generation Collection and Treatment. 31.12.2014." New Delhi: Central Pollution Control Board, 2014.

Approach towards Establishing Municipal Cadres in India. New Delhi: Ministry of Urban Development and the World Bank, 2014. https://goo.gl/Srz2f5.

"Before the National Green Tribunal Southern Zonal Bench, Chennai, Application No. 247 of 2014." September 30, 2015. http://goo.gl/SoHwxc.

Bengaluru: Way Forward—Expert Committee; BBMP Restructuring. Bengaluru: Government of Karnataka, 2015.

B.PAC 2nd Anniversary Special. Bengaluru: B.PAC, 2014.

Bhushan, Chandra, Amit Khurana, Rajeshwari Sinha, and Mouna Nagaraju. *Antibiotic Resistance in Poultry Environment: Spread of Resistance from Poultry Farm to Agricultural Field.* New Delhi: Centre for Science and Environment, 2017. https://goo.gl/dZj7kp.

Census of India, 2011. "Houselisting and Housing Census. Table HH-14: Percentage of Households to Total Households by Amenities and Assets." http://goo.gl/of7rrA.

Census of India, 2011. "Percentage of Households to Total Households by Amenities and Assets. Number of Households Not Having Latrine Facility within the Premises." http://goo.gl/rIhkYG.

Central Pollution Control Board. "State-wise Status of Common Bio-medical Waste Treatment Facilities (CBWTFs)." 2008. http://cpcb.nic.in/wast/bioimedicalwast/CBWTF_Status_2008.pdf.

Chadwick, Edwin. *Report on the Sanitary Condition of the Labouring Population and on the Means of Its Improvement.* London, 1842.

Chandigarh Master Plan—2031. http://chandigarh.gov.in/cmp_2031.htm.

Chennai City Municipal Cooperation Act, 1919 (Tamil Nadu Act 4 of 1919). https://goo.gl/guBStB.

Consolidated Annual Review Report on Implementation of Municipal Solid Wastes (Management and Handling) Rules, 2000. Annual Review Report: 2013–14. Delhi: Central Pollution Control Board, 2015, annex 3.

Constitution of 1950, part 4, directive principles of state policy. Article 40, "Organization of Village Panchayats."

A Decade of the Total Sanitation Campaign, Rapid Assessment of Processes and Outcomes. New Delhi: Water and Sanitation Program, 2010.

"Delhi-NCR Likely to Generate 95,000 MT E-wastes by 2017: ASSOCHAM." 2014. http://assocham.org/newsdetail.php?id=4633.

D-Waste. *Waste Atlas: The World's 50 Biggest Dumpsites: 2014 Report.* 2014. http://goo.gl/5kRbB8.

"The 1848 Public Health Act." UK Parliament. Accessed September 5, 2017. http://goo.gl/TKCwDo.

"Environment at a Glance 2013." OECD iLibrary. http://goo.gl/8gxz8S.

8th Five Year Plan. Vol. 2, table 1. Accessed March 31, 2016. http://planningcommission.nic.in/plans/planrel/fiveyr/8th/vol2/8v2ch13.htm.

"Environmental, Health, and Safety Guidelines for Foundries." International Finance Corporation, World Bank Group, April 30, 2007. http://bit.ly/2dtD8qD.

"Environmental Impact Assessment Study: Common Municipal Solid Waste Management Facility, Doddabidirakallu, Bengaluru." Gurgaon: AECOM India, 2015. http://kspcb.gov.in/PH/Final%20EIA%20Doddabidarakallu_23062015.pdf.

"Environmental Pollution and Impacts on Public Health: Implications of the Dandora Municipal Dumping Site in Nairobi, Kenya." Nairobi: United Nations Environment Program, c. 2010. Accessed September 28, 2017, via http://www.habitants.org/news/inhabitants_of_africas/dandora_dumping_site_the_biggest_human_rights_violation_in_kenya.

Environmental Protection Agency. *Municipal Solid Waste Generation, Recycling, and Disposal in the United States: Facts and Figures for 2012.* Accessed September 30, 2017. https://goo.gl/D7tzNh.

———. *Report on the Environment: Hazardous Waste.* Accessed November 6, 2017. https://cfpub.epa.gov/roe/indicator.cfm?i=54.

Exnora Green Pammal, *Annual Report, 2012–13.* Pammal: Exnora Green, 2013.

"First Global Strategic Workshop of Waste Pickers: Inclusive Solid Waste Management." Pune, April 27–29, 2012. https://goo.gl/JBwnCE.

"The Fuel Efficient Truck Drivers' Handbook." London: Department of Transport, Her Majesty's Stationery Office, 2009. https://goo.gl/Fsg1ai.

Global Alliance for Incinerator Alternatives / Global Anti-Incinerator Alliance website. Accessed September 5, 2017. http://www.no-burn.org/.

Government of India. *National Action Plan on Antimicrobial Resistance.* April 2017. https://goo.gl/T7iCqw.

"Government Notifies Plastic Waste Management Rules, 2016." New Delhi: Press Information Bureau, Ministry of Environment and Forests, March 18, 2016. https://goo.gl/OKEWfy.

"Hartland Landfill Facility." Capital Regional District, British Columbia. Accessed September 5, 2017. https://goo.gl/eLrYba.

"Hazardous Waste Management." Ramky Enviro Engineers. Accessed September 5, 2017. https://goo.gl/rXoCy2.

"Hazardous Waste Management." West Bengal Pollution Control Board. Accessed September 5, 2017. http://www.wbpcb.gov.in/pages/display/36-hazardous-waste-management.

Hinchey, Maurice D. "Organized Crime's Involvement in the Waste Hauling Industry." The American Mafia: The History of Organized Crime in the United States. July 24, 1986. http://mafiahistory.us/maf-hinc.html.

"How Did Bangladesh Reduce Stunting So Rapidly?" Global Nutrition Report, 2014. http://goo.gl/jUHnQ4.

India 1959: Annual Review. London: Information Service of India, 1959.

India: A Reference Annual. New Delhi: Ministry of Information and Broadcasting, 1953.

Indian Railways, Centre for Advanced Maintenance Technology. "Presentation on IR-DRDO Bio-toilet System." May 3, 2016. http://iced.cag.gov.in/wp-content/uploads/2016-17/NTP%2003/RK.pdf.

"Infant, Child and Maternal Mortality Rate." Delhi: Press Information Bureau, Government of India, Ministry of Health and Family Welfare, July 11, 2014. http://goo.gl/sLZSxc.

Inspiring Progress: Learning from Exnora Green Lammapuram's Solid Waste Management Partnerships in South Localities. Chennai: Exnora Green, 2010.

Integrated Waste Management Practices (brochure). Surat: Surat Municipal Corporation, n.d. (c. 2013).

Jeffrey, Robin. "India's Worlds of Waste." Institute of South Asian Studies Special Report, no. 28, September 17, 2015.

Maharashtra Pollution Control Board, *Annual Report, 2012–13.* Mumbai: Maharashtra Pollution Control Board, n.d. http://goo.gl/pRMdct.

"Mandate." Ministry of Urban Development. http://moud.gov.in/cms/mandate.php.

Mass Media in India 1980–81. New Delhi: Publications Division, Ministry of Information and Broadcasting, 1982.

Mehta, Balvantray G. *Report of the Team for the Study of Community Projects and National Extension Service.* 1957. http://goo.gl/CrJStl.

Ministry of Drinking Water and Sanitation. *Annual Report, 2013–14.* New Delhi: Ministry of Drinking Water and Sanitation. 2014.

Ministry of Urban Development. *Annual Report, 2014–15.* Accessed January 4, 2016. http://www.moud.gov.in/pdf/582d962fe1282English%20Annual%20Report.pdf, p. 82.

"National Inventory of Hazardous Wastes Generating Industries and Hazardous Waste Management in India." New Delhi: Central Pollution Control Board, 2009. Accessed October 5, 2017. https://goo.gl/GRsEbj.

NEWater. PUB: Singapore's National Water Agency. https://goo.gl/a752xI.

9th Five Year Plan. http://planningcommission.nic.in/plans/planrel/fiveyr/9th/default.htm.

People Research on India's Consumer Economy. "Household Survey on India's Citizen Environmental and Consumer Economy." http://www.ice360.in/en/projects/what-are-ice-360-surveys/upcoming-survey-ice3600-2016.

Phoenix Energy. "Kwinana Waste to Energy Project: Public Environmental Review. MHIEC Global WtE Plant Delivery Record." 2013. http://goo.gl/ESoJbU.

Plastic Management from Source to Resource: Engineer's Day 2011. Ahmedabad: School of Building Science and Technology, CEPT University, 2011.

"Plastics." Washington, DC: Environmental Protection Agency, March 2015. https://goo.gl/QsDZ1a.

Plastics: In a New Mould. Mumbai: Plastics Promotions Council, 2013.

"Profile of Scrap Collectors." KKPKP. Accessed September 5, 2017. http://www.kkpkp-pune.org/profile-of-scrap-collectors.html.

Project Information Document (Concept Stage)—Cairo Municipal Solid Waste Management Project—P152961. Washington, DC: World Bank, 2014. https://goo.gl/Akol4u.

"Public Private Partnerships in India." Ministry of Finance. Updated August 30, 2017. http://www.pppinindia.com/.

"Rank of Cities on Sanitation, 2009–10." Ministry of Urban Development. https://goo.gl/orz5Sc.

Recommendations to Address the Issues of Informal Sector Involved in E-waste Handling, Moradabad, Uttar Pradesh. New Delhi: Centre for Science and Environment, 2015. https://goo.gl/QMRDSG.

Reed, S., and S. T. Sheppard, eds. *Indian Year Book 1930*, Bombay: Bennett Coleman, 1930.

Report of the Commissioners Appointed to Inquire into the Sanitary State of the Army in India; with Precis of Evidence. London: Eyre and Spottiswood for Her Majesty's Stationery Office, 1863.

Report of the Working Group on Urban and Industrial Water Supply and Sanitation for 12th Five Year Plan 2012–2017. New Delhi: Planning Commission, 2011.

Rural-Urban Relationship Committee. Vol. 3. New Delhi: Government of India, Ministry of Health and Family Planning, 1966.

Samarth, Ujwala. "The Occupational Health of Waste Pickers in Pune: KKPKP and SWaCH Members Push for Health Rights." Manchester, UK: Women in Informal Employment: Globalizing and Organizing, March 2014. http://bit.ly/2e4hCc5.

Scavenging Conditions Enquiry Committee. New Delhi: Ministry of Home Affairs, Central Advisory Board for Harijan Welfare, 1960.

"The Septic Tank." Department of Health, Australian Government. Updated November 2010. http://goo.gl/bxi8TN.

"Ship Recyclers." Ship Recycling Industries Association (India). Accessed September 5, 2017. http://goo.gl/VP1Qab.

"Solid Waste Management Overview." Bruhat Bengaluru Mahanagara Palike. Accessed September 5, 2017. https://goo.gl/eXqfRv.

"Status Report on Management of Hazardous Waste in India." March 15, 1990. Accessed February 28, 2017. http://goo.gl/N6hBI3.

"Status of Sewage Treatment in India." New Delhi: Central Pollution Control Board, 2005. Accessed October 6, 2017. http://cpcb.nic.in/newitems/12.pdf.

Study on Plastic Waste Disposal through "Plasma Pyrolysis Technology." New Delhi: Central Pollution Control Board, October 2016. https://goo.gl/dYd9r3.

Telecom Regulatory Authority of India. *Annual Report, 2014–15.* New Delhi: TRAI, 2015.

Telecom Regulatory Authority of India. *The Indian Telecom Services Performance Indicators, October–December 2016.* New Delhi: TRAI, 7 April 2017.

TERI Energy Data Directory and Yearbook 2011/12. New Delhi: TERI, 2012. https://goo.gl/SOElZk.

Third Five-Year Plan, 1961–6. http://goo.gl/MEKTVk.

"Total Number of Registered Motor Vehicles in India during 1951–2012." https://data.gov.in/catalog/total-number-registered-motor-vehicles-india.

Two-Pit System. Sulabh International Social Service Organisation, https://goo.gl/EYi1T9.

UNICEF. "Nearly One Third of Children under Five in Developing Countries Are Stunted." Progress for Children, December 2007. https://goo.gl/SQi5eB.

Urban Solid Waste Management in Indian Cities. New Delhi: National Institute of Urban Affairs, 2015. https://goo.gl/yIYsbn.

World Bank, "Inadequate Sanitation Costs India the Equivalent of 6.4 Per Cent of GDP." Press release, 20 December 2010. https://goo.gl/rJmr11.

World Bank, "Motor Vehicles (per 1,000 people). Site discontinued but available at the Internet Wayback Machine. Accessed September 5, 2017. https://goo.gl/hB3Nzf.

World Bank. "Population Density (people per sq. km of land area)." http://goo.gl/s3c6aL.

Books and Articles

Acharya, Keya. "Trash Driving." *Hindu,* November 24, 2012. http://goo.gl/i8wzrR.

Advertising and Marketing. October, 15 1994.

Ahluwalia, Isher Judge, Ravi Kanbur, and P. K. Mohanty, eds., *Urbanisation in India: Challenges, Opportunities and the Way Forward.* New Delhi: SAGE, 2014.

Ahuja, Anita S., and Sachin D. Abda. "Industrial Hazardous Waste Management by Government of Gujarat." *RHIMRJ* 2, no. 5 (May 2015): 1–11. http://oaji.net/articles/2015/1250-1434252379.pdf.

Aijaz, Rumi. *Challenges for Urban Local Government in India.* Working paper no. 19, London School of Economics, August 2007. https://goo.gl/9XnVxh.

Alexander, Catherine, and Joshua Reno, eds. *Economies of Recycling: The Global Transformation of Materials, Values and Social Relations.* London: Zed Books, 2012.

Allami, Abdul Fazl. *The Ain i Akbari of Abul Fazl Allami.* Vol. 2. Translated by H. S. Jarrett. Calcutta: Asiatic Society of Bengal, 1891.

Alley, Kelly. "Idioms of Degeneracy: Assessing Ganga's Purity and Pollution." In *Purifying the Earthly Body of God: Religion and Ecology in Hindu India,* edited by Lance E. Nelson, 297–329. New York: State University of New York Press, 1998.

———. *On the Banks of the Ganga.* Ann Arbor: University of Michigan Press, 2002.

Ambedkar, B. R. *What Congress and Gandhi Have Done to the Untouchables.* Bombay: Gautam Book Centre, 1945.

Amos, Timothy. *Embodying Difference: The Making of Burakumin in Modern Japan.* Honolulu: University of Hawaii Press, 2011.

Anand, Mulk Raj. *Untouchable.* 1935. Harmondsworth: Penguin, 1988.

Anand, Nikhil. *Hydraulic City: Water and the Infrastructures of Citizenship in Mumbai.* Durham, NC: Duke University Press, 2017.

Annepu, Ranjith Kharvel. "Sustainable Solid Waste Management in India." Master's thesis, Columbia University, 2012.

Appadurai, Arjun. "Deep Democracy: Urban Governmentality and the Horizon of Politics." *Public Culture* 14, no. 1 (2002): 21–47.

Arnold, David. *Colonizing the Body: State Medicine and Epidemic Disease in Nineteenth-Century India.* Berkeley: University of California Press, 1993.

———. "Introduction: Disease, Medicine and Empire." In *Imperial Medicine and Indigenous Societies,* edited by D. Arnold. New Delhi: Oxford University Press, 1989.

Ashenburg, Katherine. *Clean: An Unsanitized History of Washing.* London: Profile Books, 2009.

Ashraf, Ajaz. "It's Safer Being a Soldier Fighting in Kashmir Than a Sewer Worker. What Does That Say About India?" Scroll.in, September 11, 2017. https://goo.gl/mzWf9C.

Avashiha, Vidhee Kiran, and Amit Garg. "Urban Infrastructure and Governance Mission under JNNURM." *Economic and Political Weekly* 51, no. 2 (January 9, 2016): 41–57.

Ayee, J., and R. Crook. *Toilet Wars: Urban Sanitation Services and the Politics of Public-Private Partnerships in Ghana.* Brighton, UK: Institute of Development Studies Working Paper, 2003.

Balch, Oliver. "Indian Law Requires Companies to Give 2% of Profits to Charity. Is It Working?" *Guardian,* April 5, 2016. https://goo.gl/uxOPBj.

Bandyopadhyay, Simanti. "Municipal Finance in India: Some Critical Issues." Working paper no. 11, International Center for Public Policy. Atlanta: Georgia State University, 2014.

Bate, Weston. *Essential but Unplanned: The Story of Melbourne's Lanes.* Melbourne: State Library of Victory and City of Melbourne, 1994.

Bauman, Zigmunt. *Wasted Lives: Modernity and Its Outcomes*. Cambridge, UK: Polity, 2004.

Baviskar, Amita. "Between Violence and Desire: Space, Power, Identity in the Making of Metropolitan Delhi." *International Social Science Journal* 55 (2003): 89–98.

Beall, Jo. "Thoughts on Poverty from a South Asian Rubbish Dump." *IDF Bulletin* 28, no. 3 (1997): 73–90.

Bhaskar, Anjor, and Poornima Chikarmane. "The Story of Waste and Its Reclaimers: Organising Waste Collectors for Better Lives and Livelihoods." *Indian Journal of Labour Economics* 55, no. 4 (2012): 595–619.

Bhaskar, R. N. "Policy Watch: Converting Waste into Energy Can Spell End of Garbage Mafia," *DNA*, August 11, 2014. https://goo.gl/zd66Bh.

Björkman, Lisa. *Pipe Politics, Contested Waters: Embedded Infrastructures of Millennial Mumbai*. Durham, NC: Duke University Press, 2015.

Bloem, Martin. "The 2006 WHO Child Growth Standards." *British Medical Journal*, 7 April 2007, 705–706.

Bonea, Amelia. *The News of Empire: Telegraphy, Journalism and the Politics of Reporting in Colonial India, c. 1830–1900*. New Delhi: Oxford University Press, 2016.

Boo, Katherine. *Behind the Beautiful Forevers*. New York: Random House, 2012.

Breman, Jan. *Footloose Labour: Working in India's Informal Economy*. Cambridge: Cambridge University Press, 1996.

Breman, Jan. "The Informal Sector." In *The Oxford India Companion to Sociology and Social Anthropology*, edited by V. Das, 1287–1317. New Delhi: Oxford University Press, 2003.

Broom, Alex, Katherine Kenny, Emma Kirby, and Mahati Chittem. "Improvisation, Therapeutic Brokerage and Antibiotic (Mis)use in India." Unpublished, 2017.

Brown, Joe, Sandy Cairncross, and Jeroen H. J. Ensink. "Water, Sanitation, Hygiene and Enteric Infections in Children." *Archives of Diseases in Childhood* 98, no. 8 (2013): 629–634.

Bryson, Cindy. A Valuable Life: Seeing Transformative Practice among Phnom Penh's Waste Pickers. PhD diss., Australian National University, Canberra, 2014.

Buradikatti, Kumar. "Waste Management Is Better in Raichur than Bengaluru: Supreme Court Panel." *Hindu*, October 19, 2015. http://goo.gl/UZszYf.

Chakrabarty, Dipesh. *Habitations of Modernity*. Chicago: University of Chicago Press, 2002.

Chaplin, Susan E. *The Politics of Sanitation in India: Cities, Services and the State*. Hyderabad: Orient BlackSwan, 2011.

Charsley, Simon. "'Untouchable': What Is in a Name?" *Journal of the Royal Anthropological Institute* 2, no. 1 (1996): 1–23.

Cheng, Kevin, Sidra Rehman, Dulani Seneviratne, and Shiny Zhang. *Reaping the Benefits from Global Value Chains*. Working paper 15/204, International Monetary Fund, September 2015. https://goo.gl/fntW5a.

Chennai Metropolitan Area. Wikipedia. Updated September 1, 2015. https://goo.gl/KqiJxo.

Chikarmane, Poornima, and Laxmi Narayan. "Organising the Unorganised: A Case Study of the Kagad Kach Patra Kashtakari Panchayat (Trade Union of Waste-Pickers)." Accessed September 5, 2017. http://www.swachcoop.com/pdf/casestudy-kagadkachpatrackashtakari.pdf.

Choudhury, Kushanava. "Raising a Stink: How People Power Forced a Waste-Management Revolution in Kerala." *Caravan*, May 1, 2017. https://goo.gl/yCcas4.

Cockayne, Emily. *Hubbub: Filth, Noise and Stench in England, 1600–1770*. New Haven, CT: Yale University Press, 2007.

Coelho, Karen, T. Venkat, and R. Chandrika. "The Spatial Reproduction of Urban Poverty: Labour and Livelihoods in a Slum Resettlement Colony." *Economic and Political Weekly* 47, nos. 47/48 (December 1, 2012): 53–63.

Coffey, Diane, Angus Deaton, Jean Drèze, Dean Spears, and Alessandro Tarozzi. "Stunting among Children: Facts and Implications." *Economic and Political Weekly* 48, no. 34 (August 24, 2013): 68–70.

Coffey, Diane, Aashish Gupta, Payal Hathi, Nidhi Khurana, Dean Spears, Nikhil Srivastav, and Sangita Vyas. "Revealed Preference for Open Defecation: Evidence from a New Survey in Rural North India." *Economic and Political Weekly* 49, no. 38 (September 20, 2014): 43–55.

———. "Understanding Exceptionally Poor Sanitation in Rural India: Purity, Pollution, and Untouchability." *Economic and Political Weekly* 52, no. 1 (January 7, 2017): 59–66.

Coffey, Diane, and Dean Spears. *Where India Goes: Abandoned Toilets, Stunted Development and the Costs of Caste.* New Delhi: HarperCollins India, 2017.

Corbin, Alain. *The Foul and the Fragrant: Odour and the French Social Imagination.* London: Picador, 1994.

Corbridge, Stuart, John Harriss, and Craig Jeffrey. *India Today: Economy, Politics and Society.* Cambridge, UK: Polity, 2013.

Cornea, Natasha, Renne Veron, and Anne Zimmer. "Clean City Politics: An Urban Political Ecology of Solid Waste in West Bengal, India." *Environment and Planning A* 49, no. 4 (2017): 728–744.

The Court. Directed by Chaitanya Tamhane. India, 2014.

Crewe, Tom. "The Strange Death of Municipal England." *London Review of Books* 38, no. 24 (2016): 6–10.

Crooks, Harold. *Dirty Business.* Toronto: James Lorimer, 1983.

———. *Giants of Garbage: The Rise of the Global Waste Industry and the Politics of Pollution Control.* Toronto: James Lorimer, 1993.

Curtis, Valerie A., Nana Garbrah-Aidoo, and Beth Scott. "Masters of Marketing: Bringing Private Sector Skills to Public Health Partnerships." *American Journal of Public Health* 97, no. 4 (2007): 634–641.

Dahiya, Bharat. "Hard Struggle and Soft Gains: Environmental Management, Civil Society and Governance in Lammapuram, South India." *Environment and Urbanization* 15, no. 1 (2003): 91–100.

Dayal, Raghu. "Dirty Flows the Ganga." *Economic and Political Weekly* 51, no. 25 (June 18, 2016): 55–65.

Debroy, Bibek, and P. D. Kaushik. *Energising Rural Development through "Panchayats."* New Delhi: Academic Foundation, 2005.

Deery, Shannon. "Melbourne Water Fined after Worker Drowned in Sewerage Channel." *Herald Sun,* February 27, 2014. http://goo.gl/qP4QJt.

Desai, Renu, Colin McFarlane, and Stephen Graham. "The Politics of Open Defecation: Informality, Body, and Infrastructure in Mumbai." *Antipode* 47, no. 1 (2015): 98–120.

Deulgaonkar, Atul. Introduction to *In Search of Dignity and Justice: The Untold Story of Conservancy Workers,* written and photographs by Sudharak Olwe. Mumbai: Bharatiya Mahila Federation [Thane Samiti], 2013.

Di Giogio, Massimiliano. "Italy's Woeful Waste Management on Trial with Il Supremo Trash King." Reuters, May 25, 2014. http://goo.gl/JJXRC1.

Dhaktode, Nitin. "Freedom from Open Defecation." *Economic and Political Weekly* 49, no. 20 (May 17, 2014): 17, 28–30.

Dhamija, Urvashi. *Sustainable Solid Waste Management.* New Delhi: Academic Foundation, 2006.

Dickey, Sarah. *Living Class in Urban India.* New Brunswick, NJ: Rutgers University Press, 2015.

Doron, Assa. "The Intoxicated Poor: Alcohol, Morality and Power among the Boatmen of Banaras." *South Asian History and Culture* 1, no. 2 (2010): 282–300.

———. *Life on the Ganga: Boatmen and the Ritual Economy of Banaras.* New Delhi: Cambridge University Press, 2013.

———. "Unclean, Unseen: Social Media, Civic Action and Urban Hygiene in India." *South Asia: Journal of South Asian Studies* 39, no. 4 (2016): 715–739.

Doron, Assa, and Robin Jeffrey. *The Great Indian Phone Book.* Cambridge, MA: Harvard University Press, 2013.

———. "Notes on Open Defecation in India." *Economic and Political Weekly,* 49, no. 49 (December 6, 2014): 72–78.

Doron, Assa, and Ira Raja. "The Cultural Politics of Shit: Class, Gender and Public Space in India." *Journal of Postcolonial Studies* 18, no. 2 (2015): 189–207.

Doshi, Sapna. "The Politics of the Evicted: Redevelopment, Subjectivity, and Difference in Mumbai's Slum Frontier." *Antipode* 45, no. 4 (2012): 844–865.

Dossani, Rafiq. *India Arriving.* New York: American Management Association, 2008.

Douglas, Mary. *Purity and Danger.* 1966. London: Ark Paperbacks, 1984.

Duffy, Daniel P. "Landfill Economics: Getting Down to Business—Part 2." Forester Network, March 16, 2016, first published 2005. http://goo.gl/t8anvh.

Dwyer, Henri, and Nickolas J. Themelis. "Inventory of U.S. 2012 Dioxin Emissions to Atmosphere." *Waste Management* 46 (December 2015): 1–5.

Echenberg, Myron. *Plague Ports.* New York: New York University Press, 2007.

Edensor, Tim. "The Culture of the Indian Street." In *Images of the Street: Planning, Identity and Control of Public Space,* edited by N. Fyfe, 201–219. London: Routledge, 1998.

Edwards, Eliuned. 2008. "Hair, Devotion and Trade in India." In *Hair: Styling, Culture and Fashion,* edited by G. Biddle-Perry and S. Cheang, 149–166. London: Bloomsbury.

Eggers, Dave. *Zeitoun.* London: Hamish Hamilton, 2009.

Ehrlich, Paul R. 1968. *The Population Bomb.* New York: Ballantine Books.

Enders, Giulia. *Gut.* Vancouver, BC: Greystone Books, 2015.

English, Angi. "Ten Properties of Wicked Problems." Center for Homeland Defense and Security for Radical Homeland Security Experimentation: Homeland Security. Accessed September 7, 2017. https://goo.gl/9egxOF.

Evans, Richard J. *Death in Hamburg: Society and Politics in the Cholera Years.* 1987. New York: Penguin, 2005.

Florence Nightingale on Health in India. Vol. 9. Edited by Gerard Vallee. Waterloo, ON: Wilfrid Laurier University Press, 2006.

Fredericks, Rosalind. "Vital Infrastructures of Trash in Dakar." *Comparative Studies of South Asia, Africa and the Middle East* 34, no. 3 (2014): 532–548.

"Fresh Kills Landfill." Wikipedia. Updated September 27, 2017. https://goo.gl/1HdJVs.

Furniss, Jamie. "Alternative Framings of Transnational Waste Flows: Reflections Based on the Egypt–China PET Plastic Trade." *Area* 47, no. 1 (2015): 24–30.

Gandhi, M. K. "Some Mussooree Reminiscences." *Harijan,* June 23, 1946, p. 198.

Gandhi, Mahatma. *Collected Works of Mahatma Gandhi.* Vol. 46. New Delhi: Publications Division, Ministry of Information and Broadcasting, 1971.

Gandhi, Sahil, and Vaidehi Tandel, "What Urbanisation Reforms Owe to K. C. Sivaramakrishnan." *Economic and Political Weekly* 52, no. 22 (June 3, 2017): 27–29.

Garrett, Laurie. *Betrayal of Trust: The Collapse of Global Public Health.* New York: Hyperion, 2001.

Garrick, E. Louis. "A Historical Context of Municipal Solid Waste Management in the United States." *Waste Management and Research* 22, no. 4 (2004): 306–322.

Garud, Piyush. "Dirt of a Nation!" January 19, 2013. https://goo.gl/1Bcq09.

George, Rose. *The Big Necessity: The Unmentionable World of Human Waste and Why It Matters.* New York: Holt Paperback, 2009.

Gertler, Paul, Manisha Shah, Maria Laura Alzua, Lisa Cameron, Sebastian Martinez, and Sumeet Patil. "How Does Health Promotion Work? Evidence from the Dirty Business of Eliminating Open Defecation." Working paper 20997, Cambridge, MA: National Bureau of Economic Research, 2015.

Ghertner, Asher. *Rule by Aesthetics: World-Class City Making in Delhi.* New York: Oxford University Press, 2015.

Ghosh, Archana, and S. Sami Ahmad. *Plague in Surat.* New Delhi: Institute of Social Sciences, 1996.

Ghosh, Dhrubajyoti. *The Trash Diggers.* New Delhi: Oxford University Press, 2017.

Gidwani, Vinay. "Remaindered Things and Remaindered Lives: Travelling with Delhi's Waste." In *Finding Delhi: Loss and Renewal in the Megacity,* edited by B. Chaturvedi, 37–54. New Delhi: Penguin Viking, 2010.

———. "Value Struggles: Waste Work and Urban Ecology in Delhi." In *Ecologies of Urbanism in India: Metropolitan Civility and Sustainability,* edited by A. Rademacher and K. Sivaramkrishnan, 184–189. Hong Kong: Hong Kong University Press, 2013.

———. "The Work of Waste: Inside India's Infra-economy." *Transactions* 40 (2015): 575–595.

———. "'Waste' and the Permanent Settlement in Bengal." *Economic and Political Weekly* 27, no. 4 (January 25, 1992): 31–46.

Gidwani, Vinay, and Amita Baviskar. "Urban Commons." *Economic and Political Weekly* 46, no. 50 (December 10, 2011): 42–43.

Gidwani, Vinay, and Bharati Chaturvedi. "Poverty as Geography." In *Urban Navigations: Politics, Space and the City in South Asia,* edited by Jonathan Shapiro Anjaria and Colin McFarlane. New Delhi: Routledge, 2011.

Gidwani, Vinay, and Julia Corwin, "Governance of Waste." *Economic and Political Weekly* 52, no. 31 (August 5, 2017): 52.

Gill, Kaveri. "Interlinked Contracts and Social Power: Patronage and Exploitation in India's Waste Recovery Market." *Journal of Development Studies* 43, no. 8 (2007): 1448–1474.

———. *Of Poverty and Plastic: Scavenging and Scrap Trading Entrepreneurs in India's Urban Informal Economy.* New Delhi: Oxford University Press, 2010.

Gille, Zsuzsa. *From the Cult of Waste to the Trash Heap of History: The Politics of Waste in Socialist and Postsocialist Hungary.* Bloomington: Indiana University Press, 2007.

Gillespie, Stuart. "Myths and Realities of Child Nutrition." *Economic and Political Weekly* 48, no. 34 (August 24, 2013): 64–67.

Gregson, Nicky, and Mike Crang. "From Waste to Resource: The Trade in Wastes and Global Recycling Economies." *Annual Review of Environment and Resources* 40 (2015): 151–176.

Gregson, Nicky, Helen Watkins, and Melania Calestani. "Inextinguishable Fibres: Demolition and the Vital Materialisms of Asbestos." *Environment and Planning A* 42 (2010): 1065–1083.

Godoy, Emilio. "The Waste Mountain Engulfing Mexico City." *Guardian,* January 9, 2012. http://goo.gl/KTuFvy.

Goklany, Tania. "How Karma Recycling Is Giving Life to E-waste." NDTV, September 23, 2015. http://goo.gl/A20PXX.

Gonzales, Eugenio M. "From Wastes to Assets: The Scavengers of Payatas." International Conference on Natural Assets, Tagatay City, January 8–11, 2003. http://www.peri.umass.edu/fileadmin/pdf/conference_papers/CDP7.pdf.

Good Hair. Dir. Jeff Stilson, 2009. https://goo.gl/DTKJdd.

Gopal, S. *The Viceroyalty of Lord Ripon 1880–1884.* London: Oxford University Press, 1953.

Gould, Harold A. "Local Government Roots of Contemporary Indian Politics." *Economic and Political Weekly* 6, no. 7 (February 13, 1971): 457–464.

"The GST Is Taking Away Ragpickers' Already-Meagre Income." *The Wire*, September 13, 2017. https://goo.gl/aozwy7.

Guerrand, Roger-Henri. "Private Spaces." In *A History of Private Life.* Vol. 4, *From the Fires of Revolution to the Great War,* edited by Michelle Perrot. Cambridge, MA: Harvard University Press, 1990.

Gupta, Dipankar. "The Importance of Being 'Rurban': Tracking Changes in a Traditional Setting." *Economic and Political Weekly* 50, no. 24 (June 13, 2015): 37–43.

Guru, Gopal. "Introduction: Theorizing Humiliation." In *Humiliation: Claims and Context,* edited by Gopal Guru, 1–19 (New Delhi: Oxford University Press, 2011).

Hammer, Jeffrey, Nazmul Chaudhury, Soma Ghosh Moulik, and Atul Pokhare. "Hygiene and Health: An Evaluation of the Total Sanitation Campaign in Maharashtra." Working paper, World Bank WSP, 2007.

Hanley, Susan B. "Urban Sanitation in Preindustrial Japan." *Journal of Interdisciplinary History* 18, no. 1 (1987): 1–27.

Harris, Gardiner. "Starving, but Not from the Lack of Food." *International New York Times,* July 12–13, 2014, 1, 6.

Harrison, Mark. *Public Health in British India.* Cambridge: Cambridge University Press, 1994.

Harriss-White, Barbara. "Inequality at Work in the Informal Economy: Key Issues and Illustrations." *International Labour Review* 142, no. 4 (2003): 459–469.

Hawkins, Gay. *The Ethics of Waste: How We Relate to Rubbish.* Lanham, MD: Rowman and Littlefield, 2006.

Hawkins, Gay, Emily Potter, and Kane Race. *Plastic Water: The Social and Material Life of Bottled Water.* Cambridge, MA: MIT Press, 2015.

Haynes, Douglas. *Rhetoric and Ritual in Colonial India.* Berkeley: University of California Press, 1991.

Haynes, Douglas E., and Nikhil Rao. "Beyond the Colonial City: Re-evaluating the Urban History of India, ca. 1920–1970." *South Asia* 36, no. 3 (2013): 317–335.

Hazari. *Untouchable: The Autobiography of an Indian Outcaste.* London: Praeger, 1971.

Helman, Christopher. "America's Biggest Landfills." *Forbes,* October 13, 2010. http://www.forbes.com/2010/10/13/los-angeles-las-vegas-business-energy-biggest-landfills.html.

Hodges, Sarah. "Chennai's Biotrash Chronicles: Chasing the Neo-liberal Syringe." Working paper 44/08, GARNET, 2008, 1–28.

———. "Medical Garbage and the Making of Neo-liberalism in India." *Economic and Political Weekly* 48, no. 48 (November 30, 2013): 112–119.

Hoelscher, Kristian. "The Evolution of the Smart Cities Agenda in India." *International Asia Studies Review* 19, no. 1 (2016): 28–44.

Hooda, A., M. Rathee, and J. Singh. "Chewing Sticks in the Era of Toothbrush: A Review." *Internet Journal of Family Practice* 9, no. 2 (2009): 1–6. http://print.ispub.com/api/0/ispub-article/4968.

INCLEN Program Evaluation Network (IPEN) Study Group, New Delhi, India. "Bio-medical Waste Management: Situational Analysis & Predictors of Performance in 25 Districts across 20 Indian States." *Indian Journal of Medical Research* 139 (2014): 141–153. https://goo.gl/1VFYaf.

Isaac, T. M. Thomas, and Richard W. Franke. *Local Democracy and Development: People's Campaign for Decentralized Planning in Kerala*. New Delhi: LeftWord, 2000.

Jackson, Lee. *Dirty Old London: The Victorian Fight against Filth*. New Haven, CT: Yale University Press, 2014.

Jagannathan, Vijay. "Cleaning the Ganga River." *Economic and Political Weekly* 49, no. 37 (September 13, 2014): 24–26.

James, C. Carkeet. *Drainage Problems of the East: Being a Revised and Enlarged Edition of "Oriental Drainage."* Bombay: Times of India Press, 1906.

———. *Further Notes on Sewage Disposal*. Bombay: Times of India Press, n.d. (c. 1900).

———. *Notes on Disposal of Sewage at the Matunga Leper Asylum*. Bombay: Times of India Press, 1901.

———. *Oriental Drainage: A Guide to the Collection, Removal and Disposal of Sewage in Eastern Cities*. Bombay: Times of India Press, 1902.

Jamil, Ghazala. "The Capitalist Logic of Spatial Segregation." *Economic and Political Weekly* 49, no. 3 (January 18, 2014): 52–58.

"Jayalalithaa Govt Scraps Free TV Scheme in Tamil Nadu." *Daily News and Analysis*, June 10, 2011. http://goo.gl/MivZPl.

Jangir, Suresh. "Garbage Wars: Villages Stand Firm against Bengaluru." *First.in*, April 12, 2016. http://goo.gl/hdsb2U.

Jeffrey, Craig, Patricia Jeffery, and Roger Jeffery. *Degrees without Freedom? Education, Masculinities and Unemployment in North India*. Stanford, CA: Stanford University Press, 2008.

Jeffrey, Robin. "Clean India! Symbols, Policies, Tensions," *South Asia* 38, no. 4 (2015): 807–819.

———. *Politics, Women and Well-Being: How Kerala Became "a Model."* 3rd ed. New Delhi: Oxford University Press, 2010.

———. *What's Happening to India?* London: Macmillan, 1986.

Jewitt, Sarah. "Poo Gurus? Researching the Threats and Opportunities Presented by Human Waste." *Applied Geography* 31 (2011): 765–766.

Jinsu, Lata. "Modi's Ganga Sutra and the Politics of Varanasi." *Down to Earth,* May 12, 2014. https://goo.gl/Mxavmd.

Jocelyn, Julian. *The History of the Royal and Indian Artillery in the Mutiny of 1857.* London: Naval and Military Press, 1915.

Jones, Rodney W. *Urban Politics in India.* Berkeley: University of California Press, 1974.

Joseph, Josy. *A Feast of Vultures.* New Delhi: HarperCollins, 2016.

Joshi, Rajkumar, and Sirajuddin Ahmed. "Status and Challenges of Municipal Solid Waste Management in India: A Review." *Cogent Environmental Science* 2 (2016): 1–18.

Kamra, Sukeshi. "Law and Radical Rhetoric in British India: The 1897 Trial of Bal Gangadhar Tilak." *South Asia: Journal of South Asian Studies* 39, no. 3 (2016): 546–559.

Kant, Ravi, Ramky Enviro Engineers. "Financial Analysis and Risk Allocation in PPPs: Public Private Partnership for Sustainable Growth. Department of Economic Affairs." 2008. http://pppinindia.com/ppp-nodal-officer-round-table.php.

Karunanathan, Mativathani. "Toothbrush and Toothpaste Use in Australia." Master of Dental Surgery thesis, University of Sydney, 1987.

Keith, A. B. *A Constitutional History of India, 1600–1935.* 2nd ed. Allahabad: Central Book Depot, 1961.

"Kerala Waste Time-Bomb Ticks Away in Kovai." *New Indian Express*, July 17, 2016. http://bit.ly/2dTYxdc.

Khaliq, Abdul, Muhammad Rhamdhani, Geoffrey Brooks, and Syed Masood. "Metal Extraction Processes for Electronic Waste and Existing Industrial Routes: A Review and Australian Perspective." *Resources* 3 (2014): 152–179.

Kim, Rockli, Ivan Mejía-Guevara, Daniel Corsi, Víctor Aguayo, S. V. Subramanian "Relative Importance of 13 Correlates of Child Stunting in South Asia: Insights from Nationally Representative Data from Afghanistan, Bangladesh, India, Nepal, and Pakistan." *Social Science and Medicine* 187 (2017): 144–154.

Kingsley, Patrick. "Waste Not: Egypt's Refuse Collectors Regain Role at Heart of Cairo Society." *Guardian*, March 28, 2014. https://goo.gl/qIXvrY.

Kochar, Rakesh. "A Global Middle Class Is More Promise than Reality." *Global Attitudes and Trends*. Pew Research Center, July 8, 2015. https://goo.gl/QaS6Tj.

Korom, Frank. "On the Ethics and Aesthetics of Recycling in India." In *Purifying the Earthly Body of God: Religion and Ecology in Hindu India*, edited by L. E. Nelson, 197–223. Albany, NY: State University of New York Press, 1998.

Krishnan, Sandhya, and Neeraj Hatekar. "Rise of the New Middle Class in India and Its Changing Structure" *Economic and Political Weekly* 52, no. 22 (June 3, 2017): 40–48.

Kumar, Dharma, and Meghnad Desai. *Cambridge Economic History of India*. Vol. 2, *c. 1751–c. 1970*. Cambridge: Cambridge University Press, 1983.

Kumar, Girish. *Local Democracy in India*. New Delhi: SAGE, 2006.

Kumar, Nita. *The Artisans of Banaras: Popular Culture and Identity, 1880–1986*. Princeton, NJ: Princeton University Press, 1988.

Kumar, Virendra, ed. *Committees and Commissions in India, 1947–73*. Vol. 11. New Delhi: Concept Publishing, 1988.

Kvarnström, Elisabeth, Joep Verhagen, Mats Nilsson, Vishwanath Srikantaiah, Karan Singh, and Shubha Ramachandran. "Honey-Suckers: Sanitation Systems without Pipes—Eco-san at Work?" C. 2011, accessed September 5, 2017. http://goo.gl/c1X2Xz.

Lamba, Sneha, and Dean Spears. "Caste, 'Cleanliness' and Cash: Effects of Caste-Based Political Reservations in Rajasthan on a Sanitation Prize." *Journal of Development Studies* 49, no. 11 (2013): 1592–1606.

Langer, Avalok. "From Rags to Ditches." *Tehelka,* April 23, 2011. https://goo.gl/tSYfHW.

Langewiesche, William. "The Shipbreakers." *Atlantic* 286, no. 2 (2000): 31–49.

Lapierre, Dominique, and Javier Moro. *Five Past Midnight in Bhopal: The Epic Story of the World's Deadliest Industrial Disaster.* New York: Warner Books, 2002.

Laporte, Dominique. *History of Shit.* Cambridge, MA: MIT Press, 1993.

"Largest Landfills, Waste Sites, and Trash Dumps in the World." *World Atlas.* Updated April 25, 2017. http://goo.gl/fWVSma.

Larkin, Brian. "The Politics and Poetics of Infrastructure." *Annual Review of Anthropology* 42 (2013): 327–343.

The Laws of Manu. Trans. W. Doniger and B. K. Smith. New Delhi: Penguin, 1991.

Laxminarayan, Ramanan, and Ranjit Roy Chaudhury. "Antibiotic Resistance in India: Drivers and Opportunities for Action." *PLOS Medicine* 13, no. 3 (2016): 1–7.

Leonard, Annie. *The Story of Stuff.* New York: Free Press, 2010.

Lewit, Eugene M., and Nancy Kerrebock. "Population-Based Growth Stunting." *Children and Poverty* 7, no. 2 (1997): 149–156.

Li, Tania. *The Will to Improve: Governmentality, Development, and the Practice of Politics.* Durham, NC: Duke University Press, 2007.

"List of Countries and Territories by Population Density." Wikipedia. Accessed October 11, 2017. https://goo.gl/8FT9Pz.

Lucas, Clay, and Aisha Dow. "Town Hall Troubles." *Age* (Melbourne), October 20, 2016.

"Mafia Obstructing Scientific Disposal of Garbage in City." *Deccan Herald,* August, 14, 2012. https://goo.gl/cS7ZPc.

Maheshwari, S. R. *Indian Administration.* 6th ed. Bombay: Orient Longmans, 2001.

"The Malagrotta Landfill and Speculation in the Galeria Valley." *Ejolt,* fact sheet 22, July 20, 2015. http://goo.gl/uehYwD.

Mankekar, Kamla. *Breaking News: A Woman in a Man's World.* New Delhi: Rupa, 2014.

Mathur, Kuldeep. *Panchayati Raj.* New Delhi: Oxford University Press, 2013.

Mathur, O. P., Debdulal Thakur, and Nilesh Rajadhyaksha. *Urban Tax Potential in India.* New Delhi: National Institute of Public Finance and Policy, 2009. https://goo.gl/wjAaUi.

McFarlane, Colin. "Sanitation in Mumbai's Informal Settlements: State, 'Slum,' and Infrastructure." *Environment and Planning A* 40, no. 1 (2008): 88–107.

McGowan, Abigail. "Ahmedabad's Home Remedies: Housing in the Re-making of an Industrial City, 1920–1960." *South Asia* 36, no. 3 (2013): 400–409.

McKenna, Maryn. "NDM-1 in India: Drug Resistance, Political Resistance." *Wired*, October 16, 2012. https://goo.gl/oENeBM.

Mehra, Preeti. "Want That Waste Paper!" *Hindu,* January 1, 2012, updated July 25, 2016. https://goo.gl/CrRiap.

Mehrotra, S. R. *The Emergence of the Indian National Congress.* New Delhi: Vikas, 1971.

Mehta, Nalin. *India on Television.* New Delhi: Harper Collins, 2008.

Melosi, Martin V. *Garbage in the Cities: Refuse, Reform and the Environment.* Revised edition. Pittsburgh: University of Pittsburgh Press, 2005.

"Memorandum on the Policy of the Government of India in Regard to Local Self-Government. 26 December 1882." In S. R. Mehrotra, *The Emergence of the Indian National Congress.* New Delhi: Vikas, 1971.

Michael, L. W., compiler. *The History of the Municipal Corporation of the City of Bombay.* Bombay: Union Press, 1902.

Mills, Chris. "The Worlds [*sic*] Largest Landfills with Photos and Stats." Owlcation, March 9, 2016. http://goo.gl/xnzfMx.

Minter, Adam. *Junkyard Planet: Travels in the Billion-Dollar Trash Trade.* New York: Bloomsbury, 2013.

Mishra, Lata, and Kunal Guha. "Stench of Money." *Mumbai Mirror,* February 7, 2016. https://goo.gl/8eiy2x.

Mohan, Dinesh. "Transport and Health: Clearing the Air." *Economic and Political Weekly* 51, no. 9 (February 27, 2016): 29–32.

Molony, J. C. *A Book of South India.* London: Methuen & Co., 1926.

Moore, Shelley. "About Toothpaste Tubes Made of Metal." eHow. Accessed September 5, 2017. http://www.ehow.com/about_4597108_toothpaste-tubes-made-metal.html.

Morante, Carmilita. "Electioneering in the Promised Land: Payatas Dumpsite, 2016." University of Nottingham Blogs, University of Nottingham, May 6, 2016.

Mosse, David. "The Anthropology of International Development." *Annual Review of Anthropology* 42 (2013): 227–246.

Mufeed, S., K. Ahmad, G. Mahmood, and R. C. Trivedi. "Municipal Solid Waste Management in India Cities." *Waste Management* 28 (2008): 459–467.

Nagarajan, Kedar. "Delhi: Waste-to-Energy Plants Face Opposition from People in Vicinity." *Indian Express,* May 30, 2016. https://goo.gl/MMsym3.

Nagle, Robin. *Picking Up: On the Streets and Behind the Trucks with the Sanitation Workers of New York City.* New York: Farrer, Strauss and Giroux, 2013.

Naipaul, V. S. *An Area of Darkness.* 1964. Harmondsworth, UK: Penguin, 1968.

Nair, Shibhu. "Mobile Stupidity." Video, 3:30, November 8, 2012. https://www.youtube.com/watch?v=4fJ6QZ24lug.

Nandgaonkar, Satish. "Photo Essay Led to Tata's Mission Dignity." *Hindu,* January 22, 2015. http://goo.gl/6JtAsE.

Nandy, Ashis. "Gandhi after Gandhi after Gandhi." *Little Magazine.* Accessed September 5, 2017. http://www.littlemag.com/nandy.htm.

Narain, Sunita. "The Undisclosed Air Pollutants." *Down to Earth,* January 31, 2017.

Narain, Sunita, and Swati Singh Sambyal. *Not in My Backyard: Solid Waste Management in Indian Cities.* New Delhi: Centre for Science and Environment, 2016.

Narayana, D. "Local Governance without Capacity Building: Ten Years of Panchayati Raj." *Economic and Political Weekly* 40, no. 26 (June 25, 2005): 2822–2832.

Natarajan, J. *History of Indian Journalism.* New Delhi: Publications Division, Ministry of Information and Broadcasting, 1955.

Nath, V. "Urbanisation in India: Review and Prospects." *Economic and Political Weekly* 28, no. 8 (February 22, 1986): 339–352.

Nehru, Jawaharlal. Speech, April 2, 1952. In *Talk of the Town,* edited by J. Pinto and R. Srivastava. New Delhi: Penguin, 2008.

Niehaus, Mark D., S. R. Moore, P. D. Patrick, L. L. Derr, B. Lorntz, A. A. Lima, R. L. Guerrant. "Early Childhood Diarrhea Is Associated with Diminished Cognitive Function 4 to 7 Years Later in Children in a Northeast Brazilian Shantytown." *American Journal of Tropical Medicine and Hygiene* 66, no. 5 (2002): 590–593.

Norris, Lucy. "The Limits of Ethicality in International Markets: Imported Second-Hand Clothing in India." *Geoforum* 67 (2015): 183–193.

———. *Recycling Indian Clothing: Global Contexts of Reuse and Value.* Bloomington: Indiana University Press, 2010.

Oldenburg, Philip. *Big City Government in India: Councillor, Administrator and Citizen in Delhi.* Tucson: University of Arizona Press for the Association for Asian Studies, 1976.

Olivelle, Patrick. "Hair and Society: Social Significance of Hair in South Asia Traditions." In *Hair: Its Power and Meaning in Asian Cultures,* edited by A. Hiltebeitel and B. D. Miller, 11–50. New York: State University of New York Press, 1998.

O'Reilly, Kathleen, Richa Dhanju, and Abhineety Goel. "Exploring 'The Remote' and 'The Rural': Open Defecation and Latrine Use in Uttarakhand, India." *World Development* 93 (2017): 193–205.

O'Reilly, Kathleen, Richa Dhanju, and Elizabeth Louis. "Subjected to Sanitation: Caste Relations and Sanitation Adoption in Rural Tamil Nadu." *Journal of Development Studies,* November 1, 2016. http://dx.doi.org/10.1080/00220388.2016.1241385.

"Orissa State Level: Background Paper." Bhubaneshwar: KIIT School of Rural Management, 2011. http://urk.tiss.edu/images/pdf/Orissa-State-level-Background-Paper.pdf.

Packard, Vance. *The Waste Makers.* 1960. Brooklyn, NY: Ig Publishing, 1988.

Panagarhiya, Arvind. "Does India Really Suffer from Worse Child Malnutrition than Sub-Saharan Africa?" *Economic and Political Weekly* 48, no. 10 (May 4, 2013): 98–111.

Patel, Almitra. "Waste-Management Miracle in Warangal, Oct 2012." Accessed September 5, 2017. http://goo.gl/MKJXEU.

"Peepoo, a Bag That Could Solve India's Toilet Woes." *Deccan Herald,* March 11, 2011. https://goo.gl/NYtaOa.

Pellow, David N. *Resisting Global Toxics: Transnational Movements for Environmental Justice.* Cambridge, MA: MIT Press, 2007.

Penner, Barbara. *Bathroom.* London: Reaktion Books, 2013.

Phadke, Shilpa, Sameera Khan, and Shilpa Ranade. *Why Loiter?* New Delhi: Penguin, 2011.

Pinto, Jerry, and Rahul Srivastava, eds. *Talk of the Town.* New Delhi: Penguin, 2008.

Piplai, Tapas. "Automobile Industry: Shifting Strategic Focus." *Economic and Political Weekly* 36, no. 30 (July 28, 2001): 2892–2897.

Prasad, Chandra Bhan. "Markets and Manu: Economic Reforms and Its Impact on Caste in India." Working paper 08-01, Center for the Advanced Study of India, University of Pennsylvania, 2008.

Prashad, Vijay. "The Technology of Sanitation in Colonial Delhi." *Modern Asian Studies* 35, no. 1 (2001): 113–155.

Premchand. *Deliverance and Other Stories.* Translated by David Rubin. 1931. New Delhi: Penguin, 1988.

Prendergast, Andrew J., and Jean H. Humphrey. "The Stunting Syndrome in Developing Countries." *Paediatrics and International Child Health* 34, no. 4 (2014): 250–265.

"Providing Safe and Sustainable Water for All." Veolia. Accessed September 28, 2017. https://veolia.in/about-us/about-us/history.

Rajadhyaksha, Ashish, and Paul Willemen. *Encyclopaedia of Indian Cinema.* Revised edition. New Delhi: Oxford University Press, 1999.

Rajivlochan, Meeta. "Swachh Bharat's Success Lies in Trusting the Town Councils." *Hindustan Times,* December 9, 2015. https://goo.gl/FJrtQf.

Ram, N. S. Mohan, "Recycling End of Life Vehicles," *Seminar,* no. 690 (February 2017): 45–49.

Ramana, Mridula. *Western Medicine and Public Health in Colonial Bombay 1845–1895.* Hyderabad: Orient Longman, 2002.

Ramesh, Jairam. "A Toilet for Everyone." *India Today,* June 6, 2014. https://goo.gl/vNKSdW.

Rana, Rishi, Rajiv Ganguly, and Ashok Kumar Gupta. "An Assessment of Solid Waste Management System in Chandigarh City, India." *Electronic Journal of Geotechnical Engineering* 20, no. 6 (2015): 1547–1572.

Rao, S. L., and I. Natarajan. *Indian Market Demographics: The Consumer Classes.* New Delhi: Global Business Press, 1996.

Rathje, William, and Cullen Murphy. *Rubbish! The Archaeology of Garbage.* Tucson: University of Arizona Press, 2001.

Redfield, Peter. "Bioexpectations: Life Technologies as Humanitarian Goods." *Public Culture* 24, no. 1 (2015): 157–184.

Reno, Joshua O. *Waste Away: Working and Living with a North American Landfill.* Berkeley: University of California Press, 2016.

Robinson, Jennifer. "Apex Landfill: There's No Place like Home for Las Vegas Garbage." *Las Vegas Review Journal,* April 21, 2013. https://goo.gl/FPTYHm.

Rohra, Sunali, and Barnik Maitra. "The Urban Capacity Conundrum." *Financial Express,* May 20, 2015. https://goo.gl/FxfwKr.

Rosenberg, Charles E. *The Cholera Years: The United States in 1832, 1849 and 1866.* 1962. Chicago: University of Chicago Press, 1987.

Rothermund, Dietmar. *An Economic History of India.* London: Routledge, 1993.

Royte, Elizabeth. *Garbage Land: On the Secret Trail of Trash.* New York: Back Bay Books, 2006.

Rucevska, I., C. Nellemann, N. Isarin, W. Yang, N. Liu, K. Yu, S. Sandnæs, K. Olley, H. McCann, L. Devia, L. Bisschop, D. Soesilo, T. Schoolmeester, R. Henriksen, R. Nilsen. *Waste Crime—Waste Risks: Gaps in Meeting the Global Waste Challenge; a Rapid Response Assessment.* UN Environmental Program, 2015. https://goo.gl/iwGMRG.

"Runners Exposed to High Pollution Levels during Delhi Marathon." *Down to Earth,* November 30, 2016, pp. 18–44.

Russell, R. V. *Tribes and Castes of the Central Provinces.* Vol. 1. London: Macmillan, 1916.

Sachs, Noah M. "Garbage Everywhere." *Atlantic,* June 20, 2014. https://goo.gl/vuee6z.

Sahu, Geetanjoy. "Workers of Alang-Sosiya: A Survey of Working Conditions in a Ship-Breaking Yard, 1983–2013." *Economic and Political Weekly* 49, no. 50 (December 13, 2014): 52–59.

Sambyal, Swati Singh. "Trashing the Ragpicker." *Down to Earth,* April 30, 2016, pp. 16–17.

"The Sanitary Commissioner with the Government of India." *British Medical Journal,* November 11, 1911, pp. 1294–1295.

Sandesara, Utpal, and Tom Wooten. *No One Had a Tongue to Speak: The Untold Story of One of History's Deadliest Floods.* Amherst, NY: Prometheus Books, 2011.

Sandhu, Kiran. "Between Hype and Veracity: An Analysis of Privatization of Solid Waste Management Services, Amritsar City, India." Paper presented at the 5th International Conference on Solid Waste Management, Bengaluru, November 2015.

Sarkar, S. "Sewers and Sewer Networks." August 28, 2015. https://goo.gl/szmIHc.

Sedlak, David. *Water 4.0: The Past, Present and Future of the World's Most Vital Resource.* New Haven, CT: Yale University Press, 2014.

Sen, Amartya. "Social Exclusion: Concept, Application and Scrutiny." Social Development paper no. 1. Asian Development Bank, Manila, June 2000.

Sengupta, Sushmita. "On Green Track." *Down to Earth,* November 15, 2013. https://goo.gl/91JviS.

Sengupta, Sushmita, Snigdha Das, and Rashmi Verma. "Mission Madness." *Down to Earth,* July 24, 2017. https://goo.gl/ysaUjb.

Shah, Ghanshyam. *Public Health and Urban Development: The Plague in Surat.* New Delhi: SAGE, 1997.

Shah, Ghanshyam, Harsh Mander, Sukhadeo Thorat, Satish Deshpande, and Amita Baviskar. *Untouchability in Rural India.* New Delhi: Sage, 2006.

"Shanghai Laogang Engineered Sanitary Landfill Phase IV." Veolia. Accessed September 5, 2017. http://goo.gl/2h7fvz.

Shapiro, Fred. "Quotes Uncovered: Who Said No Crisis Should Go to Waste?" *Freakonomics* (blog), August 13, 2009. https://goo.gl/4R11JB.

Sharma, Mukul. "Brahmanical Activism As Eco-Casteism: Reading the Life Narratives of Bindeshwar Pathak, Sulabh International, and 'Liberated' Dalits." *Biography* 40, no. 1 (2017): 199–221.

Shinoda, Takashi. *Marginalization in the Midst of Modernization: Sweepers in Western India.* New Delhi: Manohar, 2005.

Silverstein, Yoshi. "The 'Mountain of Crap' Becomes a Park." *The Dirt: Uniting the Built and Natural Environments,* October 3, 2015. https://goo.gl/gVFxnb.

Singh, Bhasha. *Unseen: The Truth about India's Manual Scavengers.* Translated by R. Talwar. Hindi edition, 2012. New Delhi: Penguin, 2014.

Singh, K. S. *People of India: The Scheduled Castes*. Vol. 2. Delhi: Oxford University Press for Anthropological Survey of India, 1993.

Sivaramakrishnan, K. C. *Governance of Megacities: Fractured Thinking, Fragmented Setup*. New Delhi: Oxford University Press, 2015.

———. *Re-visioning Indian Cities: The Urban Renewal Mission*. New Delhi: Sage, 2011.

———. "Revisiting the 74th Constitutional Amendment for Better Metropolitan Governance. *Economic and Political Weekly* 48, no. 13 (March 20, 2013): 86–94.

Slade, Giles. *Made to Break: Technology and Obsolescence in America*. Cambridge, MA: Harvard University Press, 2006.

Solanki, Durgesh. "Cast(e)ing Life: The Experience of Living in Peripheral Caste Quarters." In *Peripheral Visions in the Globalizing Present: Space, Mobility and Aesthetics*, edited by Esther Pareen, Hanneke Stuit, and Astrid Van Weyenberg, 109–125. Leiden, Netherlands: Brill, 2016.

Spears, Dean. "How Much International Variation in Child Height Can Sanitation Explain?" Working paper, Princeton Research Program in Development Studies, 2013.

Spears, Dean, and Sneha Lamba. "Effects of Early-Life Exposure to Sanitation on Childhood Cognitive Skills: Evidence from India's Total Sanitation Campaign." *Journal of Human Resources* 51, no. 2 (2016): 298–327.

Srinivas, Tulasi. "Flush with Success: Bathing, Defecation, Worship, and Social Change in South India." *Space and Culture* 5, no. 4 (2002): 368–386.

Srivastav, Nikhil. "Why Open Defecation in India Will End Only with the Annihilation of Caste." *Scroll.in*, September 11, 2016. https://goo.gl/qkbTgg.

Srivastava, Sanjay. *Entangled Urbanism: Slum, Gated Community and Shopping Mall in Delhi and Gurgaon*. New Delhi: Oxford University Press, 2015.

Srivastava, Vinay Kumar. "On Sanitation: A Memory Ethnography." *Social Change* 44, no. 2 (2014): 275–290.

Sruthijith, K. K. "Newsprint Price Hikes Forcing Publishing Cos to Rejig Practices." *LiveMint,* March 12, 2008. https://goo.gl/lVZsyI.

Sterndale, Reginald Craufuird. *Municipal Work in India: Hints on Sanitation, General Conservancy and Improvement in Municipalities, Towns, and Villages.* Calcutta: Thacker, Spink, 1881.

Subramanian, Meera. "The Burning Garbage Heap That Choked Mumbai." *New Yorker,* February 26, 2016. http://goo.gl/9gghyH.

Subramanian, S. "The Poverty Line: Getting It Wrong Again . . . and Again." *Economic and Political Weekly* 49, no. 47 (November 22, 2014): 66–70.

Suchitra, M. "Stench in My Backyard." *Down to Earth,* September 15, 2012. http://www.downtoearth.org.in/coverage/stench-in-my—backyard-38970.

Sundaram, Ravi. *Pirate Modernity: Delhi's Media Urbanism.* London: Routledge, 2010.

Sunny, Shiv. "Delhi's Ghazipur Landfill Collapse: 2 Dead as Mountain of Trash Sweeps Many into Nearby Canal." *Hindustan Times*, September 2, 2017. https://goo.gl/PvdxXZ.

Tarlo, Emma. *Entanglement: The Secret Lives of Hair.* London: Oneworld, 2016.

Tatham, David. *Winslow Homer and the Pictorial Press.* Syracuse, NY: Syracuse University Press, 2003.

Thakur, Joydeep. "Today It Is Ghazipur, Tomorrow It Can Be Bhalswa or Okhla in Delhi, Say Experts." *Hindustan Times*, September 1, 2017. https://goo.gl/ReE7cQ.

Tharakan, Michael. "Gandhian and Marxist Approaches to Decentralised Governance in India: Points of Similarity." *Social Scientist* 40, nos. 9 / 10 (2012): 47–60.

Thorat, Sukhadeo. "On Economic Exclusion and Inclusive Policy." *Little Magazine* 6, nos. 4–5: 8–17.

Tinker, Hugh. *The Foundations of Local Self-Government in India, Pakistan and Burma*. London: Athlone Press, 1954.

Tiwari, Manish. "Titanic Junkyard." *Down to Earth*, March 15, 2008. http://archive.ban.org/library/down_to_earth.html.

Tiwari, Rashmi, and Sanatan Nayak. "Drinking Water, Sanitation and Waterborne Diseases." *Economic and Political Weekly* 52, no. 23 (June 10, 2017): 136–140.

Tong, Xin, and Jici Wang. "The Shadow of the Global Network: E-waste Flows to China." In *Economies of Recycling: The Global Transformation of Materials, Values and Social Relations,* edited by Catherine Alexander and Joshua Reno, 98–116. London: Zed Books, 2012.

Tripathi, Tulika. "Safai Karmi Scheme of Uttar Pradesh: Caste Dominance Continues." *Economic and Political Weekly* 47, no. 37 (September 15, 2012): 26–29.

Tsing, Anna L. *The Mushroom at the End of the World: On the Possibility of Life in Capitalist Ruins.* Princeton, NJ: Princeton University Press, 2015.

"2014 Badaun gang rape allegations." Wikipedia. Accessed October 6, 2017. https://en.wikipedia.org/wiki/2014_Badaun_gang_rape_allegations.

Vaidya, Chetan, and Brad Johnson. "Ahmedabad Municipal Bond." *Economic and Political Weekly* 36, no. 30 (July 28, 2001): 2884–2891.

Vallee, Gerard, ed. *Florence Nightingale on Health in India.* Waterloo, ON: Wilfrid Laurier University Press, 2006.

van der Geest, Sjaak. "Akan Shit: Getting Rid of Dirt in Ghana." *Anthropology Today* 14, no. 3 (1998): 8–12.

Varghese, Abraham. "The Mystery Plague." *Esquire* (UK) 5, no. 2 (1995): 31–36.

Vivek, P. S. *The Scavengers: Exploited Class of City Professionals.* Mumbai: Himalaya Publishing House, 1998.

———. "Scavengers: Mumbai's Neglected Workers." *Economic and Political Weekly* 35, no. 42 (October 14, 2000): 3722–3724.

Wachira, Muchemi. "Heaps of Garbage Chokes [*sic*] Nairobi City." *Daily Nation,* December 29, 2015. http://goo.gl/yQHzWu.

Walsh, Edward J., and Rex Warland. *Don't Burn It Here: Grassroots Challenges to Trash Incinerators.* University Park, PA: Penn State Press, 1997.

Waltner-Toews, David. *The Origin of Feces.* Toronto: ECW Press, 2016.

Wang, Zhaohua, Bin Zhang, and Dabo Guan. "Take Responsibility for Electronic-Waste Disposal." *Nature,* August 3, 2016. https://goo.gl/mPTf8q.

Weber, Thomas. *Hugging the Trees: The Story of the Chipko Movement.* New Delhi: Viking, 1988.

Weinstein, Lisa. *The Durable Slum: Dharavi and the Right to Stay Put in Globalizing Mumbai.* Minneapolis: University of Minnesota Press, 2014.

Wilson, Bezwada. Foreword to *Unseen: The Truth about India's Manual Scavengers,* by B. Singh, translated by R. Talwar. New Delhi: Penguin, 2014.

Wohl, Anthony S. *Endangered Lives: Public Health in Victorian Britain.* London: J. M. Dent, 1983.

Wu, Amy. "Good Product, Bad Package." *Guardian,* July 18, 2014. http://goo.gl/Yhsq5a.

Xinzhong, Yu. "The Treatment of Night Soil and Waste in Modern China." In *Health and Hygiene in Chinese East Asia,* edited by A. K. Che Leung and C. Furth, 51–71. Durham, NC: Duke University Press, 2010.

Xu, Yamin. "Policing Civility on the Streets: Encounters with Litterbugs, 'Nightsoil Lords,' and Street Corner Urinators in Republican Beijing." *Twentieth-Century China* 3, no. 2 (2005): 28–71.

Xue, Yong. "'Treasure Nightsoil as If It Were Gold': Economic and Ecological Links between Urban and Rural Areas in Late Imperial Jiangnan." *Late Imperial China* 26, no. 1 (2005): 41–71.

Yates, Michelle. "The Human-as-Waste, the Labor Theory of Value and Disposability in Contemporary Capitalism." *Antipode* 43, no. 5 (2011): 1679–1695.

Zhu, Da, P. U. Asnani, Christian Zurbrugg, Sebastian Anapolsky, and Shyamala K. Mani. *Improving Municipal Solid Waste Management in India: A Sourcebook for Policy Makers and Practitioners.* Washington, DC: World Bank Group, 2008.

Media Sources

"After Una Atrocity, Dalits Protest and Refuse to Dispose of Carcasses in Gujarat." *Hindu,* July 30, 2016. https://goo.gl/EP8VUx.

"Alang Yard Dismantles Record Ships in 2011–12. *Business Standard,* April 9, 2012. http://goo.gl/z1VjB3.

Bhatnagar, Gaurav Vivek. "Okhla Waste-to-Energy Plant Using Experimental Chinese Technology Back in Limelight." *The Wire,* April 26, 2016. https://goo.gl/Z4iFpu.

"Bhim Yatra." Safai Karmachari Andolan, December 10, 2015. http://www.safaikarmachariandolan.org/Bhim-Yatra.html.

Biswas, Soutik. "Do India's Stray Dogs Kill More People than Terror Attacks?" *BBC News,* May 6, 2016. https://goo.gl/8SZJc2.

"BJP's Next Mission: End Manual Scavenging." *Hindu,* April 3, 2015. http://goo.gl/TzTjZi.

Brown, William. "Delhi's Dilemma: What to Do with Its Tonnes of Waste?" *Aljazeera,* November 29, 2016. https://goo.gl/fKdqki.

"Can Incinerators Help Manage India's Growing Waste Management Problem?" *Economic Times,* September 9, 2015.

"Cashing In on Fly Ash." *Hindu BusinessLine,* August 4, 2006. https://goo.gl/IIZMxH.

"Centre to Popularise Municipal Bonds." *Hindu,* September 6, 2016. https://goo.gl/XBdIRz.

"Child Health and Nutrition." *Child Line 1098.* Accessed September 5, 2017. http://goo.gl/bmUblc.

"Colgate-Palmolive (India) Gains after Gujarat Unit Starts Producing Toothpaste." *Business Standard,* May 23, 2014. http://goo.gl/RttxFO.

"Controversial Durham Energy-from-Waste Incinerator a Year Behind Schedule." *Star* (Toronto), January 5, 2016. http://goo.gl/tHKEST.

"Cops Take on Auto Mafia, Raid Godown in Sotiganj." *Times of India,* January 31, 2015. http://goo.gl/p4yKma.

"CPI(ML) Activist Lynched for Objecting to Rajasthan Officials Taking Photos of Women Defecating." *The Wire,* June 17, 2017. "18 Stories High and Still Burning, Fire at Landfill Exposes India's Growing Trash Crisis." *Los Angeles Times,* March 23, 2016. http://lat.ms/22Ji1SJ.

"Eliminating Manual Scavenging—The Honey-Sucker Approach." *RainwaterHarvesting* (blog). November 10, 2011. https://goo.gl/vHdMEg.

"Environment Ministry Announces New Rules for Disposal of Hazardous Waste." *Economic Times,* April 3, 2016. http://goo.gl/UTlyEB.

"Ewaste Up as More Dump Old Television Sets for Flat Screen." *Times of India,* June 13, 2014. http://goo.gl/gNSH1c.

"Garbage Piles Up across City as Sanitation Workers Continue Strike." *New Indian Express,* July 12, 2015. http://goo.gl/LWWNUo.

Good Garbage. Directed by Shosh Shlam and Ada Ushpiz [in Arabic]. 2013.

Gowda, Aravind. "Bengaluru Garbage Mafia Issues Threat to Residents." *India Today,* December 5, 2015. https://goo.gl/sQCbKd.

Gupta, Surojit. "Time Indian Cities Woke Up to Municipal Bonds." *Times of India,* July 20, 2013. https://goo.gl/aNkm5I.

Henry, Nikhila. "Research Scholar Hangs Self after Expulsion from Central University." *Hindu,* January 17, 2016. https://goo.gl/d5SSIJ.

"Hundreds of Sanitation Workers Carrying Bodies of 4 Colleagues Storm Collectorate." *Nagpur Today,* March 16, 2016. http://goo.gl/ZvAolg.

"Import and Export of Paper and Cardboard, an International Comparison in 2015." *Statista,* https://goo.gl/RNtqHB.

"India's New Rulers." *Hinduism Today,* November 1999. https://goo.gl/DuqyWY.

"India's Top Companies for Sustainability and CSR 2016." *futurescape.* Accessed October 8, 2017. https://goo.gl/ozWPY6.

Iqbal, Mohammed. "The Case of Delhi's Missing Dustbins." *Hindu,* December 4, 2014. https://goo.gl/p6qfXb.

"Junk Old Car, Get 50% Excise Cut on New?" *Times of India,* January 18, 2016. http://goo.gl/KPVKgI.

Kandhari, Ruhi. "Drinking Sewage in Varanasi." *Thethirdpole.net,* October 12, 2015. https://www.thethirdpole.net/2015/10/12/drinking-sewage-in-varanasi/.

Kristof, Nicholas. "Half the Kids in This Part of India Are Stunted." *New York Times,* October 15, 2015. http://goo.gl/IpGfuP.

Laschon, Eliza. "Contract Inked for $400m Kwinana Thermal Waste Facility in WA." ABC News, February 16, 2016. http://goo.gl/qBXQZA.

Mahadevan, G. "Mobile Incinerator Brought to Trivandrum Remains Inoperational." *Hindu,* December 10, 2012. http://goo.gl/RHTyIe.

Mahesh, Koride. "Waste Management Project: Greater Hyderabad Civic Body in Dilemma as Workers Oppose Move." *Times of India,* February 13, 2014. https://goo.gl/o1l21T.

Messenger, Ben. "First Integrated End-of-Life Vehicle Recycling Facility for India by 2018." *Waste Management World,* August 11, 2016. https://goo.gl/zjzhPM.

Narayanan, Vivek. "Four Die of Asphyxiation in Restaurant Septic Tank at Chennai Hotel." *Hindu,* January 20, 2016. https://goo.gl/Tfp2ml.

Nijish, T. P., and Aswin J. Kumar. "Mobile Incinerator Deal Heads for a Legal Fight." *Times of India,* October 9, 2013. http://goo.gl/I4O8xq.

"Number of Ships in the World Merchant Fleet as of January 1, 2015, by Type." *Statista,* http://goo.gl/CwP4v6.

"Number of Vehicles Scrapped in the U.S. from 2002 to 2014 (in million units)." *Statista,* 2016. http://goo.gl/92H53V.

"The Park Plan." Freshkills Park: The Freshkills Park Alliance. Accessed September 5, 2017. http://goo.gl/Foo9y1.

"Ragpickers Battle Toxic Fumes and Hunger as Deonar Fire Smolders." *Times of India,* February 2, 2016. http://bit.ly/2e7k82u.

"The Rapunzel Machine." Video, 01:07, June 26, 2015. http://www.dailymotion.com/video/x2vdw61.

"Rate of Stunting Dropping Fast." *Daily Star,* November 4, 2015. http://www.thedailystar.net/frontpage/rate-stunting-dropping-fast-166978.

"Republic Services, Inc." 2014 Fortune 500. Updated March 31, 2014. http://fortune-500.silk.co/page/Republic-Services—Inc.

"Rs 94 Crore Spent on Ads of Swachh Bharat Mission in 1 Year." *Economic Times,* July 8, 2015. http://goo.gl/4XGVwk.

Rodrigues, Malika. "Sachet Up the Ramp." *Economic Times,* March 13, 2002. https://goo.gl/WertbV.

Safai Karmachari Andolan website. Accessed September 5, 2017. http://safaikarmachariandolan.org/contactus.html.

Satymev Jayate, "Don't Waste Your Garbage." Season 2, episode 3, 2014. http://www.satyamevjayate.in/dont-waste-your-garbage.aspx.

"70% of Indian Sewage Treatment Plants Dysfunctional: Javadekar." *Times of India,* November 21, 2014. https://goo.gl/CL5Oe6.

"Sewage Treatment in Pune Region Gives State the Jitters." *Times of India,* October 17, 2015. https://goo.gl/htUqRd.

"Ship Breaking in Bangladesh," Young Power in Social Action. Accessed September 5, 2017. https://goo.gl/pnvDaq.

"Six Quotes from PM Modi on Swachh Bharat Abhiyan." *India Today,* October 2, 2014. https://goo.gl/xSCmhn.

"Slurry Dumping Leading to Destruction of Mangrove." *Hindu,* December 14, 2015. http://goo.gl/uPWXOe.

Tadepalli, Siddharth. "The Filthy Tale of Jawahar Nagar." *Times of India,* October 1, 2015. https://goo.gl/8Gjhxy.

Tomczyk, Karolina. "Paper Prices Remain Soft Despite Supply Cuts." *Spend Matters,* July 28, 2016. http://spendmatters.com/2016/07/28/95660/.

"'Tony' Projects: Council in Firing Line." *Times of India,* January 16, 2016. http://goo.gl/wWYofE.

"Toothpaste Industry: An Overview. *Allprojectreports.com.* Accessed September 5, 2017. http://goo.gl/AlI8jK.

"Toothpaste Market in India to 2017." *Wattpad,* June 17, 2014. https://goo.gl/Bw9GWa.

Trivedi, Divya. "A Blot upon the Nation." *Hindu,* March 30, 2012. https://goo.gl/frMklW.

"20 Years Down the Line What Ails the Urban Local Bodies." *Down to Earth,* June 1, 2012. https://goo.gl/fcLDio.

Wakin, Daniel J. "Rabbis' Rules and Indian Wigs Stir Crisis in Orthodox Brooklyn." *New York Times,* May 14, 2004. https://goo.gl/uYimN7.

Wilson, Carla. "Victoria House Prices Surge to Another High." *Times-Colonist,* June 1, 2016. http://goo.gl/H2F3Qp.

Ugly Indian, "Why Is India So Filthy?" TEDxBangalore. Video, 17:33, October 27, 2104. https://www.youtube.com/watch?v=tf1VA5jqmRo.

"Vidya Balan Campaigns for Sanitation in UP, Bihar." *Indian Express,* August 26, 2015. https://goo.gl/zT9EkV.

"Witness: Hair India." Al Jazeera English. Video, 45:09, January 31, 2010. https://goo.gl/zsccr3.

ACKNOWLEDGMENTS

In the Preface, we thanked the family members who put up with us. Here we try, inadequately, to record the debts we owe to a great many people who shared their skills and knowledge with a pair of curious generalists.

We both have special gratitude toward old friends and advisers: Dipesh Chakrabarty, Nalin Mehta, V. Thiruppugazh, P. Vijaya Kumar, Khyrunnisa A., and Shukla and Kailash Nath. Along the waste path we were encouraged and helped by Susan Chaplin, Peter Friedlander, Gay Hawkins, Craig Jeffrey, Kama Maclean, Dilip Menon, Ira Raja, Kate Sullivan, Philip Taylor, Thomas Weber, and Ian Woolford, Owen Bullock imposed discipline on an early draft of the manuscript, Lee Li Kheng in Singapore drew admirable maps, and Mark Carter in Melbourne turned statistics into graphs.

We were very fortunate to benefit from the specialists who joined the workshop on waste organized by the Institute of South Asian Studies in Singapore in July 2015 and who helped us before and after: Ravi Agarwal (Toxics Link, New Delhi), Harsha Anantharaman (Transparent Chennai), Bharati Chaturvedi (Chintan, New Delhi), Shubhagato Dasgupta (Centre for Policy Research), M. S. Goutham Reddy (Ramky Enviro Engineers, Hyderabad), Amy Ho (Environmental Sustainability, National University of Singapore), Shibu Nair (Zero Waste, Thiruvananthapuram), Praveen Ravi (Athena Infonomics, Chennai), and Fadil Sapaat (National Environmental Agency, Singapore).

At Harvard, we are grateful to reviewers who made valuable suggestions about the manuscript and to the editorial team, especially Kate Brick and Sharmila Sen, who willingly shared our fascination with waste and improved the manuscript with inspired suggestions and crisp admonitions. We are also grateful to Mary Ann Short and Brian Ostrander for astute editing and welcome fact-checking.

Doron thanks:
In Australia, friends who read versions of the manuscript and offered insightful comments are Alex Broom, Jonathan Ben-Tal, Meera Ashar, Philip Taylor, Annie McCarthy, and Francesca Merlan. Colleagues at the Australian National University who helped are Kavesh Muhamad, Alan Ramsey, Andy Kipnis, Matt Tomlinson, Kirin Narayan, and Ken George. In New Zealand, I thank Harry Allen, Joy Florence, and fellow garbologist Graeme MacRae.

In Delhi, Neha Tiwari and Ali Taqi (Zabaan), Mr. D. C. Solanki (DCS Hair International), and Rupan and the Raja family for their kind hospitality, support, and knowledge. I also thank Amita Baviskar, Charu Gupta, Mukul Sharma, and Akanksha Babar.

In Kerala, Pardhan K. S., Paul, Sue, and Lesley.

In Mumbai, Akanksha Awal, friends at Tata Institute of Social Studies, Jayshankar and Anjali Monteiro, Faiz Ullah, and Deepak Sewant.

In Pune, Kush Jha, many SWaCH members, Maitreyi Shankar, and Sangita.

In Varanasi, Ajay Pinku Pandey provided generous support and insights; also Rakesh Singh, Deepak Kumar, Navneet Raman, Petra Manefeld, and boatmen friends.

In Kangra, Didi Contractor, Sourabh Padhke, and Catherine Schuetze.

In Israel, Raya Doron, Udi, Ishai, Enosh, Guy, Adi, and Rachel, whose knowledge of economies of recycling paved the way for many garbage encounters; friends and colleagues who provided generous support include Nir Aviely, Ronit Ricci, Ornit Shani, Fredrik Galtung, David Shulman, Yigal Bronner, Ronie Parciack, and Tal Amit.

In Sweden, Göran Skoglund from Filbornaverket Waste to Energy Plant, Helsingborg; and also Kristina Myrvold and Harprit Singh and colleagues in Swedish South Asia Studies Network.

In the Netherlands, Frank Nagtegaal and family, Dennis Rodgers, Katarzyna Cwiertka, and colleagues in the Garbage Matters project (Leiden).

In the United Kingdom, Michael Dwyer, Rachel Dwyer, Chris Pinney, Nandini Gooptu, Barbara Harriss-White, Alice Street, and Jamie Cross.

In the United States, Jenny Huberman, Lawrence Cohen, and Frank Korom.

Jeffrey thanks:

In Australia, Talis Polis, who has performed the role of general reader uncomplainingly and meticulously for thirty years.

Also Jonathan Balls, Surjeet Dhanji, Harry Fischer, Kate Hocking, Salim Lakha, Judy Morton, Ian Rae, Katrina Sharpe, Pawan Singh, R. F. I. Smith, Pradeep Taneja, Vijaya Vaidyanath, and Shabbir Wahid.

In Singapore, Deeparghya Mukherjee, S. Narayan, Amitendu Palit, Ronojoy Sen, Vinod Rai, Dipinder Randhawa, and other colleagues at the Institute of South Asian Studies. Also, Chong Kuek On, Vincent Teo Hup Ee, and Alfred Hee for tours of their facilities.

In Victoria, British Columbia, Kase and Shirley Roodbol for introduction to the Hartland Landfill Facility, a contender for the world's most beautifully situated landfill, and David and Dawn McLean.

In Grenville, Quebec, Ian Young.

In New Delhi, Bezwada Wilson, Pradeep Khandelwal, Manish Gupta, Kanak Tiwari, Dr. Meenakshi Gopinath, and S. Anand.

In Surat, M. K. Das, R. J. Patel, Dr. Vikas Desai, E. H. Pathan, Nimisha Doctor, Sudhan Jha, and Vimal Trivedi.

In Ahmedabad, Dr. Guruprasad Mohapatra, Prashant A. Pandya, Yashpal Prabhakar, Naresh R. Rajput, Rakesh Soni, Dr. Mona Aiyer, Dr. Anil Ray, Ajay Katuri, and Tridip Suhrud.

In Bhavnagar and Alang, Rohit Agrawal, Alap Gia, Haresh Parmar, P. D. Vyas, and Chinthan Kalthia.

In Hyderabad, Subodh Kundamutham, Ravi Kant, Khader Saheb, Somesh Kumar, Sujeet Govindaraju, Bonagiri Srinivas, G. Ramprakash, Harry Samson, and Jogarao Bhamidipati.

In Raichur, S. Kanth, Sharanabasappa Patted, and Rukkesh Doddamani.

In Bengaluru, Dr. A. Ravindra, Amit Chaudhary, Revathy Ashok, Kalpana Kar, Nalini Shekar, Praveen Kumar, Prince Devasagayam,

P. Viswanath, Arun Mugesh, B. Veerabhadrappa, V. Ravichandar, Nupur Tandon, N. S. Ramakanth, and Praveen Kumar G.

In Chennai and environs, Dharmesh Shah, Dr. Mangalam Balasubramanian, Deepa Karthykeyan, Dr. Chandrakant B. Kamble, P. Selvaraj, and Sheela Santha Nair.

In Arcot, S. Parijatham.

In Mamallapuram, Dr. Kalpana Sankar.

In Kolkata and Haldia, Aftabuddin Ahmed, Md Algamgir, Suvojit Bagchi, Snehangshu Chakraborty, and Saikat Ray.

In Mumbai, Faiz Ullah and Nikhil Titus (who together led him up Mount Deonar), Darryl D'Monte, Jyothi Mhabsekhar, Uttam Gade, Lina Mathias, Dr. Shaileshkumar Darokar, Anahita Mukherji, Debartha Banerjee, and Lata Narayan.

In Allahabad, Sara Rai and M. Aslam.

INDEX